PHARMACEUTICAL DESIGN AND DEVELOPMENT

ELLIS HORWOOD SERIES IN PHARMACEUTICAL TECHNOLOGY
incorporating Pharmacological Sciences

Series Editor: Michael H. Rubinstein, Professor of Pharmaceutical Technology, School of Pharmacy, Liverpool John Moores University
Series Consultant: Professor C.G. Wilson, J.P. Todd Professor of Pharmaceutics, Strathclyde University

Titles published (still in print) and in press

Armstrong & James	**UNDERSTANDING EXPERIMENTAL DESIGN AND INTERPRETATION IN PHARMACEUTICS**
Cartwright & Matthews	**PHARMACEUTICAL PRODUCT LICENSING: Requirements for Europe**
Cartwright & Matthews	**INTERNATIONAL PHARMACEUTICAL PRODUCT REGISTRATION: Quality, Safety, Efficacy**
Clark & Moos	**DRUG DISCOVERY TECHNOLOGIES**
Cole	**PHARMACEUTICAL PRODUCTION FACILITIES: Design and Application**
Cole, Hogan & Aulton	**PHARMACEUTICAL COATING TECHNOLOGY**
Cook	**POTASSIUM CHANNELS: Structure, Classification, Function and Therapeutic Potential**
Damaini	**SULPHUR-CONTAINING DRUGS AND RELATED ORGANIC COMPOUNDS: Volumes 1-3, Parts A and B**
D'Arcy & McElnay	**PHARMACY AND PHARMACOTHERAPY OF ASTHMA**
Denyer & Baird	**GUIDE TO MICROBIOLOGICAL CONTROL IN PHARMACEUTICS**
Doods & Van Meel	**RECEPTOR DATA FOR BIOLOGICAL EXPERIMENTS: A Guide to Drug Selectivity**
Ford & Timmins	**PHARMACEUTICAL THERMAL ANALYSIS: Techniques and Applications**
Glasby	**DICTIONARY OF ANTIBIOTIC-PRODUCING ORGANISMS**
Hardy et al.	**DRUG DELIVERY TO THE GASTROINTESTINAL TRACT**
Harvey	**DRUGS FROM NATURAL PRODUCTS: Pharmaceuticals and Agrochemicals**
Hider & Barlow	**POLYPEPTIDE AND PROTEIN DRUGS: Production, Characterization, Formulation**
Ioannides & Lewis	**DRUGS, DIET AND DISEASE, Volume 1: Mechanistic Approaches to Cancer**
Izquierdo & Medina	**NATURALLY OCCURRING BENZODIAZEPINES: Structure, Distribution and Function**
Junginger	**DRUG TARGETING AND DELIVERY: Concepts in Dosage Form Design**
Krogsgaard-Larsen & Hansen	**EXCITATORY AMINO ACID RECEPTORS: Design of Agonists and Antagonists**
Kourounakis & Rekka	**ADVANCED DRUG DESIGN AND DEVELOPMENT**
Labaune	**HANDBOOK OF PHARMACOKINETICS: The Toxicity Asssessment of Chemicals**
Macheras, Reppas & Dressman	**BIOPHARMACEUTICS OF ORALLY ADMINISTERED DRUGS**
Martinez	**PEPTIDE HORMONES AS PROHORMONES**
Rainsford	**ANTI-RHEUMATIC DRUGS: Actions and Side Effects**
Ramabhadran	**PHARMACEUTICAL DESIGN AND DEVELOPMENT: A Molecular Biological Approach**
Ridgway Watt	**TABLET MACHINE INSTRUMENTATION IN PHARMACEUTICS: Principles and Practice**
Roth et al.	**PHARMACEUTICAL CHEMISTRY, Volume 1: Drug Synthesis**
Roth et al.	**PHARMACEUTICAL CHEMISTRY, Volume 2: Drug Analysis**
Rubinstein	**PHARMACEUTICAL TECHNOLOGY Controlled Drug Release, Volume 1:**
Russell & Chopra	**UNDERSTANDING ANTIBACTERIAL ACTION AND RESISTANCE**
Taylor & Kennewell	**MODERN MEDICINAL CHEMISTRY**
Theobald	**RADIOPHARMACEUTICALS: Using Radioactive Compounds in Pharmaceutics and Medicine**
Vergnaud	**CONTROLLED DRUG RELEASE OF ORAL DOSAGE FORMS**
Washington	**PARTICLE SIZE ANALYSIS IN PHARMACEUTICS AND OTHER INDUSTRIES**
Washington et al.	**PHARMACOKINETIC MODELLING USING STELLA ON THE APPLE MACINTOSH (TM)**
Wells	**PHARMACEUTICAL PREFORMULATION**
Wells & Rubinstein	**PHARMACEUTICAL TECHNOLOGY Controlled Drug Release, Volume 2**
Wells & Rubinstein	**PHARMACEUTICAL TECHNOLOGY Tableting Technology, Volume 2**
Wilson & Washington	**PHYSIOLOGICAL PHARMACEUTICS**
Woolfson & McCafferty	**PERCUTANEOUS ANAESTHESIA**

PHARMACEUTICAL DESIGN AND DEVELOPMENT
A Molecular Biology Approach

T. V. RAMABHADRAN

ELLIS HORWOOD
NEW YORK LONDON TORONTO SYDNEY TOKYO SINGAPORE

First published 1994 by
Ellis Horwood Limited
Campus 400, Maylands Avenue
Hemel Hempstead
Hertfordshire, HP2 7EZ
A division of
Simon & Schuster International Group

Printed and bound in Great Britain by
Bookcraft, Midsomer Norton

Library of Congress Cataloging-in-Publication Data

Available from the publisher

British Library Cataloguing in Publication Data

A catalogue record for this book is available from
the British Library

ISBN 0-13-553884-X

1 2 3 4 5 98 97 96 95 94

Table of contents

A colour section appears between pages 24 and 25

Preface

The spectacular developments in molecular biology and biotechnology over the past fifteen years have profoundly impacted the design and development of pharmaceuticals. It is certain that almost everyone involved in the discovery and development of drugs will encounter these concepts at some point hereafter. The aim of this book is to bring together, under one cover, the variety of ways in which recent discoveries in molecular and cell biology are influencing the existing processes of drug development and also spawning new technologies unimaginable heretofore.

In undertaking the daunting task of covering this wide range of concepts, many of them outside of my specialization, the foremost question I had to address was that of the intended readership. Originally, the idea for this book evolved from a half-day workshop which was developed for the INTERPHEX-USA meeting in 1989. Therefore, pharmacologists and pharmaceutical scientists and managers, ranging from those in R&D activities to those involved in clinical studies and regulatory affairs, formed the initial group to whom this book was addressed. This is the rationale for devoting an entire chapter to the basic concepts in molecular biology. Subsequently, I have written to expand the readership to other groups. I believe that advanced undergraduate and graduate students in all areas of biomedical sciences contemplating careers in the pharmaceutical and biotechnology industries will find the material useful. This book should be particularly useful to students in undergraduate programs offering specialized degrees in biotechnology. In addition, I have also aimed to make this book useful to non-scientists, notably pharmaceutical and biotechnology executives, as well as investment managers and attorneys who wish to gain an appreciation for the technologies they administer or deal with in an advisory capacity. Further, practicing physicians who encounter biotechnology-derived drugs and/or treatment modalities in the clinic are likely to find this book useful. Lastly, it is my hope that this book will merit the attention of specialists in biotechnology, in areas outside of their field of specialization.

In addressing the book to such a broad audience, I have begun each chapter with a historical perspective of the developments followed by a brief overview of the topics covered in further detail within the chapter. Where appropriate, the chapters include case studies on salient examples of the concepts discussed. Readers with limited interest in scientific details may prefer to read the initial section and move to the specific examples discussed towards the end of each chapter. I have included many references to the current literature in biotechnology for the benefit of students and researchers who may wish to pursue specific topics in further detail; the Appendix included to update the chapters contains new and/or useful information published between the compilation of the manuscript and its typesetting. Where available, review articles have been cited, as these include prioritized references to the original articles. In the spirit of focusing on the concepts, no deliberate attempt has been made to address scientific priorities or to associate names of scientists with recent breakthrough discoveries. I hope that I will be forgiven for this violation of this general scientific norm.

Writing a book of this range, over an extended period, especially by a single individual, is impossible without the support and encouragement of a large group of colleagues, well-wishers, and some institutions. I thank all of them for their encouragement and support. I am grateful to the Pharmaceutical Manufacturers Association, Amgen Corporation, Eli Lilly Company and Arthur D. Little Decision Resources Inc. for generously providing useful information and literature. Most of the graphics in the book are owed to Paul Fracasso's artistic abilities guided by his scientific capabilities. Advice and illustrations from members of the Structural Chemistry Group of Miles Pharmaceuticals Inc., Drs Robert Tilton, Sarah Heald, and Arthur Robbins, have been invaluable; further, I am indebted to Dr Suresh Katti of this group for critical reading and advice on the material covered in Chapter 5, one of the areas farthest removed from my expertise. Almost all of the material herein was written during the two years I spent in the stimulating environment of Dr Paul Greengard's laboratory at the Rockefeller University. Among members of the Greengard lab, I am greatly indebted to my colleague and friend Dr Sam Gandy for his constant encouragement, which played a very vital part in the successful completion of this book. I thank Sue Horwood of Ellis Horwood for her initial interest, continued encouragement, gentle prodding, and patient handling of deviations from the promised schedule. I am also grateful to my wife, Rajani, for her constant encouragement, and for proofreading the drafts of all chapters. I thank Dr Clarence Hiskey for his critical reading and comments on the early chapters. As much as I am grateful to the persons named above, I take sole responsibility for all errors and omissions found in this book.

Finally, the sacrifice of my wife, Rajani, and that of my sons, Sanjeev and Sachin, by their tolerance of my spending the weekends which were rightfully theirs, hunched over the computer, has been central to this protracted project. Therefore I dedicate this book to them, as well as to my late mother, Lakshmy, and my father, Venkatachalam, to whom I am perennially indebted.

Guilford, CT
June 1993

T. V. Ramabhadran

1

Introduction and historical perspective

The decade of the 1970s witnessed two seminal and revolutionary advances in biological sciences which have impacted the future of the design and the development of pharmaceuticals in an unprecedented manner. The emergence of DNA cloning technologies, known commonly as recombinant DNA (rDNA) technology, and the methodologies for the production of monoclonal antibodies, called hybridoma technology, were the centerpieces of the revolution which was the culmination of decades of basic research in molecular biology, cell biology, and immunology. These developments in biology, referred to commonly as "biotechnology", were facilitated by several preceding and concomitant developments in the chemical technologies of peptide synthesis, automated microsequencing of proteins, and gene synthesis. Many novel technological advances and improvements in older methods have since occurred in the wake of these two major breakthroughs, and several others have been impelled to develop by the opportunities and needs created by the new developments. Advances in instrumentation and methods for structure determination with the help of powerful computers are also contributing to the exploitation of the biotechnological progress for pharmaceutical drug development. The aim of this book is to describe these technologies as they impact on the development of drugs directly as well as through their impact on the development of diagnostics and animal models, which in turn facilitate drug design and development.

Major advances in the development of pharmaceuticals during the decades preceding the 1970s and in the nineteenth century were the result of advances in pharmacology, analytical chemistry and synthetic organic chemistry. Studies of the effects of naturally occurring substances on biological systems combined with the ability to analyze the structure of such agents, and to produce synthetic equivalents and derivatives in the chemistry laboratory gave birth to the pharmaceutical industry, which at this time is composed of several multinational corporations with total annual sales of several billion dollars.

A concept central to pharmaceutical development was the postulation of the presence in biological systems of "receptor substances" or "receptors" to which drugs would bind with specificity, thus eliciting their responses. The receptor concept was propounded by Langley, who studied the action of curare on the neuromuscular junction, and by Ehrlich from his studies of antigen–antibody interactions and the binding of dyes to cells. In this era, the receptor substances or receptors were treated as ''black boxes'' and their properties were inferred by their interaction with a series of related compounds, efficiently supplied by the organic chemists. Thus, the development of pharmaceuticals has relied heavily on the laborious process of ''synthesize and screen'' and this approach has led to many important drug substances. Although the synthetic and analytical capabilities provided for the synthesis of an unprecedented number of low-molecular-weight compounds of defined structure as test candidates, the receptors to which they bound were not amenable to structural analysis owing to their comparatively large size. Isolation and characterization of receptors using biochemical techniques has been relatively slow and laborious.

The new technologies of recombinant DNA and monoclonal antibodies address the receptor side of the drug development equation. The ability to obtain detailed structures of the receptors and their macromolecular ligands using molecular biological analysis of the gene sequences, production of receptors in large quantities for structural analyses, and development of specific antibody reagents to analyze their presence in organs and tissues have opened new vistas for drug development and for refinement of older drugs.

DRUG RECEPTORS

Drugs produce their biological effects through interaction with molecular constituents of cells. With a few exceptions, such as antacids and metal ion chelating agents which interact with small molecules, most drugs interact with cellular macromolecules, namely proteins, nucleic acids, carbohydrates, lipids, and combinations of these. Among these, proteins, owing to their diversity and the key roles in cellular metabolism, form the predominant class of drug receptors. Many drugs currently in use are targeted against proteins as exemplified by inhibitors of metabolic enzymes such as dihydrofolate or acetylcholinesterase. Natural ligands for many physiological receptors in the cell are themselves proteins. The earliest and the greatest impact of biotechnology has been concentrated on proteins.

Among other cellular macromolecules, nucleic acids, mainly DNA, are the receptors for a variety of chemotherapeutic agents used in the treatment of cancers. New therapeutic approaches targeting nucleic acids are under development in the wake of the detailed understanding of gene expression provided by the molecular biological tools entailed through recombinant DNA. Carbohydrates are the receptors for a host of plant lectins, and the lipids are receptors for agents such as general anesthetics. Recent independent developments in the analysis of cellular carbohydrates, which are often linked to proteins, promise new opportunities for drug development: this area, known as ''glycobiology'', is also benefiting from recent developments in biotechnology. Similarly, greater understanding of cell biology in recent times has revealed the importance of lipids and lipid conjugates in cell function. These molecules play important structural roles in anchoring proteins to membranes. Lipids and lipid derivatives are also involved as intracellular effectors in the pathways of transduction of extracellular signals.

Protein receptors and ligands

The earliest and the most obvious benefit to accrue from biotechnology was the ability to produce an unlimited supply of therapeutic proteins available heretofore only in small quantities. Use of proteins as therapeutics predates the developments in biotechnology. For example, use of human growth hormone, antihemophilia factor VIII, and immunoglobulin fractions extracted from human sources was well established prior to the advent of recombinant DNA techniques. However, the sources for their production were limited. More importantly, the safety of the products was a major concern because of contamination by human pathogens. Presence of the human immunodeficiency virus, HIV, in the factor VIII preparations derived from human blood, and of the slow-acting infectious agent causing Creutzfeldt–Jakob disease in growth hormone prepared from human cadavers have had devastating consequences on the patient populations using these proteins therapeutically. Recombinant materials, although not entirely without new safety issues, allow for the production of these proteins free of pathogens. In addition to these first-line therapeutics, availability of proteins in virtually unlimited quantities has spurred on their use in other areas of drug development. These applications, listed in Table 1.1, are discussed in greater detail in the following chapters.

Table 1.1. Applications of proteins in pharmaceutical development

- THERAPEUTICS
  - Replacement therapy
  - Augmentation
  - Vaccines
  - Chimeric proteins with novel activities
- ASSAYS FOR RANDOM, MASS SCREENING
  - Low-molecular-weight active compounds
- STRUCTURE-BASED RATIONAL DRUG DESIGN
  - Low-molecular-weight active compounds
  - Engineering of novel proteins
- DIAGNOSTIC APPLICATIONS
  - Enzymes and antibodies

Protein drugs have been used extensively in replacement therapies in cases where the patient is unable to produce the required protein in sufficient quantities as in the case of insulin in type I diabetics. Alternatively, external administration of some proteins, to augment quantities naturally produced by the body, can be therapeutically beneficial as with the use of interferon formulations in the treatment of cancers and certain viral infections. The ability to produce large quantities of proteins with directed changes in the primary sequence can be exploited to produce smaller segments of proteins with improved therapeutic potential as in the case of subunit and peptide vaccines. In addition, protein chimeras with novel activities can also be produced as discussed in Chapter 3. In all these cases, the protein drug is the ligand for endogenous receptors.

Most cell-surface macromolecules which relay extracellular signals to the interior of the cell and produce intracellular responses are proteins. Their production in desired quantities and in desired cell systems is being used to produce highly defined, and often safer, screening systems for drug development as in the case of surface components and crucial metabolic enzymes of the human immunodeficiency virus (HIV). These aspects of biotechnology are discussed in detail in Chapter 4. Further, the availability of unlimited supplies of pure proteins, coupled with advances in theoretical concepts and laboratory techniques for the determination of their structures, provides new opportunities for the rational design of drugs, to supplant or to focus the random screening approach which has been the mainstay of drug development. A valuable adjunct to the structural studies is the ability to produce specific protein variants "on demand" using the powerful and elegant technique of site-directed mutagenesis. The concepts and advances in this area are discussed in Chapter 5. Proteins are used as reagents in the diagnostic tests notably as antigens and antibodies. Production of proteins in large quantities and with higher purity provides avenues for the development of sensitive diagnostic kits as in the case of immunological and biochemical detection of infection with HIV. Such applications are discussed in Chapter 8. Fig. 1.1 schematically depicts the typical uses of proteins in drug discovery and development.

Nucleic acids receptors and ligands

Nucleic acids, predominantly DNA, are the target receptors for many chemotherapeutic agents used in the treatment of cancer. These agents interact with DNA in a non-specific manner interfering with the capacity of DNA to specify the correct proteins and to replicate itself. Recent developments in the use of nucleic acids in pharmaceutical development are listed in Table 1.2. Advances in molecular biology and biotechnology have led to the accumulation of sequence information on hundreds of human genes and also to the development of methodologies for the specific modulation of the expression of selected genes using synthetic DNA of defined sequence. Methods are being developed for the selective destruction of specific nucleic acid molecules and for the inhibition of their expression into proteins in somatic cells. Another major application of nucleic acids is in gene therapy, where the deficiency of a particular protein is corrected by the incorporation of the appropriate gene into a specific cell population of the patient. The introduction of genes into the germline of mice and other laboratory animals is being used to develop animal models for diseases such as Alzheimer's, for which no convenient animal models exist. These animal models are extremely valuable for the testing of drugs, especially in cases where no animal models exist. Chapters 6 and 7 detail these applications of nucleic acids.

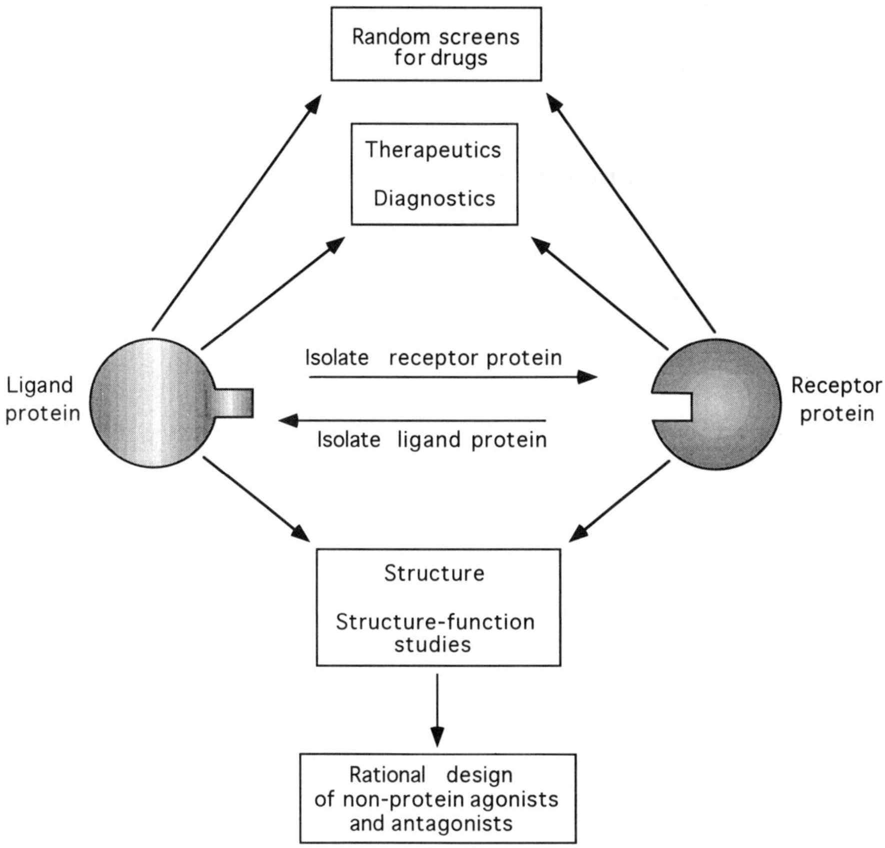

Fig. 1.1. Applications of proteins in drug discovery and development.

Nucleic acids are also valuable as diagnostic reagents. In combination with the recently developed amplification method, polymerase chain reaction (PCR), nucleic acid probes allow the detection of trace amounts of a specified nucleic acid sequence. Thus, the presence of the DNA of pathogens can be ascertained with great sensitivity and rapidity. Further, these tools permit the analysis and the detection of gene defects in individual patients, and aid in the tailoring of therapeutic strategies. These applications are discussed in Chapter 8.

Table 1.2. Applications of nucleic acids in pharmaceutical development

- AID TO PRODUCTION OF PROTEINS
  - Gene isolation
  - Gene synthesis
  - DNA sequencing
- SPECIFIC INHIBITION OF GENE EXPRESSION
  - Antisense nucleic acid drugs
- GENE THERAPY
  - Complete genes
  - Vectors for gene delivery
- TRANSGENIC ANIMALS
  - Complete genes
  - Tissue-specific regulatory elements
- DIAGNOSTIC APPLICATION
  - Gene probes

An ambitious effort is now under way to determine the sequence of the entire human genome comprising some three billion base pairs using the nucleic acid technologies and advanced computer technologies. The complete nucleotide sequence is expected to contribute to an unprecedented understanding of human diseases and to appropriate therapeutic approaches. However the utility, the specific approaches, and the cost–benefit questions are still being debated. This and other frontier issues are discussed in Chapter 9.

Other receptors and ligands

While proteins and nucleic acids are the macromolecules directly amenable to manipulation through biotechnological processes, growth of research in these areas is contributing to the development of therapeutic strategies aimed at the carbohydrate and lipid moieties. The recent field of "glycobiology" is focused on the structure and function of cellular carbohydrates. Although development of glycobiology is based primarily on technical advances indigenous to carbohydrate chemistry, its application is propelled by the biological information rapidly emerging through the applications of biotechnology (Karlsson, 1991). Sugar clusters or oligosaccharides are often linked to proteins. An understanding of the structure–function relation of glycoproteins is beginning to reveal diagnostic and therapeutic approaches aimed at the carbohydrate components of the cellular machinery (Hodgson, 1991). Similar avenues for drug development are provided by the detailed understanding of protein–lipid interactions, and the function of lipid-linked proteins and glycolipids. Lipids have been shown to play critical roles in the subcellular localization of proteins, the assembly of macromolecular complexes, and the activation of key enzymes in signal transduction in cellular pathways (Hoffman, 1991). Glycolipids are also involved in initiating and maintaining cellular responses to extracellular stimuli. Thus lipids and enzymes involved in their metabolism also present promising opportunities for drug development. These areas are beyond the scope of this book and are not treated under individual heads, but discussion pertaining to these topics is interspersed with appropriate chapters.

BIOTECHNOLOGY INDUSTRY

Commercialization of the discoveries in genetic engineering and monoclonal antibody technology began in the late 1970s. A handful of small biotechnology companies was founded through the collaboration of academic scientists and venture capitalists. Large pharmaceutical companies whose drug discovery programs were oriented chemically were slow to take to the biologically oriented approach. However, some companies such as Eli Lilly bought early into the technology through contractual agreements with the biotech companies, and others followed suit. Genentech was the first biotechnology company to make a spectacular public stock offering on Wall Street in 1980, and since that time hundreds of companies have been formed. At the present time, a high proportion of the international biotechnology effort is concentrated in the US. Of the 737 companies from 25 countries listed in the ''1992 Genetic Engineering News Guide to Biotechnology Companies'', the highest number, 547, are in the US, with the United Kingdom having the next highest, 56 (*Genetic Engineering News*, 1991). A more recent report puts the number of biotechnology companies in the US at 742, with a majority of these focusing on the development of therapeutics (Dibner, 1991).

Many small biotech companies that started in the late 1970s and 1980s were initially focused on improved methods for the production of proteins which were well established as therapeutics. Thus, insulin, human growth hormone, and factor VIII were early targets of pharmaceutical biotechnology. Interferon, the antiviral protein, because of reports of its antitumor effects also became a protein of intense interest to the biotechnology industry. Attention then turned to other less-established natural proteins which were available in small amounts such as the clot-dissolving protein, tissue plasminogen activator and cell growth factors. Involvement of the large pharmaceutical houses was beneficial and crucial to the development of the protein therapeutics because of their overall experience and broader capabilities in clinical testing and in dealing with regulatory issues. Being a new class of drugs produced through methods unused heretofore, governmental regulatory agencies had to evolve new criteria and standards for efficacy and, more importantly, safety of these products. As a source of guidance to the biotech industry, several ''points to consider'' documents dealing with the different aspects of the biological drug approval process have been developed by the Food and Drug Administration (FDA) in the US.

Today, practically, every major pharmaceutical company has some in-house research efforts in biotechnology and many have gained access to select technologies through alliances with or ownership of smaller biotechnology companies. New biotech companies, focused on further developments brought on by the initial wave, have arisen during the 1980s (Dibner, 1991). Biotechnology has come to be an integral part of pharmaceutical R&D. The blending of the traditional pharmaceutical industry practices with the biotechnology industry has created newer approaches to the development of drugs using established methods of synthetic chemistry.

PRODUCTS AND MARKETS

During the early years, the dazzle and the promise of the new technology made it attractive to financial markets. It also placed high expectations on the biotechnology companies. The lofty expectations created in investment circles generally by promotional hype were often at odds with scientific realities. This is best exemplified by the unlimited promise and the limited profits generated early on with interferons and more recently with tissue plasminogen activator, tPA. Unlike the products of the computer revolution to which biotechnology is often compared, the products for human healthcare were more complex to bring to the market. These factors led to unfulfilled expectations and resultant disenchantment with the prospects of biotechnology's impact on the pharmaceutical industry. However many of these doubts seem to have been laid to rest as is evident from the first wave of products in the market and in clinical trials. The interest of the financial community in biotechnology is on the rise, although warm and cold spells of confidence based on the success or failure of individual products are commonplace (Spalding, 1993). At the time of writing, over a hundred "biotech" drugs are in various stages of clinical development, and over a dozen have won FDA approval. They can be divided into three major categories: blood products, immunotherapeutics, and infectious disease products (Roth, 1991). Among the categories, blood products appear to be poised to take on the major share of revenues. Table 1.3 is a list of currently approved protein drugs and the indications for their use, published by the Pharmaceutical Manufacturers Association (PMA Survey Report, 1991). Three more drugs have been approved in 1992, to bring the total of FDA-approved biotech drugs to 19, comprising 12 categories of proteins (Shamel and Keough, 1993). However, as a large number of genetically engineered protein drugs are approaching the market, a backlog appears to be building at the FDA in the US (Gibbons, 1991; Copmann, 1991). This is expected to delay the appearance of new drugs in the market with the attendant financial consequences which are expected to impact the biotechnology industry. In response to these concerns, the FDA has announced reforms which include the use of outside contractors to speed up the review process (Metheny, 1992).

Table 1.3. Approved biotechnology-derived therapeutics in the US (1992)

Trade name	Protein	Indication
1. Actimmune	Interferon gamma-1b	Chronic granulomatous disease
2. Activase	Tissue plasminogen activator	Acute myocardial infarction Acute pulmonary embolism
3. Alferon N	Interferon alfa-n3	Genital warts
4. Engerix-B	Hepatitis B vaccine	Hepatitis B immunization
5. Epogen	Erythropoietin alfa	Anemia of chronic renal failure
6. Humatrope	Human growth hormone	Growth hormone deficiency
7. Humulin	Human insulin	Diabetes
8. Intron A	Interferon alfa-2b	Hairy cell leukemia
9. Leukine	GM-CSF	Autologous bone marrow transplant
10. Neupogen	rG-CSF	Chemotherapy-induced neutropenia
11. Procrit	Erythropoietin alfa	Anemia of chronic renal failure
12. Prokine	GM-CSF	Autologous bone marrow transplant
13. Proleukin*	Interleukin-2	Metastatic kidney cancer
14. OncoscintCR/OV*	Monoclonal antibody	Detection of colorectal and ovarian cancers
15. Orthoclone OKT3	Monoclonal antibody	Acute kidney transplant rejection
16. Protropin	Human growth hormone	Growth hormone deficiency
17. Recombinate*	Factor VIII	Hemophilia A
18. Recombivax HB	Hepatitis B vaccine	Hepatitis B vaccination
19. Roferon-A	Interferon alfa-2a	Hairy cell leukemia, AIDS-related Kaposi's sarcoma

Compiled from the Pharmaceutical Manufacturers' Association (PMA) Report on ''Biotechnology Medicines in Development'' 1991; **BioWorld Today*, January 14, 1993. Also see Appendix.

Estimates of the 1991 and 1992 US biotechnology drug sales are around 1.7 to 3 billion dollars (Roth, 1991; Bylinsky, 1991; Shamel and Keough, 1993), and include the proteins shown in Table 1.3. This total sales figure pales in comparison to the market size of the traditional pharmaceutical US sales, which runs to around $50 billion (O'Reilly, 1991). In 1990, the sale of Glaxo's Zantac alone produced 1.3 billion dollars in the US (2.4 billion worldwide), and the five top selling drugs raked up over 3 billion dollars in US sales. By this criterion, biotechnology products have a long way to go. However, these comparisons pit the performance of the fledgling biotechnology industry, which is only a decade old, against that of the century-old traditional pharmaceuticals. Nonetheless, optimistic predictions have been made for the future market share of biotechnology-derived products. It is predicted that the US sales of "biotech" drugs would be over 5 billion dollars by 1996, with a compounded annual growth rate of 48.9% between 1988 and 1995, and is predicted to reach 23 billion dollars in the year 2000 (Dibner, 1991). Another, more recent estimate predicts a lower, 9 billion dollar, sales figure for the year 2002 (Shamel and Keough, 1993). It is estimated that the biotech industry will achieve worldwide sales in the 30 to 70 billion dollar range by the year 2000.

A recent study comparing the clinical success rates of biopharmaceuticals and conventional drugs indicates a higher clinical success rate and shorter approval times for biopharmaceuticals (Bienz-Tadmor *et al.,* 1992). Further, the cost of discovery and development of a protein drug compares favorably with that for chemical drugs. For example, the discovery and development cost of the protein drug Epogen at 150 million dollars is well below the average cost of discovering and developing a chemical drug, which is estimated to be around 231 million dollars. However, it is estimated that, at least at the present time, the average research cost for biotechnology products is nearly twice that for conventional chemical drugs. The spending per employee is also considerably higher for the biotech companies, reflecting the research-intensive nature of the industry. In 1990, biotechnology companies spent $71,639 per employee compared to $18,909 spent by traditional pharmaceutical companies. On average, biotech firms spent about 46% of their revenues on research against the 10% figure for pharmaceutical companies.

The sales projections described above deal with the direct sales volumes of therapeutic or diagnostic products from biotechnology. Future contributions of biotechnology to drug development will include the creation of well-defined test systems. These may be in the form of providing pure proteins for structure determination, and in the form of enzymes, whole cell systems, and transgenic animals for testing of candidate drugs. These contributions, although not appearing in sales charts of biotechnology products, will add to the sales of newer chemical drugs. In addition, the new technologies of nucleic acid therapies and gene technologies are likely to produce new drugs and therapeutic modalities whose market potential and marketing strategies are difficult to define at this time.

LEGAL AND SOCIAL ASPECTS OF BIOTECHNOLOGY

Protection of intellectual property through patents forms a vital part of entrepreneur and investor confidence in any industrial endeavor. Until 1990, 3378 biotechnology patents were issued in the US, with an average waiting period of 25.6 months, which is significantly longer than the 18 months required for all patents (PMA Survey Report, 1991). Of these, 1321 patents were healthcare related. The influx of patent applications coupled with the newness of the technology appears to have resulted in an overall slowing of the patenting process (Manbeck, 1991). Biotechnology patenting strategies were based on previous experience of the patenting of pharmaceuticals. However, the concept of patentability has required redefinition when applied to many biotechnological situations. Questions have been raised regarding the patentability of DNA sequences (Aldhous, 1991; also see Chapter 9), and of new animals created through recombinant DNA manipulations (Meyer, 1991).

The product development pipelines of many companies overlap, leading to patent disputes. Many patent litigations have already been fought or are currently in the courts relating to patent rights and infringements in the context of protein drug manufacture and other technologies (Ratner, 1991; Bluestone, 1991a; Bluestone, 1991b). It is certain that others will be fought in these and other newly developing areas.

Aside from the patenting, and regulatory issues relating to product safety, the techniques of the biotechnology industry have raised many ethical issues, and also societal concerns related to environmental safety (Miller, 1991; Davis, 1991). However, the situation relating to most of pharmaceutical biotechnology, at least with regards to protein drugs, *in vitro* assay systems, and diagnostics, is simpler compared to other areas of rDNA applications which involve the deliberate release of engineered plants, bacteria, and viruses into the environment. Nonetheless, some of the same concerns have been raised with respect to the containment of engineered organisms used in pharmaceutical production on the grounds of worker safety and possible release at production sites. Ethical and philosophical questions relating to gene therapy (Culliton, 1991) and to transgenic animal technology, questioning man's right to change the genetic composition of other species, have been raised. Many of these issues, raised usually by environmental and animal rights' activists, have in many instances led to delays in approval of certain procedures involving genetically engineered products and organisms (Stewart, 1991; Brooks and Johnson, 1991). Fortunately, their impact on the development of pharmaceutical biotechnology, at least in the US, has not been seriously adverse. But in Europe, the regulatory policies for biotechnology have been, and continue to be, much more restrictive (Shackley and Hodgson, 1991; Dixon, 1993), resulting in many European multinational pharmaceutical companies basing their biotechnology operations in the US.

As has been the case with conventional drugs, therapeutic proteins produced by biotechnology are also open to misuse as in the cases of the use of human growth hormone and erythropoietin by athletes to enhance their athletic performance. Their being identical to their counterparts produced in the body makes their detection in routine tests nearly impossible (Spalding, 1991). These concerns are also being addressed by the manufacturers of such drugs.

All things considered, it is fair to state confidently that, over the past two decades, biotechnology has matured and has entrenched itself as an integral part of pharmaceutical discovery and development. The results seen in the first two decades of biotechnology demonstrate the power of the technology, and the current rapid pace of developments predicts many new and heretofore unimaginable applications. These developments will have an impact on the practice of medicine and on the pharmaceutical industry in presently unpredictable but exciting ways which will carry well into the twenty-first century and after.

GENERAL READING

Brooks, H. and Johnson, R. B. (1991). Comments: public policy issues. In *The Genetic Revolution: Scientific Prospects and Public Perceptions.* B. D. Davis, ed. (Baltimore: The Johns Hopkins University Press), pp. 266–282.

Bylinsky, G. (1991). Biotech firms tackle the giants. *Fortune* August 12, 78–82.

Davis, B.D. (Ed.) (1991). *The Genetic Revolution: Scientific Prospects and Public Perceptions* (Baltimore: The Johns Hopkins University Press).

DiPalma, J.R. (1965). Introduction; brief history. In *Drill's Pharmacology in Medicine.* J.R. DiPalma, ed. (New York: McGraw-Hill), pp. 1–5.

Goldstein, A., Aronow, L., and Kalman, S.M. (1974). Molecular mechanisms of drug action. In *Principles of Drug Action: the Basis of Pharmacology.* (New York: John Wiley & Sons), pp. 1–127.

Kevles, D.J. and Hood, L. (Eds) (1992). *The Code of Codes: Scientific and Social Issues in the Human Genome Project* (Cambridge, Massachusetts: Harvard University Press).

Miller, H.I. (1991). Regulation. In *The Genetic Revolution: Scientific Prospects and Public Perceptions.* B. D. Davis, ed. (Baltimore: The Johns Hopkins University Press), pp. 196–211.

O'Reilly, B. (1991). Drugmakers. *Fortune* July 29, 48–63.

Ross, E.M. (1990). Pharmacodynamics: Mechanism of drug action and relationship between drug concentration and effect. In *Pharmacological Basis of Therapeutics.* A.G. Gilman, T. W. Rall, A. S. Nies, and P. Taylor, eds (New York: Pergamon Press), pp. 33–48.

Roth, S. (1991). Biopharmaceutical products, trends, and growth forecast for the 1990s. *Genetic Engineering News* February, 5–30.

Spalding, B.J. and McCormick, D. (1991). R & D spending still soaring. *Bio/Technology* **9,** 690–692.

Stewart, R.B. (1991). Regulatory Law. In *The Genetic Revolution: Scientific Prospects and Public Perceptions.* B. D. Davis, ed. (Baltimore: The Johns Hopkins University Press), pp. 212–238.

Tietelman, R. (1989). *Gene Dreams: Wall Street, Academia, and the Rise of Biotechnology* (New York: Basic Books).

Weatherall, M. (1990). *In Search of a Cure* (Oxford: Oxford University Press).

REFERENCES

Aldhous, P. (1991). Human genome project: tit for tat patents? *Nature* **353,** 785.

Bienz-Tadmor, B., Dicerbo, P.A., Tadmor, G., and Lasgna, L. (1992). Biopharmaceuticals and conventional drugs: clinical success rates. *Bio/Technology* **10,** 521–525.

Bluestone, M. (1991a). Centocor and Xoma square off: do patent trials hurt more than help? *Bio/Technology* **9,** 910.

Bluestone, M. (1991b). Lawyers, lawyers everywhere: will Kodak foil Cetus's PCR sale. *Bio/Technology* **9,** 1028.

Brooks, H. and Johnson, R.B. (1991). Comments: public policy issues. In *The Genetic Revolution: Scientific Prospects and Public Perceptions.* B. D. Davis, ed. (Baltimore: The Johns Hopkins University Press), pp. 266–282.

Bylinsky, G. (1991). Biotech firms tackle the giants. *Fortune* August 12, 78–82.

Copmann, T.L. (1991). Science is not the barrier to innovation in biotechnology medicine. In *PMA Survey Report: Biotechnology Medicines in Development* (Washington, DC: Pharmaceutical Manufacturers Association), p. 16.

Culliton, B.J. (1991). Gene therapy on the move. *Nature* **354,** 429.

Davis, B.D. (1991). Summary and comments: the scientific chapters. In *The Genetic Revolution: Scientific Prospects and Public Perceptions.* B.D. Davis, ed. (Baltimore: The Johns Hopkins University Press), pp. 239–265.

Dibner, M.D. (1991). Tracking trends in U.S. biotechnology. *Bio/Technology* **9,** 1334–1337.

Dixon, B. (1993). Who's who in European antibiotech? *Bio/Technology* **11,** 44–48.

Genetic Engineering News (1991). 1992 Genetic Engineering News Guide to Biotechnology Companies. *Genetic Engineering News* November/December, 16–42.

Gibbons, A. (1991). Biotech pipeline: bottleneck ahead. *Science* **254,** 369.

Hodgson, J. (1991). Carbohydrate-based therapeutics. *Bio/Technology* **9,** 609–613.

Hoffman, M. (1991). Playing tag with membrane proteins. *Science* **254,** 650–651.

Karlsson, K-A. (1991). Glycobiology: a growing field for drug design. *TiPs* **12,** 265–272.

Manbeck, H. F., Jr. (1991). Patenting biotechnology inventions: a patent and trademark office perspective. In *PMA Survey Report: Biotechnology Medicines in Development* (Washington, DC: Pharmaceutical Manufacturers Association), p. 15.

Metheny, B. (1992). FDA reforms advocated by White House council near completion. *Genetic Engineering News* January, 3–25.

Meyer, S.J. (1991). Legal issues in biotechnology: patenting. In *Recombinant DNA Technology and Applications.* A. Prokop, R.K. Bajpai, and C. Ho, eds. (New York: McGraw-Hill), pp. 583–598.

Miller, H.I. (1991). Regulation. In *The Genetic Revolution: Scientific Prospects and Public Perceptions.* B.D. Davis, ed. (Baltimore: The Johns Hopkins University Press), pp. 196–211.

O'Reilly, B. (1991). Drugmakers. *Fortune* July 29, 48–63.

PMA Survey Report (1991). *Biotechnology Medicines in Development* (Washington, DC: Pharmaceutical Manufacturers Association).

Ratner, M. (1991). EPO, factor VIII shockers. *Bio/Technology* **9,** 327.

Roth, S. (1991). Biopharmaceutical products, trends, and growth forecast for the 1990s. *Genetic Engineering News* February, 5–30.

Shackley, S. and Hodgson, J. (1991). Biotechnology regulation in Europe. *Bio/Technology* **9,** 1056–1061.

Shamel, R.E. and Keough, M. (1993). Biopharmaceuticals: towards the year 2000. *Genetic Engineering News* **13,** January 1, 4–5.

Spalding, B.J. (1991). Black-market biotechnology: athletes abuse EPO and HGH. *Bio/Technology* **9,** 1050–1053.

Spalding, B.J. (1993). Biotech sector rides on Synergen's shoulders. *Bio/Technology* **11,** 17–18.

Stewart, R.B. (1991). Regulatory Law. In *The Genetic Revolution: Scientific Prospects and Public Perceptions*. B.D. Davis, ed. (Baltimore: The Johns Hopkins University Press), pp. 212–238.

2

Molecular and cell biological foundations of biotechnology

The term "biotechnology" has been used in different contexts to signify a variety of technological endeavors. Defined as the exploitation of biological systems for human benefit, biotechnology is ancient, dating back to agricultural and fermentation activities that are as old as human civilizations. More recent definitions of biotechnology include the development and production of antibiotics as well as improvement of producer strains by mutagenesis and selection (Miller, 1991). However, as widely used in the pharmaceutical industry and financial circles today, as well as in the context of this book, biotechnology refers predominantly to two revolutionary advances in biological sciences which occurred in the 1970s, and their ramifications. The basic components of biotechnology under this definition are commonly known as "recombinant DNA" (rDNA) technology or "genetic engineering", which involves the manipulation of genetic material of cells to produce and modify proteins, and "hybridoma" technology which involves the production of unlimited amounts of monospecific antibodies. The aim of this chapter is to review the basic principles of rDNA and hybridoma technologies in order to provide the necessary background for the following chapters. It is also intended as an "extended glossary" or a rapid refresher. In-depth coverage of these topics is beyond the scope of this book and several excellent references on these topics are cited for further reading. A note of caution is in order however; for almost every generalization of mechanisms in molecular and cell biology, there are exceptions which underscore the rule. In the context of this chapter, clarity of the concepts is emphasized over detailed accuracy. Relevant extensions of the concepts discussed here are presented at appropriate locations in the subsequent chapters in "boxes".

PRINCIPLES OF RECOMBINANT DNA

Proteins: the targets of DNA manipulations

The central goal of almost all DNA or gene manipulations is to influence protein products encoded by the genes. Proteins are a major component of all cells, accounting for nearly half their dry mass, whether they be bacterial or mammalian. They form the structural components of a cell and are also the catalysts for the execution of biochemical reactions within cells. Proteins also play key roles in intercellular and intracellular communications. Thus it is possible to alter the chemical reactions in a cell and its state by augmenting or suppressing the expression of specific proteins. The tools of rDNA technology permit the manipulation of desired cellular proteins and the creation of directed alterations in the sequence of natural proteins by manipulating the specific DNA sequences which direct their production.

Composition of proteins

Proteins are long, unbranched polymers of small monomeric units known as amino acids which have an average molecular weight of about 110 daltons per monomer. With a few rare exceptions, proteins are composed of twenty L-amino acids. The basic structure of an amino acid is shown in Fig. 2.1. The side chains represented by the R group impart distinguishing physicochemical properties to the amino acids. The twenty common amino acids, and the three- and the one-letter abbreviations used commonly in the literature are listed in Table 2.1A.

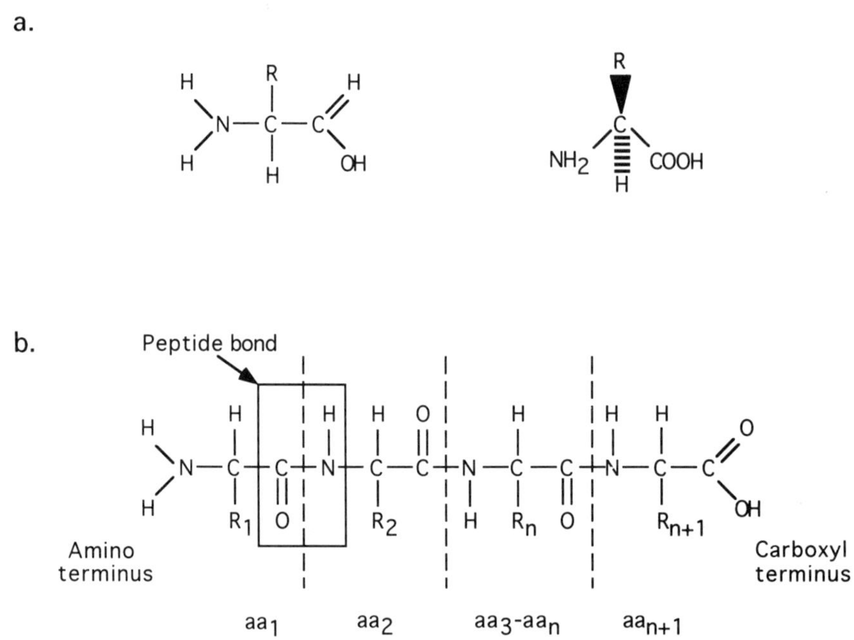

Fig. 2.1. a. Basic chemical structure and stereochemistry of L-amino acids. b. Polymeric structure of proteins and peptides constructed from monomeric units.

Also listed in Table 2.1A is the average frequency of occurrence of each amino acid determined from the sequences of 25,814 proteins representing 7,348,950 amino acids compiled by the National Biomedical Research Foundation (NBRF) database (Appendix III, Gribskov and Devereux, 1991). Amino acids are usually classified into two broad groups: polar or hydrophilic and non-polar or hydrophobic, based on the properties of the side group which determines the interaction of the region of the polypeptide incorporating the particular amino acid, with water. The acid–base property is one of the easily discernible properties conferred by the side chains. Thus, amino acids are also classified as acidic, basic, or neutral depending on the ionization properties of the side groups. The ionized groups contribute the charges necessary for the electrostatic interactions involved in the function of proteins. The side chains of the twenty amino acids and their characteristics are shown in Table 2.1B.

Table 2.1A. Amino acids in proteins

Amino acid	Three-letter code	One-letter code	Relative abundance
Alanine	Ala	A	7.60
Arginine	Arg	R	5.23
Asparagine	Asn	N	4.36
Aspartic acid	Asp	D	5.21
Cysteine	Cys	C	1.89
Glutamine	Gln	Q	4.17
Glutamic acid	Glu	E	6.32
Glycine	Gly	G	7.19
Histidine	His	H	2.28
Isoleucine	Ile	I	5.29
Leucine	Leu	L	9.17
Lysine	Lys	K	5.81
Methionine	Met	M	2.29
Phenylalanine	Phe	F	3.97
Proline	Pro	P	5.20
Serine	Ser	S	7.15
Threonine	Thr	T	5.87
Tryptophan	Trp	W	1.31
Tyrosine	Tyr	Y	3.21
Valine	Val	V	6.49

Table 2.1B.

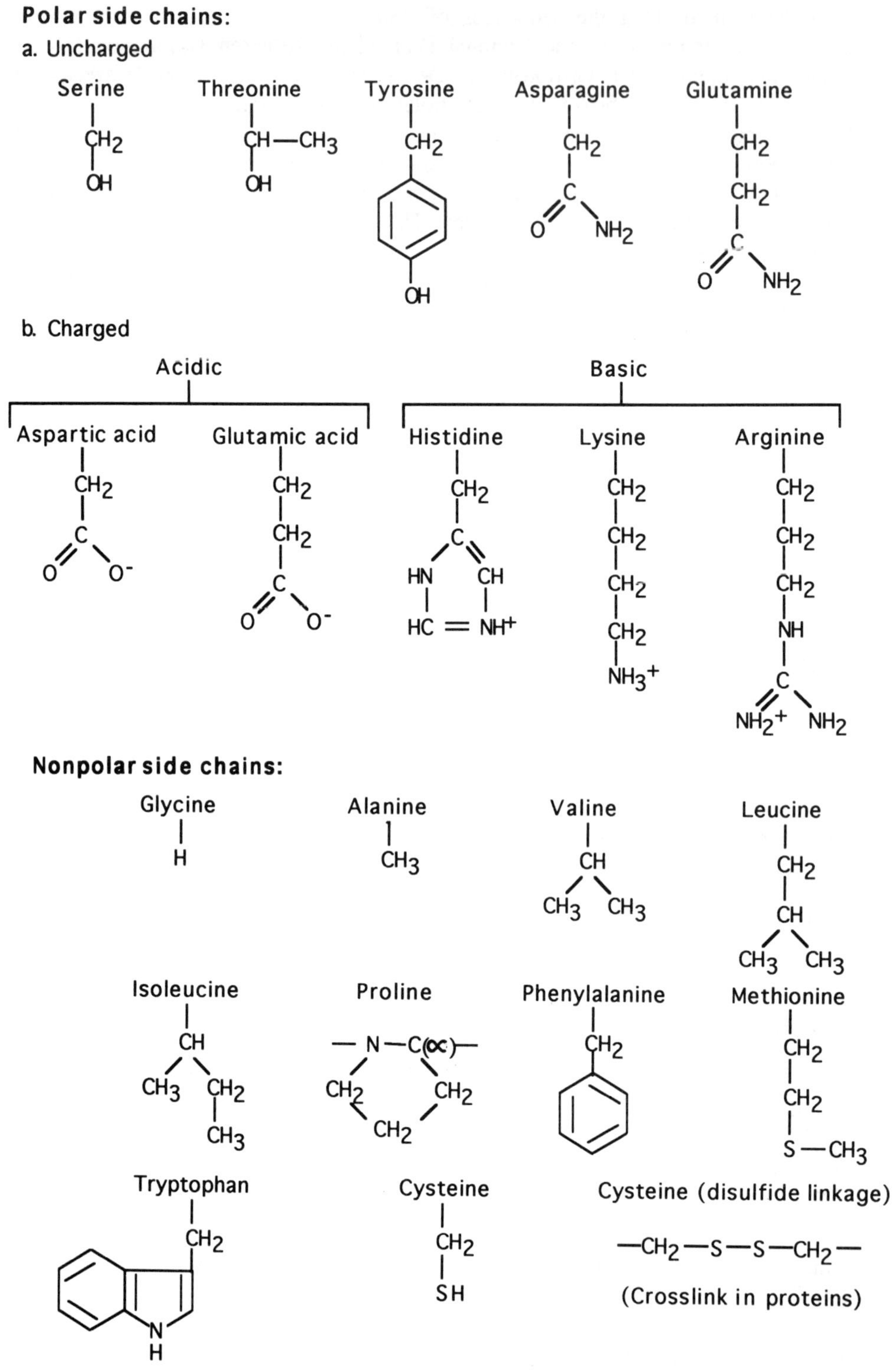
Polar side chains:
a. Uncharged
Serine
Threonine
Tyrosine
Asparagine
Glutamine
b. Charged
Acidic
Basic
Aspartic acid
Glutamic acid
Histidine
Lysine
Arginine
Nonpolar side chains:
Glycine
Alanine
Valine
Leucine
Isoleucine
Proline
Phenylalanine
Methionine
Tryptophan
Cysteine
Cysteine (disulfide linkage)
—CH2—S—S—CH2—
(Crosslink in proteins)

Primary structure of proteins

Proteins are linear polymers of random assortments of the twenty basic amino acids listed in Table 2.1A, and are composed of variable numbers of monomeric units. The molecular weights of proteins range from a few thousand daltons or less (for peptides or oligopeptides) to several thousand daltons (for polypeptides). For example, the thyrotropin-releasing hormone, TRH, is composed of 3 amino acids; somatostatin, a peptide hormone, is composed of 14 amino acids; insulin is made up of 51 amino acids; the human growth hormone is made up of 191 amino acids; and coagulation factor VIII is composed of 2332 amino acids. Amino acids in proteins are linked by amide linkages or peptide bonds formed between the carboxyl group of an amino acid and the amino group of the succeeding amino acid as shown in Fig. 2.1b, leaving free an amino group at one end and a carboxylic acid group at the other end of the chain. By convention, numbering of the amino acid residues in the protein begins at the free amino terminus.

The twenty basic units of differing chemical properties, their random order and variable abundance in the polymer, and the variable length of proteins provide a tremendous diversity to proteins as a class. For example, there are 400 possible dipeptides (20×20) and 8000 (20^3) possible tripeptides, and the numbers become astronomical (20^{100}) when even moderately small proteins of as few as 100 amino acids are considered. Superimposed on this diversity are further modifications such as intrachain and interchain disulfide linkages, which are covalent linkages between cysteines, and other covalent modifications of the sidechains of individual amino acids (discussed below). The linear amino acid sequence together with further covalent modifications is known as the ''primary structure'' of a protein.

Secondary, tertiary, and quaternary structures

The linear sequence of amino acids in a protein, under appropriate environmental conditions, confers upon the protein a distinct three-dimensional structure necessary for its activity. The chemical forces which determine the structure involve ionic, hydrophobic and van der Waals' interactions, and hydrogen bonds. Depending on the local amino acid sequence, the polypeptide backbone assumes a regular structure or exists as a random coil. The regular structural motifs assumed by a polypeptide chain are cylindrical, alpha-helical structures or sheet-like structures known as beta sheets or beta strands. Such local structures within a protein together make up its ''secondary structure''. Once formed, the secondary structural motifs interact with other such regions, distant in the linear sequence, to produce a folded protein. The outcome of these regional interactions is the ''tertiary structure'' of the protein. Furthermore, many active proteins and enzymes are composed of a group of either similar or dissimilar protein subunits. The interactions that occur between subunits, i.e. interchain interactions, lead to the structure of the protein complex termed the ''quaternary structure''. These definitions are outlined in the schematic Fig. 2.2. In the current scientific literature, several representations are used to depict a folded protein, each suited to emphasize a particular aspect of the structure. A typical example of the commonly used representations of protein structure, as applied to a small protein of 99 amino acids, the protease of the HIV virus discussed at length in Chapter 5, is shown in Fig. 2.3.

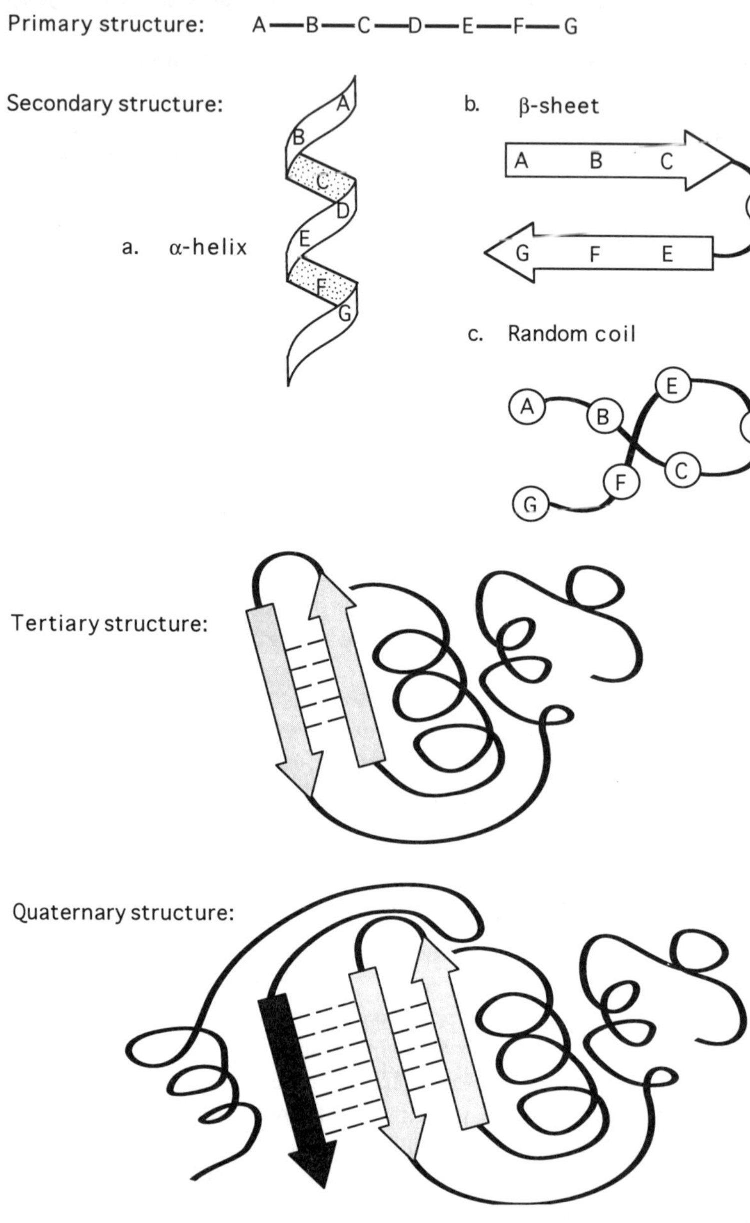

Fig. 2.2. Structural features of proteins.

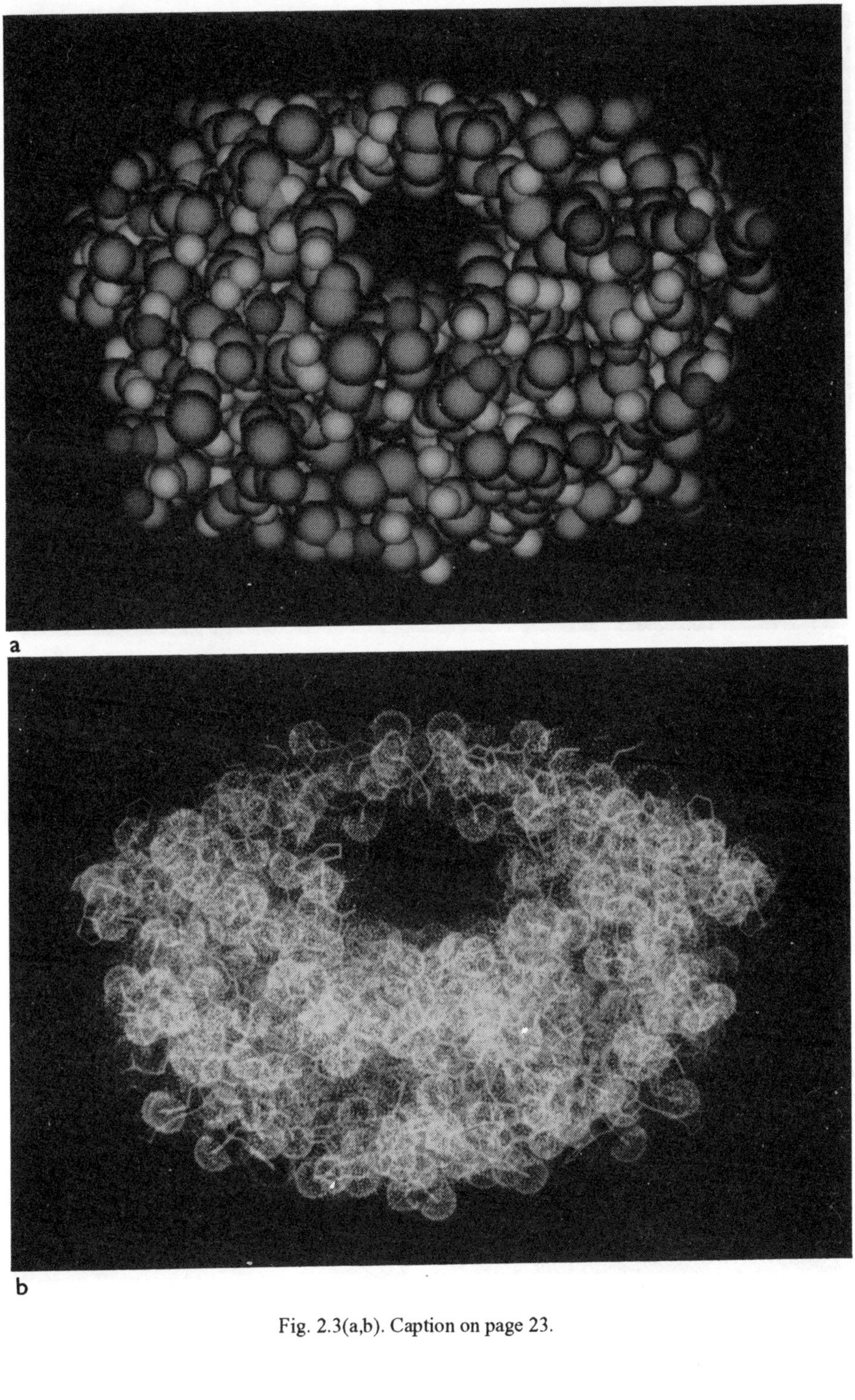

a

b

Fig. 2.3(a,b). Caption on page 23.

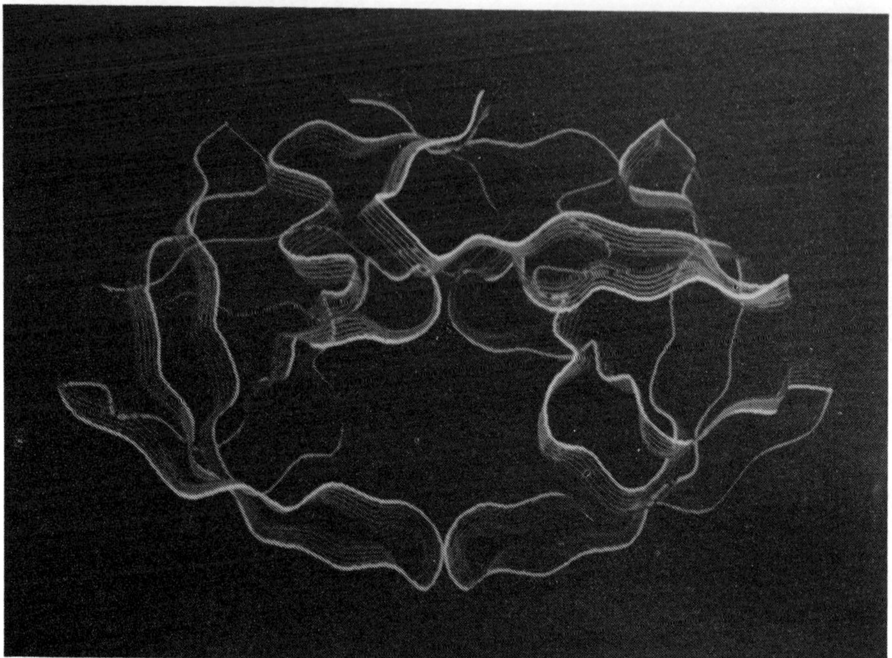

c

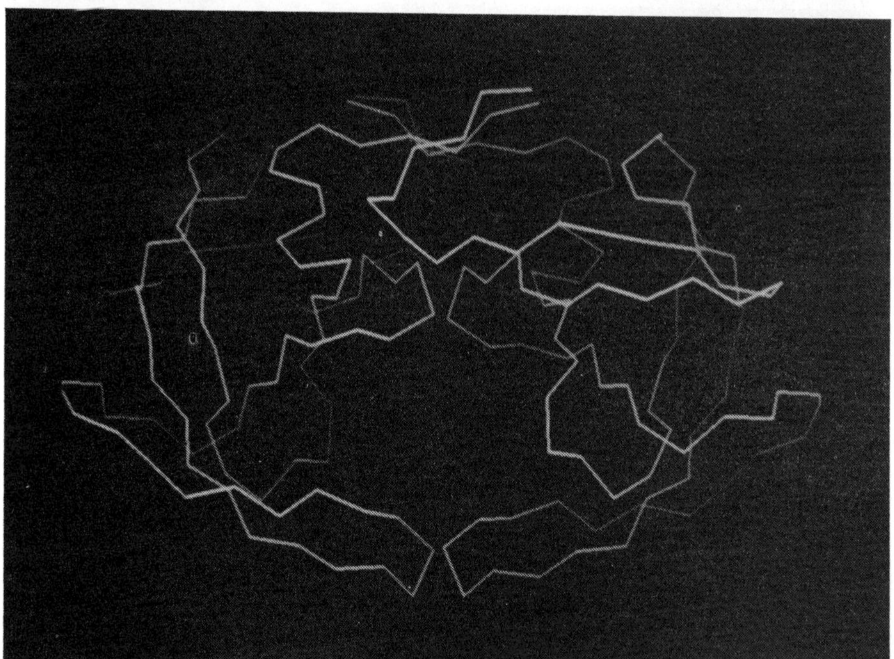

d

Fig. 2.3(c,d). Caption on page 23.

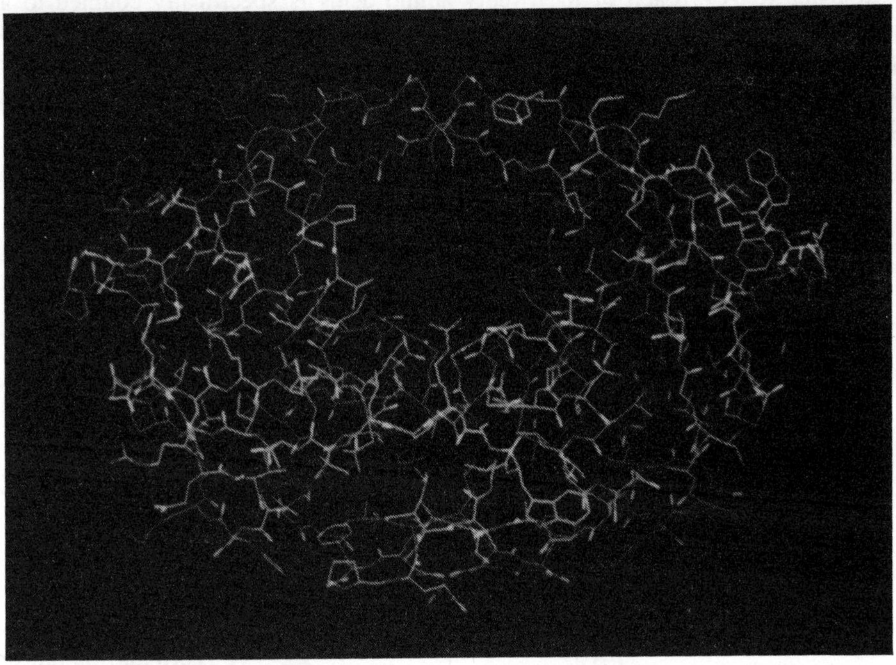

Fig. 2.3. (See colour section.) Common representations of protein structure. The 99 amino acid protease of the human immunodeficiency virus (HIV), which functions as a homodimer, is shown in different representations: a. space-filling representation with atoms designated as solid spheres; b. van der Waals (VDW) sphere dot surface representation indicating the atomic surface but allowing underlying chemical bonds to be seen; c. ribbon diagram representation indicating the path traced by the amino acids that define the protein; d. Cα stick figure connecting the positions of the α-carbon atom of each amino acid by virtual bonds, illustrating the overall trace and fold of the protein; e. all-atom representation with atomic centers connected by lines indicating chemical connectivity. (Courtesy of Dr Robert F. Tilton, Miles Pharmaceuticals Inc. Computer-generated images using co-ordinates determined by Wlodawer *et al.* (1989) *Science* **24,** 616–621.)

Synthesis of proteins

The chemical polymerization of even a moderately sized protein of a hundred amino acids in the laboratory is extremely laborious, and the yields of active product can often be low to zero (Kent and Parker, 1988). Cells accomplish this task by using an intricate mechanism which involves catalytic machinery composed of proteins, nucleic acids and their complexes, and synthesize polypeptide chains that are composed of hundreds of amino acids. This process is depicted in Fig. 2.4, and is described in the sections below. The basic components of the cellular protein synthesis apparatus, in all known biological systems, are ribosomes, which are aggregate structures containing over fifty distinct proteins, and three distinct molecules of nucleic acid known as ribosomal ribonucleic acid (ribosomal RNA or rRNA). The amino acids are ‘‘brought’’ to the ribosomes, "the assembly bench", by an RNA molecule known appropriately as "transfer RNA". Each of the twenty amino acids is specifically coupled to a set of transfer RNAs (discussed below) which catalyze their incorporation into appropriate locations in the linear sequence of polypeptide chains. Several other intracellular proteins known as "initiation and elongation factors" are also required for protein synthesis.

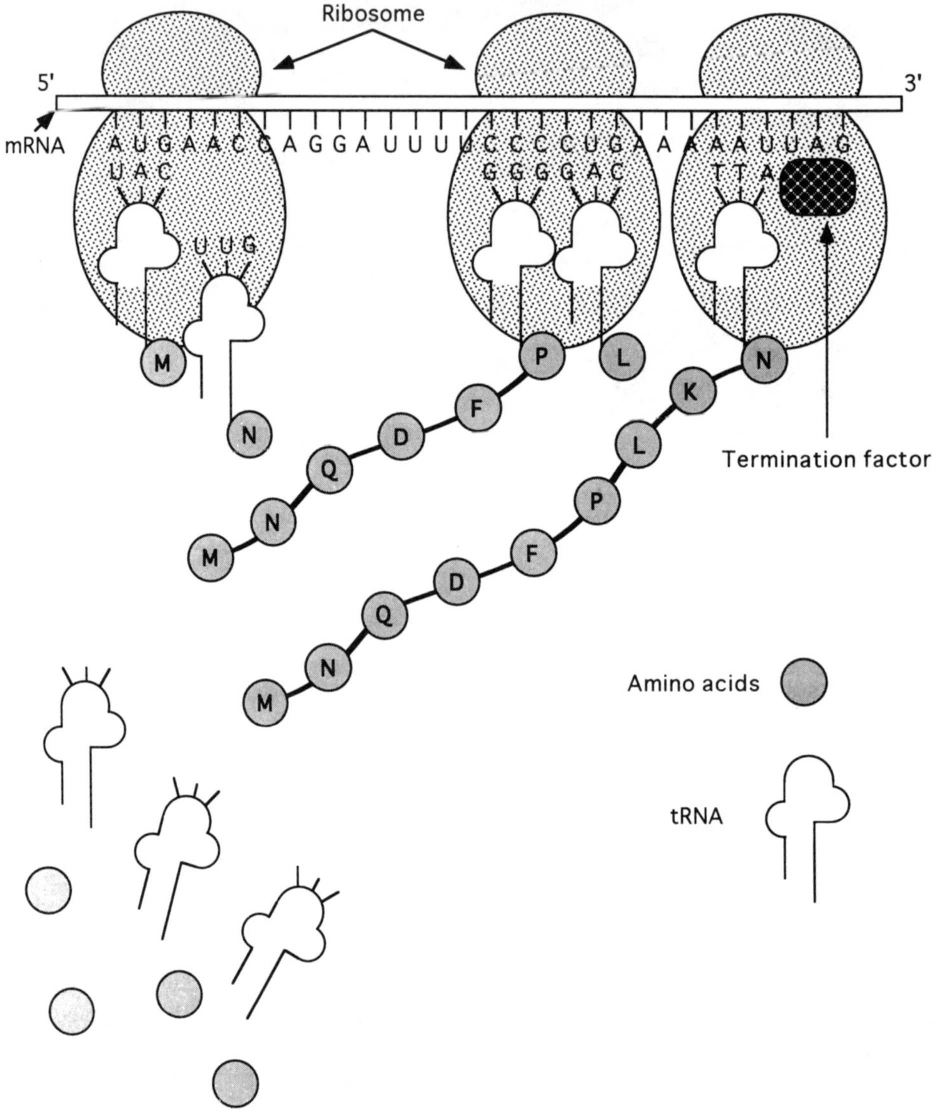

Fig. 2.4. Mechanism of cellular protein synthesis — "translation" of mRNA.

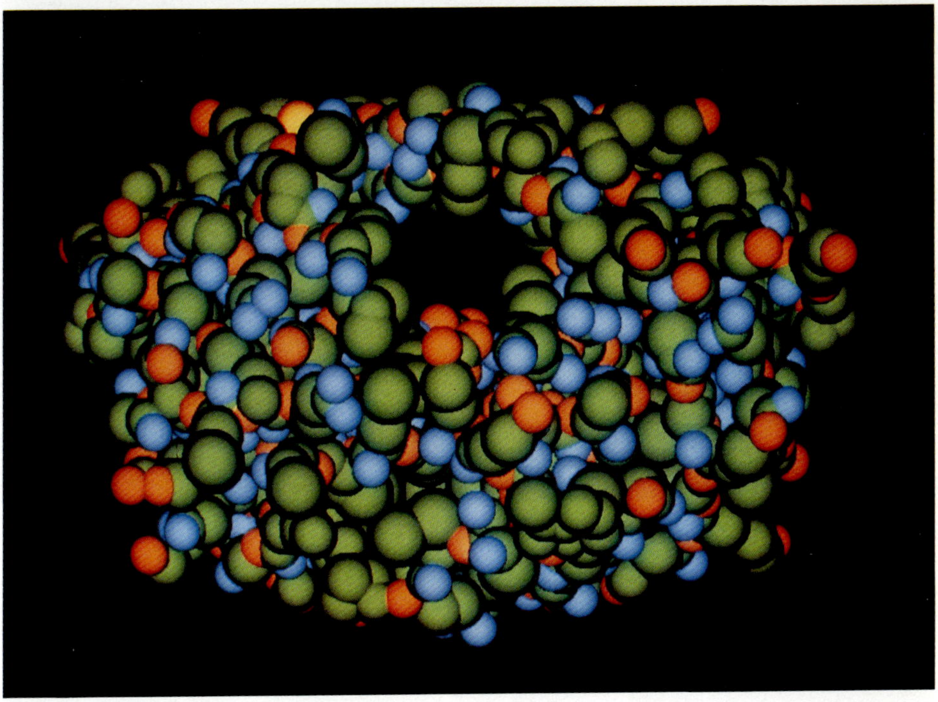

a.

Fig. 2.3. Common representations of protein structure. The 99 amino acid protease of the human immunodeficiency virus (HIV), which functions as a homodimer, is shown in different representations: a. space-filling representation with atoms designated as solid spheres; b. van der Waals (VDW) sphere dot surface representation indicating the atomic surface but allowing underlying chemical bonds to be seen; c. ribbon diagram representation indicating the path traced by the amino acids that define the protein; d. Cα stick figure connecting the positions of the α-carbon atom of each amino acid by virtual bonds, illustrating the overall trace and fold of the protein; e. all-atom representation with atomic centers connected by lines indicating chemical connectivity. (Courtesy of Dr Robert F. Tilton, Miles Pharmaceuticals Inc. Computer-generated images using co-ordinates determined by Wlodawer *et al.* (1989) *Science* **24,** 616–621.)

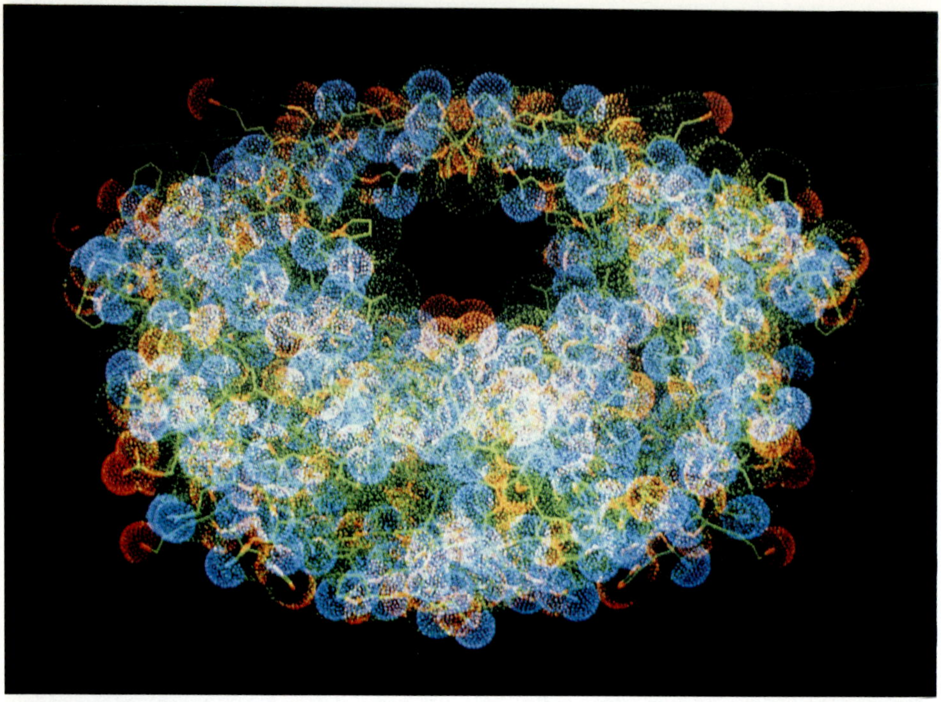

b.

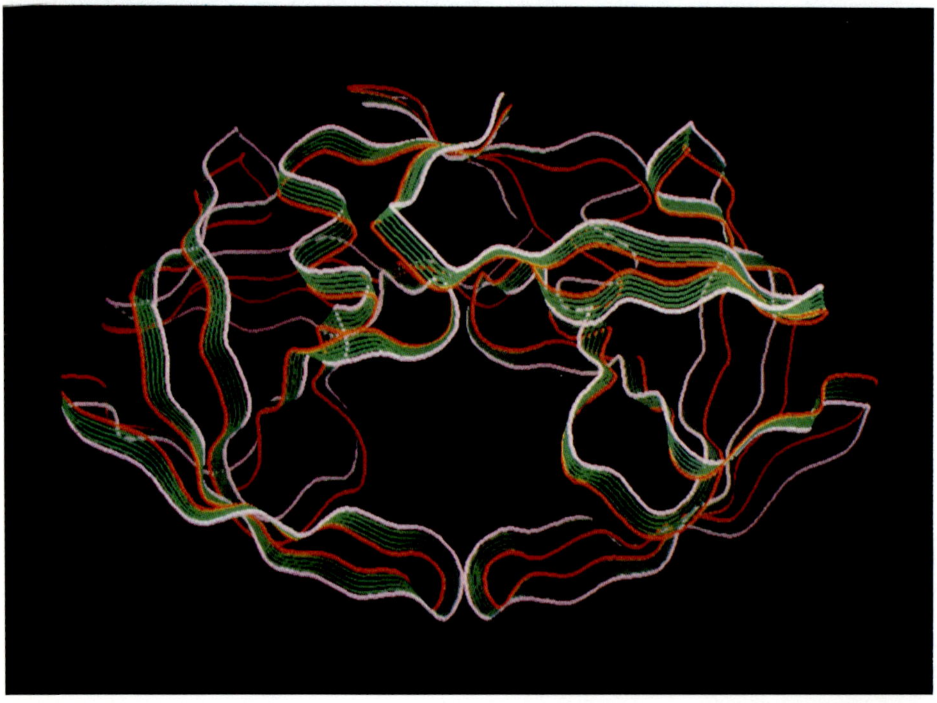

c.

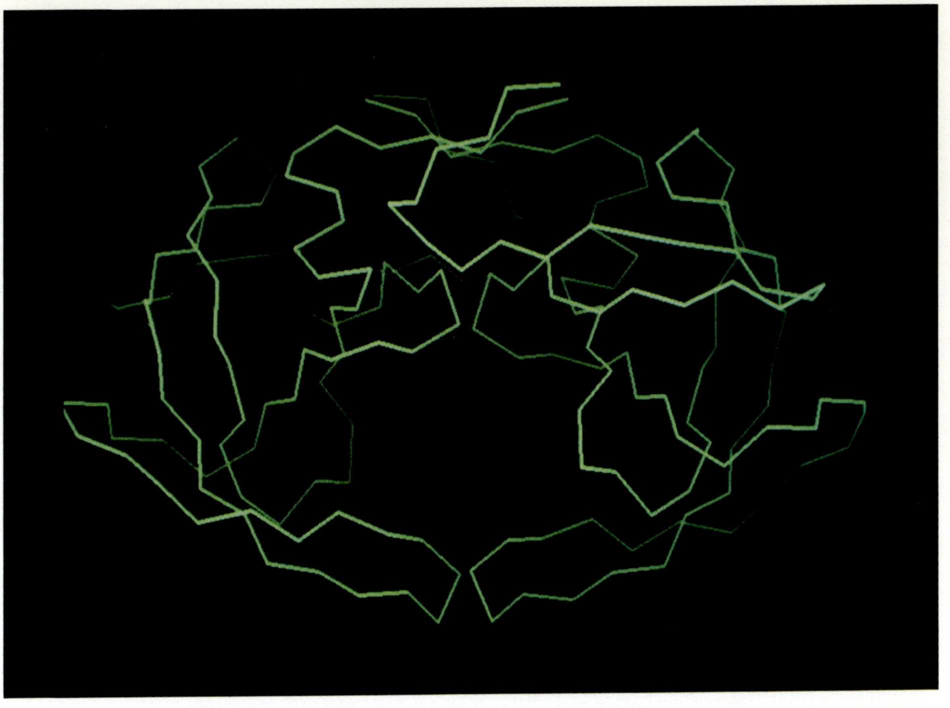

d.

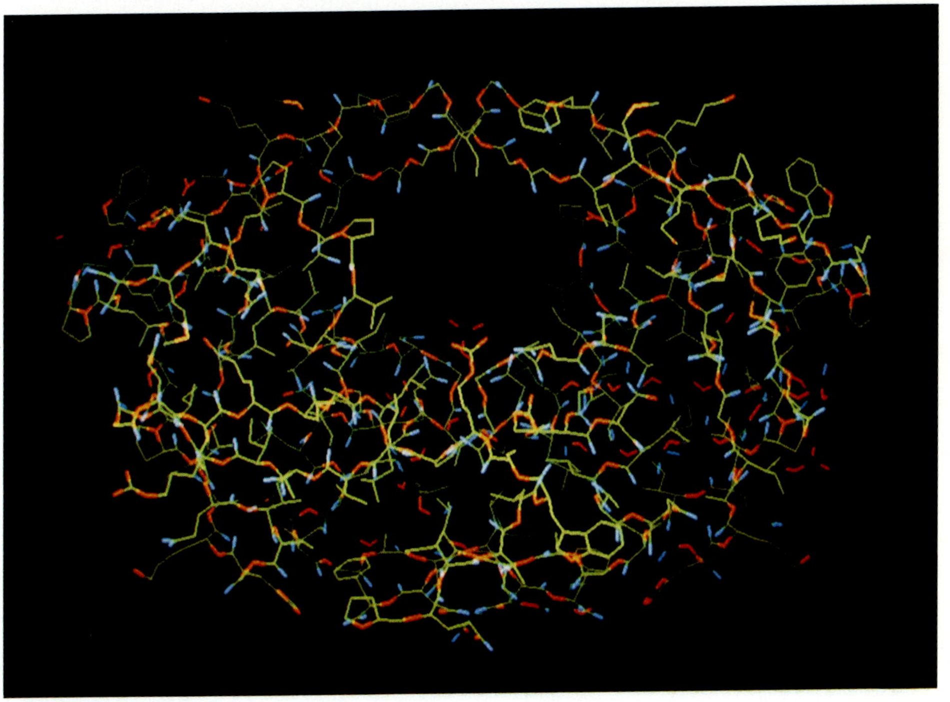

e.

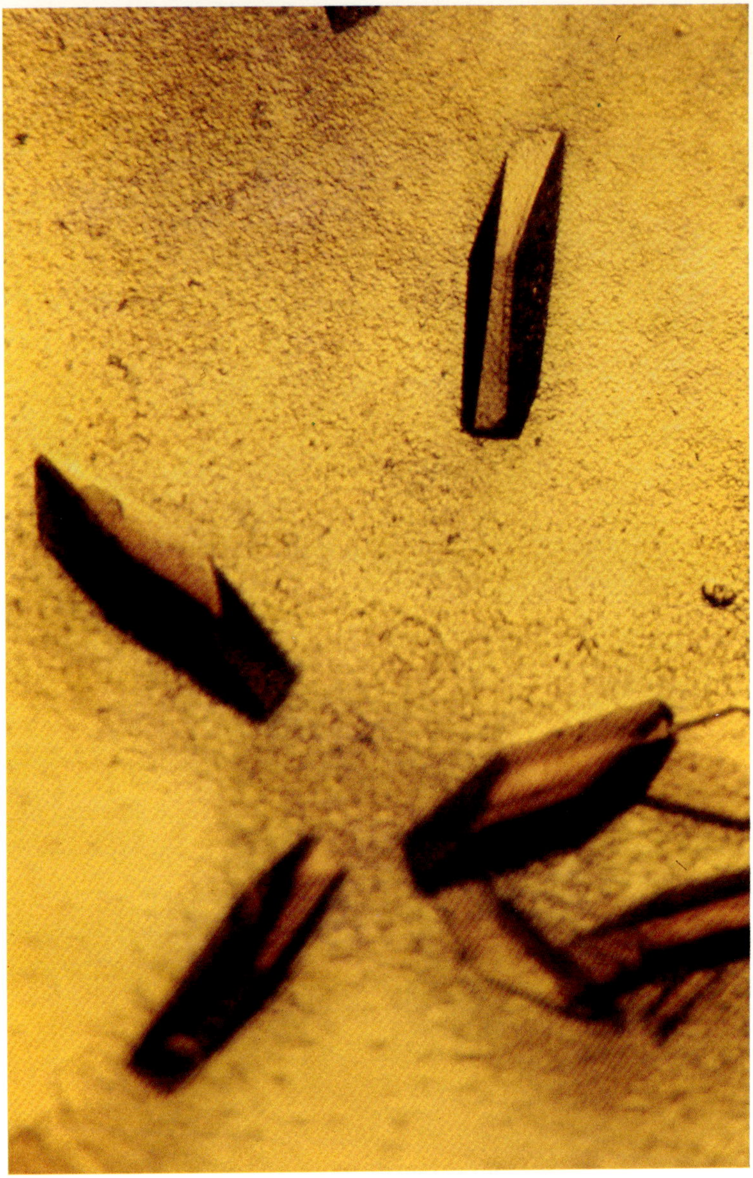

A.

Fig. 5.3. Protein structure determination by X-ray diffraction. A. Crystals of porcine heart aconitase composed of 754 amino acids. The orthorhombic crystals shown are about 0.5 mm in the longest dimension. B. Film showing the diffraction pattern obtained from the above crystal. These data were used to obtain a 2.7 Å resolution structure shown in two representations in panels C and D. Panel C shows the tracing of the protein backbone, with the small molecule (in red and yellow) in the central region depicting the iron-containing cofactor of the enzyme. Panel D shows the space-filling representation. (Courtesy of Dr Arthur H. Robbins, Miles Pharmaceuticals Inc. For details see: A.H. Robbins and C.D. Stout (1989). *Proteins: Structure, Function, and Genetics* **5**, 289–312.)

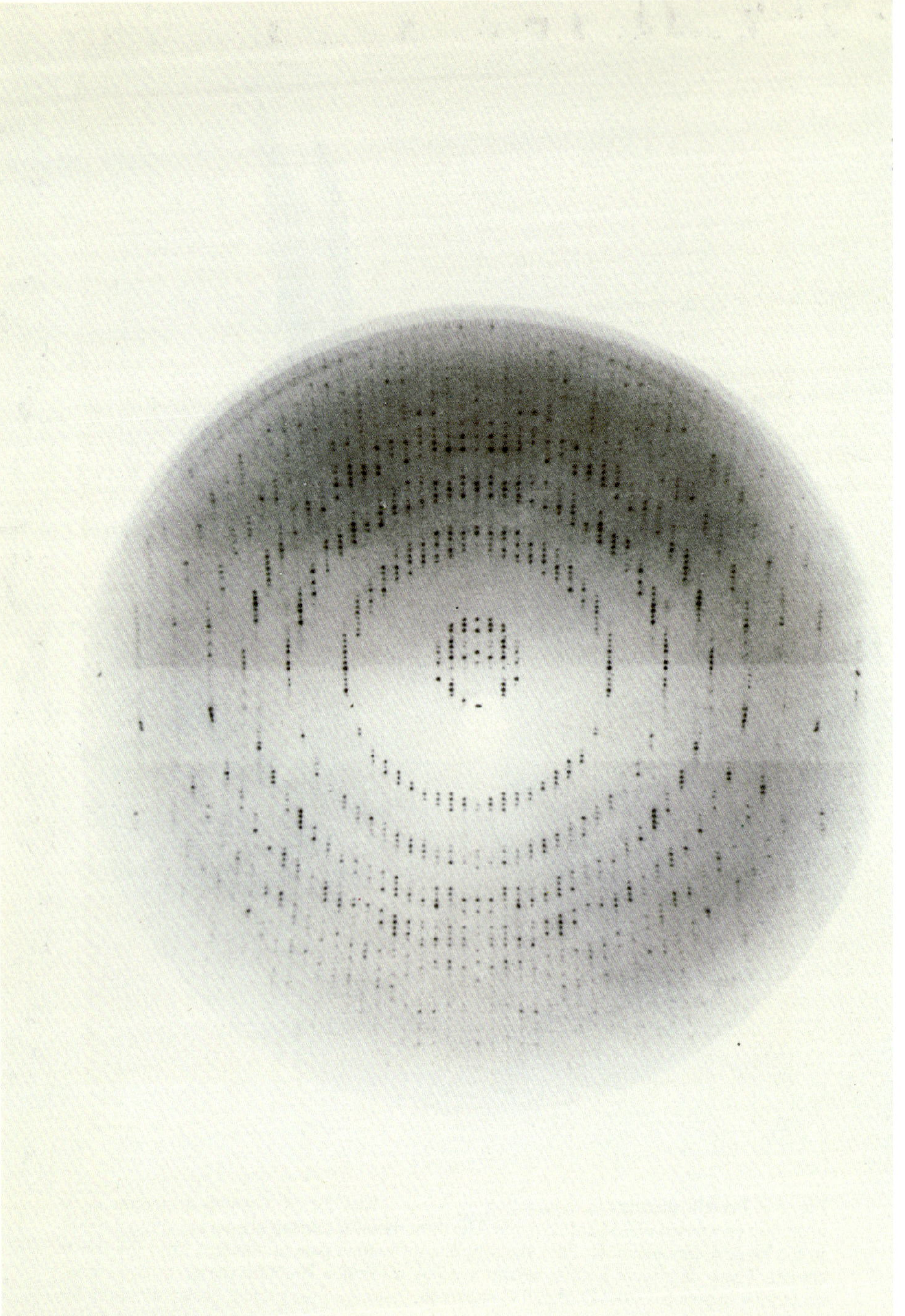

B.

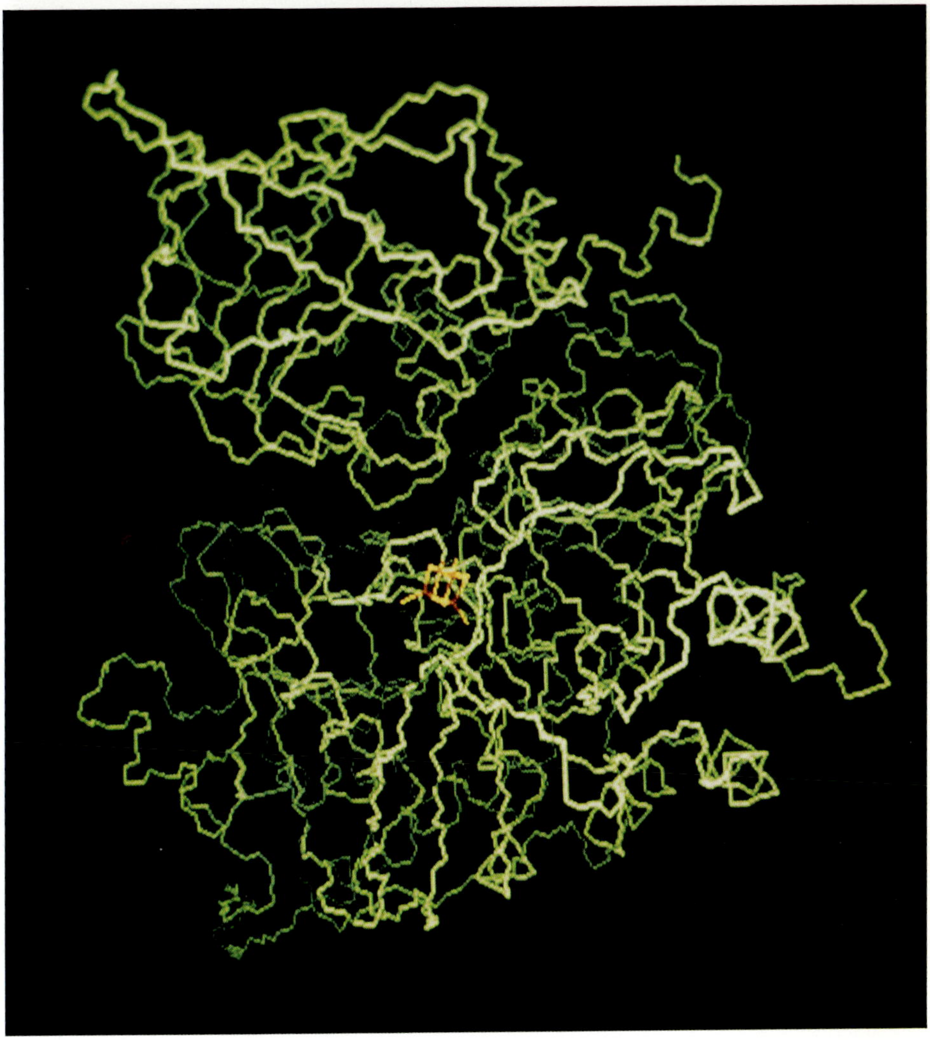

C.

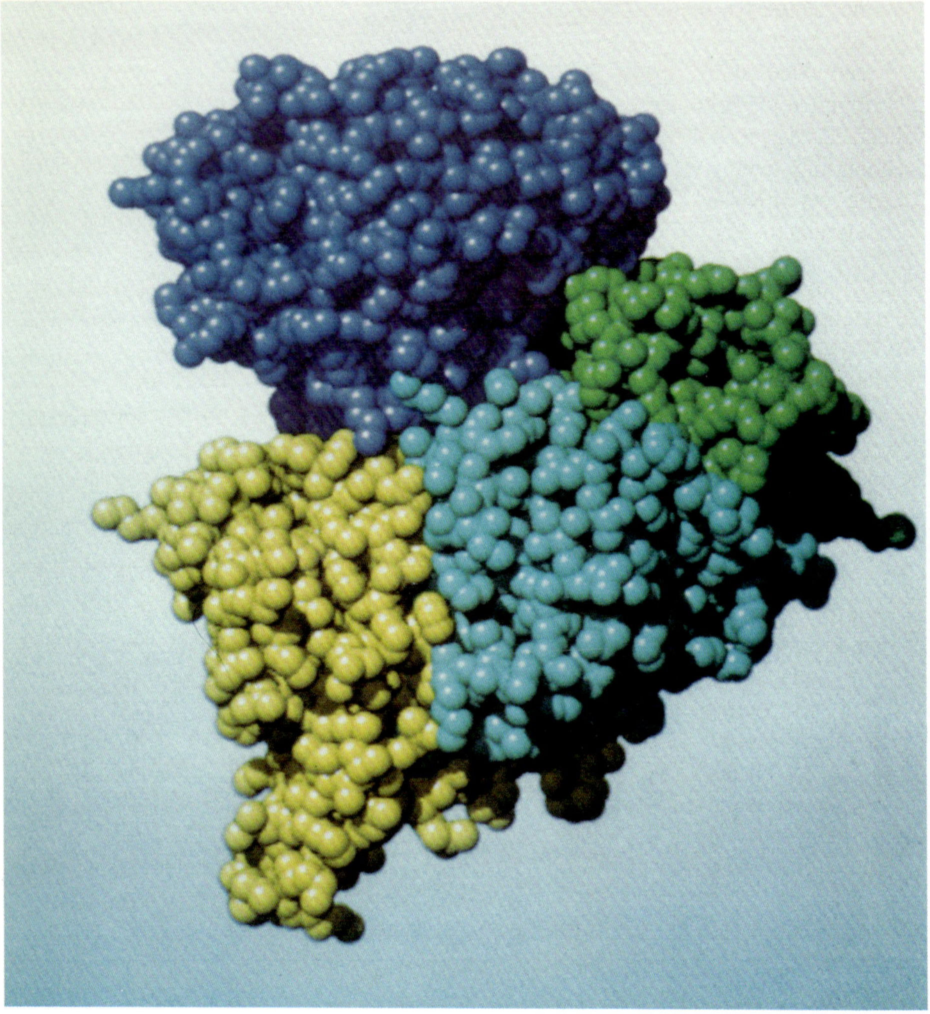

D.

A unique messenger RNA for each protein

The components of the protein synthesis machinery described above are used for the synthesis of all proteins. The identity of a particular protein being synthesized is specified by a nucleic acid known as messenger ribonucleic acid or mRNA. As the name suggests, the mRNA is a macromolecule which "transmits" to the ribosomal machinery, a copy of the information or "message" encoding the linear sequence of a protein. This information is stored in a segment of deoxyribonucleic acid (DNA) known as the "gene" for the protein being synthesized. Several identical "messages" are produced from one copy of the corresponding gene, resulting in the amplification of information arriving at the ribosome via mRNA. The enzymatic process of production of RNA copy of a DNA segment is known as "transcription".

Information in mRNA; the genetic code

Nucleic acids, both DNA (deoxyribonucleic acid) and RNA (ribonucleic acid), are linear polymers of four bases linked to a sugar–phosphate backbone as shown in Fig. 2.5a. The differences between DNA and RNA reside in the sugar moiety forming the backbone, and in one of the four bases: whereas the sugar in RNA is ribose, it is deoxyribose in DNA; both molecules contain bases adenine (A), guanine (G), and cytosine (C) but whereas the fourth base in RNA is uracil (U), its counterpart in DNA is a methylated form of uracil, thymine (T).

Because nucleic acids are made of four bases, the genetic code (the information for protein sequence stored in DNA and transcribed into mRNA) is a code with four alphabets. Specifying twenty amino acids using a four-base alphabet requires the use of multiple bases to denote any given amino acid. A two-letter code has the capacity to specify only 16 (4×4: one of the four bases in each of the two positions) amino acids, which is clearly insufficient of code for the twenty amino acids. A three-letter code has the coding capacity for 64 ($4 \times 4 \times 4$), which is greater than the twenty required to code all the amino acids. It has been proved experimentally that nature uses a three-letter code to encode protein information in nucleic acids. Furthermore, the code is non-overlapping, i.e. each amino acid, and that amino acid alone, being specified by a distinct triplet of bases. In other words, changing the bases of a triplet causes a change in only one amino acid which the triplet specifies in the protein. The 64 triplets are called codons, and these are used to specify the twenty amino acids and the signals for stopping polymerization of the chains called "stop" codons. Obviously, most amino acids are coded by more than one triplet and therefore the code is "degenerate". Table 2.2 lists the amino acids and the corresponding codons. Note that some amino acids (methionine and tryptophan) are represented by only a single codon, while others (leucine and serine) are specified by six different codons. Three codons are used to specify polymerization stop or chain termination.

The process by which the ribosomes convert the nucleic acid code into the amino acid sequence is appropriately called "translation", and the protein synthesis machinery is called the "translational apparatus" of the cell. A single mRNA is translated by several ribosomes before it is degraded. Thus a single mRNA molecule gives rise to several molecules of the protein it encodes, causing an amplification of gene expression similar to the situation discussed earlier in the transcription of a gene into several mRNA copies.

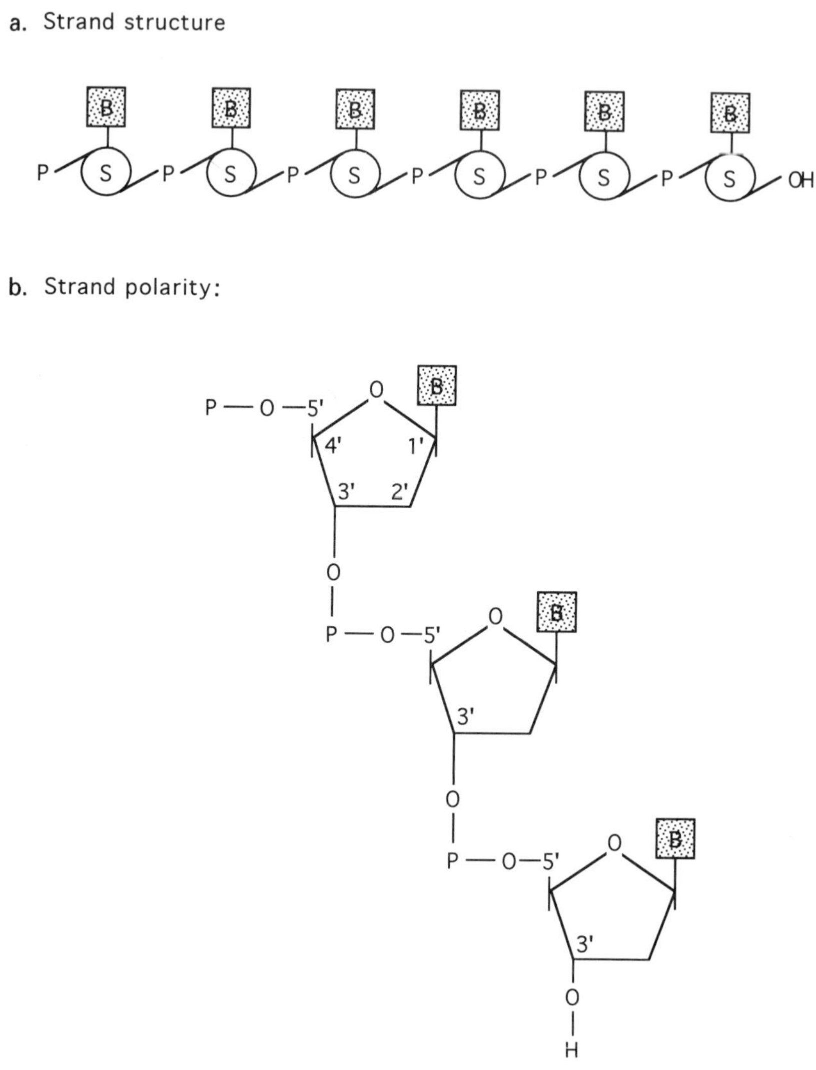

Fig. 2.5. Polymeric structure of nucleic acids. a. Linear structure. b. Basis of strand polarity in double-stranded nucleic acids.

Table 2.2. Amino acids and their codons in mRNA

Amino acid	Codons in mRNA
Ala	GCA GCC GCG GCU
Arg	AGA AGG CGA CGC CGG CGU
Asn	AAC AAU
Asp	GAC GAU
Cys	UGC UGU
Gln	CAA CAG
Glu	GAA GAG
Gly	GGA GGC GGG GGU
His	CAC CAU
Ile	AUA AUC AUU
Leu	UUA UUG CUA CUC CUG CUU
Lys	AAA AAG
Met	AUG
Phe	UUC UUU
Pro	CCA CCC CCG CCU
Ser	AGC AGU UCA UCC UCG UCU
Thr	ACA ACC ACG ACU
Trp	UGG
Tyr	UAC UAU
Val	GUA GUC GUG GUU
STOP	UAA UAG UGA

The genetic code is universal. All biological systems (or nearly all) use the same code. This principle has important consequences to the developments in rDNA. Thus, the code in messenger RNAs of a human cell can be translated by bacterial protein synthesis machinery into a protein of the same sequence as in the human cell. Production of human proteins in bacteria and other organisms would be immensely difficult, if not impossible, if each organism had a different genetic code.

Within the messenger RNA, the codons are arranged contiguously in the same linear order as the corresponding amino acids in the protein. In addition to the contiguous coding information, the message contains extra stretches of bases flanking the coding stretch on either side which are not translated, and hence are called "untranslated sequences" or UTRs. Some of these extra bases have regulatory roles in translation and in stabilizing the message against degradation. The starting point for polymerization of a protein is signaled by the presence of an AUG codon (for methionine) in the mRNA. A message usually contains several AUG triplets within the coding sequence and in the UTRs. Ribosomes recognize the appropriate AUG codon that denotes the beginning of the protein by recognizing the surrounding RNA sequence, and start the polypeptide chain synthesis. This process is known as "initiation of translation", and the AUG codon involved is known as the "initiation codon". Thus the first amino acid in all proteins is methionine, which is often removed once the protein is made.

Once protein synthesis is initiated, amino acids are added to the peptide chain corresponding to each triplet in the mRNA until the ribosome encounters a termination or stop codon, whereupon the polypeptide chain is released from the ribosome, and assumes its final configuration. A ribosome covers about 50 bases of an mRNA, which is usually hundreds of bases long. Thus, several ribosomes translate an mRNA consecutively and simultaneously at any instant as shown in Fig. 2.4. A group of ribosomes translating a message is called a "polyribosome".

Transfer RNA: the adapter

Incorporation of amino acids into a polypeptide chain occurs through the involvement of a class of small RNA molecules known as transfer RNA or tRNA. For each codon in mRNA, there is a corresponding tRNA to which the amino acid specified by the codon is covalently attached. Since multiple codons specify the same amino acid (degenerate code), a given amino acid may be linked to a set of tRNAs.

tRNAs interact with the corresponding codons in mRNA by complementary pairing of the bases of a particular codon and three contiguous bases known as "anticodon" present in the tRNA specific for that codon as shown in Fig. 2.4.. (The complementary base-pairing phenomenon, a central mechanism in nucleic acid function, is discussed in detail in the section below on DNA.) The anticodon sequence is the key feature that distinguishes different tRNA species. The high specificity of base-pairing allows translation of the nucleic acid code into protein sequence with very high fidelity.

DNA, the mastertape

All the information coding for every protein in an organism is contained in its DNA in units called genes. The DNA content of almost every cell in a multicellular organism is the same and contains all the information needed to create the entire organism.

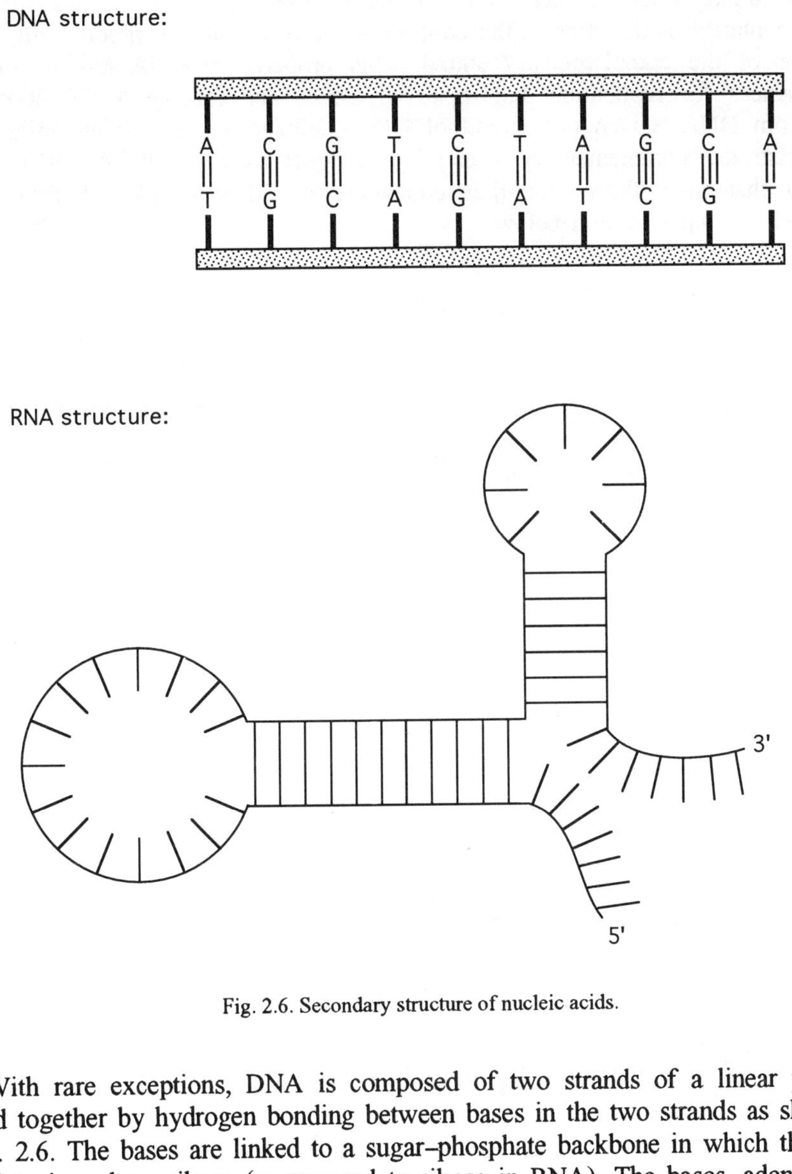

Fig. 2.6. Secondary structure of nucleic acids.

With rare exceptions, DNA is composed of two strands of a linear polymer held together by hydrogen bonding between bases in the two strands as shown in Fig. 2.6. The bases are linked to a sugar–phosphate backbone in which the sugar moiety is a deoxyribose (as opposed to ribose in RNA). The bases, adenine (A), guanine (G), cytosine (C), and thymine (T), are linked to the deoxyribose. A and G are known as purines, and C and T are known as pyrimidines. The hydrogen bonds that hold the strands of DNA together are very specific. Purines on one strand are always paired with pyrimidines on the complementary strand. Further specificity is introduced by the strict pairing of A (purine) with T (pyrimidine) forming two hydrogen bonds, and of G (purine) with C (pyrimidine) forming three hydrogen bonds (Fig. 2.6). This pairing is uninterrupted along the length of the two strands like a zipper, giving DNA its rod-like shape. Because of the complementarity of the strands, the base sequence of one strand predicts the base sequence of the complementary strand. This property of DNA has important consequences for replication and repair of DNA, and for the transcription of RNA from DNA. Given one strand of DNA, cellular polymerase enzymes can polymerize the complementary strand by using it as the template. It is this property that also allows for the sequencing of DNA in the laboratory as described in a later section below.

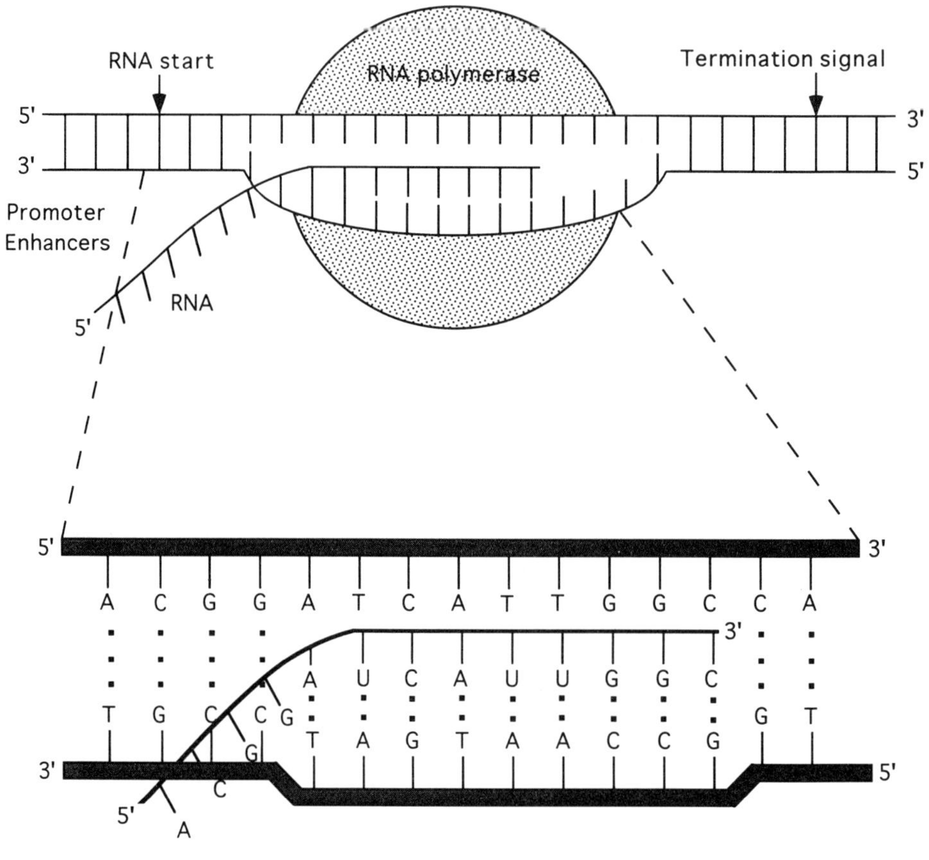

Fig. 2.7. Mechanism of RNA synthesis — transcription.

A strand of DNA has a polarity arising from the nature of the sugar–phosphate linkage. The hydroxyl group in the 3 position of the base linked–deoxyribose moiety is bonded via the phosphate group to the 5 position hydroxyl of the following deoxyribose as shown in Fig. 2.5b, giving the backbone a free phosphate group on one end and a free hydroxyl group on the other. These positions on the deoxyribose are denoted as 5 prime (5′) and 3 prime (3′) to distinguish them from the numbering of the atoms of the base attached to the deoxyribose (a similar polarity also occurs in RNA). In double-stranded DNA, the complementary strands have opposite polarities and are hence referred to as antiparallel strands. In many biological situations, the free ends of a DNA strand are covalently linked to form circular molecules. For example, plasmids described in cloning applications in a later section are covalently closed circular DNA molecules.

The specific hydrogen bonding between bases is an important feature of the structure and function of nucleic acids, both DNA and RNA. RNA is produced by copying one of the strands of DNA by using the complementarity of base pairing (see Fig. 2.7). In addition, single-stranded RNA molecules, notably tRNA and rRNA, are also stabilized by base pair interactions between complementary bases in the distant parts of the molecule as shown in Fig. 2.6. Thus, tRNAs, which are about 75 nucleotides in length, are stabilized by several base pairings and assume a "clover leaf" structure. In RNAs, A pairs with U (Uracil) which replaces T of DNA.

Base pairing interaction between the nucleic acid strands forms the rationale for nucleic acid-based diagnostic and therapeutic technologies described in the subsequent chapters.

Transcription: copying of RNA

DNA → RNA → protein is known as the central dogma of molecular biology. Thus RNA, derived from DNA by the process termed "transcription", is an obligate intermediate in the production of proteins. As discussed above, DNA contains the coding information for every protein expressed in every cell of an organism. In the human genome, this is estimated to be between 50,000 and 100,000 genes, amounting to about 0.3 billion base pairs of DNA. Mammalian cells contain far more DNA, nearly 3 billion base pairs. Therefore, a large fraction of a mammalian cell's DNA does not code for proteins. While the function of this "non-coding" DNA is not fully understood, some of the "extra" DNA in the proximity of the protein coding sequences is used for the control of transcription. The process of transcription is outlined in Fig. 2.7. Stretches of DNA known as "promoters" and "enhancers", which are themselves not transcribed, direct the positioning of the transcribing enzyme, RNA polymerase, to begin the copying of one of the DNA strands into RNA. A complementary copy of this strand of DNA is created by the enzyme using the base pairing principles discussed earlier. DNA sequences at the distal end of the gene instruct the polymerase to stop further polymerization, at which point the RNA chain is released.

A stretch of DNA containing the coding information of a protein and the regulatory sequences required for its expression is known as the gene for the protein. Since all the regulatory sequences do not appear in the RNA copy of the gene, the RNA copy is always smaller than the gene from which it is transcribed.

In addition to the RNA polymerase which is required for all transcription, several protein factors, known as "transcription factors", modulate the transcription of specific genes. Thus, for example, the gene for albumin is transcribed in a liver cell but not in other tissues, while the gene for growth hormone is transcribed in a set of pituitary cells known as somatotrophs but is not even transcribed in other cells of the pituitary. Similarly, antibody genes are expressed at high levels in mature B lymphocytes, but not in other cells and tissues. This "tissue-specific" expression is mediated by transcription factors which are expressed and/or activated in the particular cell type. The promoter regions of the regulated genes contain sequences capable of interacting with the transcription factors (McKnight, 1991). Many promoters are regulated by sets of external stimuli such as heat, heavy metals, and steroid hormones. Promoters contain sequence motifs which are essential for such regulation through their interaction with the appropriate transcription factors. Thus, in view of the specific DNA–protein interactions involved, transcription factors and their target sequences in the promoter are possible targets for development of drugs which act by activating or silencing the expression of the gene or genes involved in a disease.

Processing of RNA: introns

In simple situations encountered in prokaryotes such as bacteria, a stretch of DNA is copied into a collinear RNA molecule, and is immediately available to the ribosomes for translation. Every base in the RNA transcribed from the DNA arrives at the translation machinery. However, this is not the case in higher eukaryotic cells, where transcription occurs within the nucleus and the resultant mRNA is transported to the cytoplasm to be translated by ribosomes. In the process of synthesis and transport, the primary transcription product undergoes maturation and evolves as the message suitable for translation.

One of the key steps in mRNA maturation is the removal of "introns", which are sequences in DNA which contain no protein coding information but are nonetheless interspersed within the region of DNA coding for a particular protein, interrupting the continuity of the coding information into segments known as "exons", as shown in Fig. 2.8a. The sequence of one of the intron–exon junctions occurring in the human growth hormone gene is shown as an example in Fig. 2.8b. Removal of introns is obligatory for the translation of the message in the correct frame by ribosomes. The mechanism of intron removal which is a part of RNA maturation is known appropriately as "splicing". It is performed by a complex nuclear machinery composed of RNA and proteins, resulting in the accurate removal of the intervening introns from the primary RNA transcript or the pre-mRNA. Splicing results in the uninterrupted assembly of exons to produce a continuous run of codons.

Although not all animal and plant cell genes contain introns, they are present in the majority. A single gene may contain multiple introns, some of which can be extremely large, contributing thousands of bases to a gene. In many cases, the final coding stretch of DNA represented by the processed mRNA derived from it may be more than an order of magnitude smaller than the gene itself. The messenger RNA for coagulation factor VIII is a typical example. The coding sequence for this protein, composed of 2351 codons (including a 19 amino acid secretion signal) or 7053 nucleotides, is interspersed in the genome in a stretch of DNA 186,000 bases long as 26 segments or exons ranging from 69 to 3106 bases. The final messenger RNA, inclusive of the 5′ and 3′ noncoding sequences, is 9000 bases in length. The coding sequence in DNA is interrupted by 25 introns, the largest of which is 32,400 bases in length (Gitschier *et al.,* 1984).

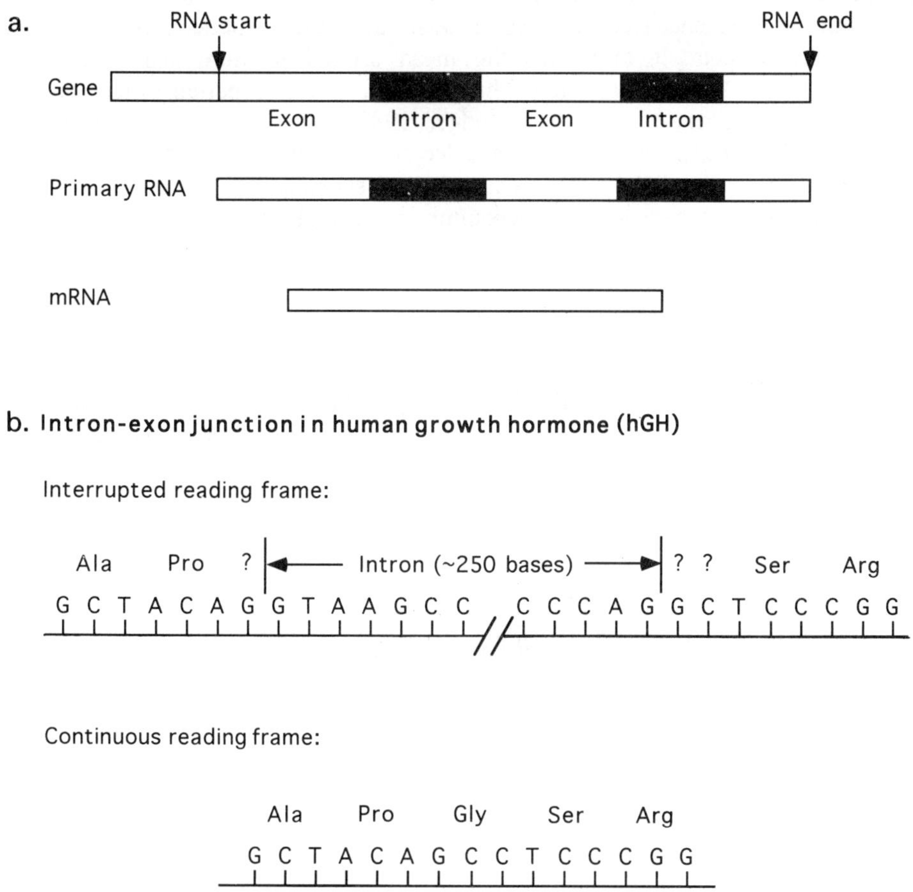

Fig. 2.8. RNA splicing: a. removal of introns from primary RNA transcript; b. consequence of introns and requirement of their removal for translation.

The primary transcription product of a gene containing multiple introns can be spliced in alternate patterns to derive distinct mRNAs and proteins from the same DNA sequence (Maniatis, 1991). This alternate splicing is used in nature in many instances, and in some cases the combinatorial splicing patterns lead to several distinct messages. A simple case of alternate splicing which occurs in the expression of the calcitonin gene resulting in calcitonin production in the parathyroid glands and the production of calcitonin gene-related peptide (CGRP) in the brain is shown in Fig. 2.9 (Royer and Kemper, 1990). A single primary RNA is processed to yield two different mRNAs coding for two proteins with identical amino termini but with either calcitonin or CGRP at the carboxyl terminus. The respective peptides are released from the precursor by proteolysis. Interestingly, CGRP was discovered at the mRNA level and the peptide was synthesized based on the sequence predicted by the mRNA. Its function was unknown. Subsequent studies have shown that the peptide has important physiological effects. It influences the mean arterial pressure and heart rate, depending on the route of injection. This peptide has been reported to have a role in the differentiation of neurons (Mudge, 1989). This discovery is a prime example of how rDNA approaches have led to the identification of new protein activities at the gene level. Other examples of serendipitous discovery of new activities from DNA sequence are becoming increasingly common.

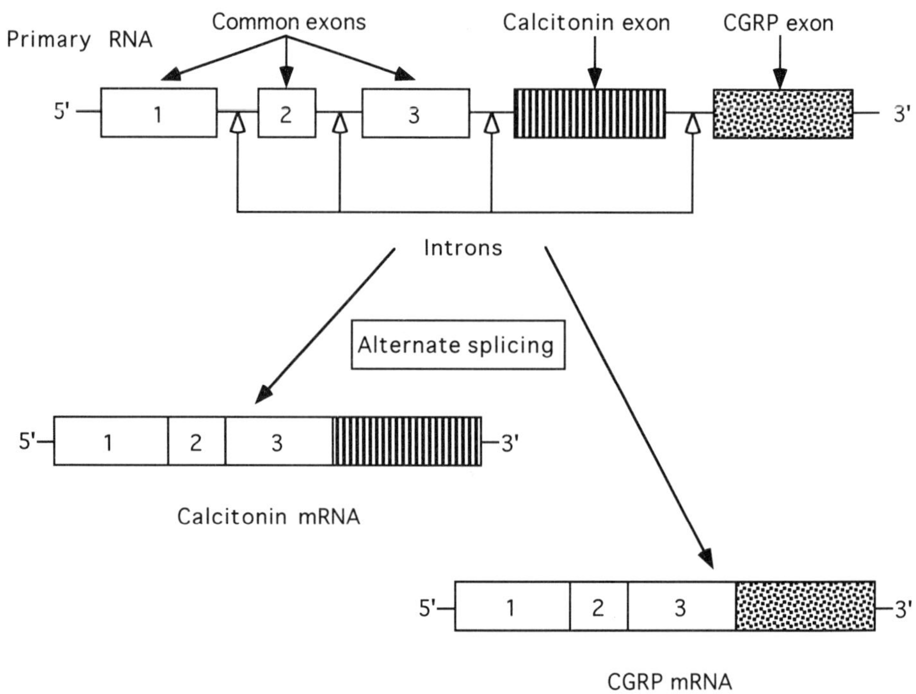

Fig. 2.9. Alternate splicing of calcitonin–gene RNA to produce two different mRNA encoding precursor proteins containing either calcitonin or CGRP peptides.

A further complex example of alternate splicing is found in the derivation of mRNA from the rat muscle troponin gene, where 64 distinct mRNAs are derived from a single gene containing 18 exons by combinatorial alternate splicing which is precisely regulated in a developmental stage-specific and in a tissue-specific manner (Nadal-Ginard, 1990).

The function of introns within genes is not established, but the introns in many cases appear to separate the coding information for the functional domains of a protein. It is hypothesized that the arrangement of information for functional modules separated by stretches of noncoding sequences allows the shuffling of the modules between different genes to form new combinations leading to the creation of novel proteins during evolution. The implications of the domain structure of proteins to the development of new protein entities using rDNA methods are discussed in detail in Chapter 3.

Reverse transcription and cDNA

The major direction of information flow in biological systems is from DNA to RNA to protein. However, there are instances in which RNA is copied into a complementary DNA strand by the process dubbed "reverse transcription" by the enzyme known as the "reverse transcriptase". This mechanism is used by retroviruses including the HIV virus, whose infectious particles contain RNA as the genetic material. The virus particles contain a virally encoded reverse transcriptase which, following infection, copies the viral RNA into DNA. The resultant DNA copy is incorporated into the genome of the infected cell.

Reverse transcriptase has been an important tool in the development of rDNA technology, for the production of complementary DNAs or "cDNAs" corresponding to the messenger RNAs. As described in a previous section, a gene or its primary RNA transcript is much larger than the mRNA which is derived from it. A copy of the mRNA in the DNA-form, synthesized using reverse transcriptase, is known as the "cDNA" of the message, and differs from the gene in lacking all of the introns, as shown in Fig. 2.10. mRNAs are highly unstable molecules *in vivo* and are also susceptible to degradation during isolation and storage. Because of their chemical composition and single-stranded nature, it is also not possible to manipulate RNAs using restriction endonucleases and other enzymes used in cloning. The availability of the mRNA information as a stable cDNA copy permits the manipulation of the coding sequence using the tools of rDNA technology. Owing to their smaller size relative to the genes they correspond to, manipulation of cDNA is less cumbersome.

Mutations: heritable changes in DNA

Codons in the DNA determine the amino acids incorporated into a protein. Changes in the codons, be they substitution, deletion or insertion of bases, change the primary sequence of the protein product, often with attendant deleterious consequences to the cell or the organism. In addition, base changes in the regulatory regions of DNA which are not transcribed and/or translated can also influence the level, timing, and location of expression of proteins. Changes in

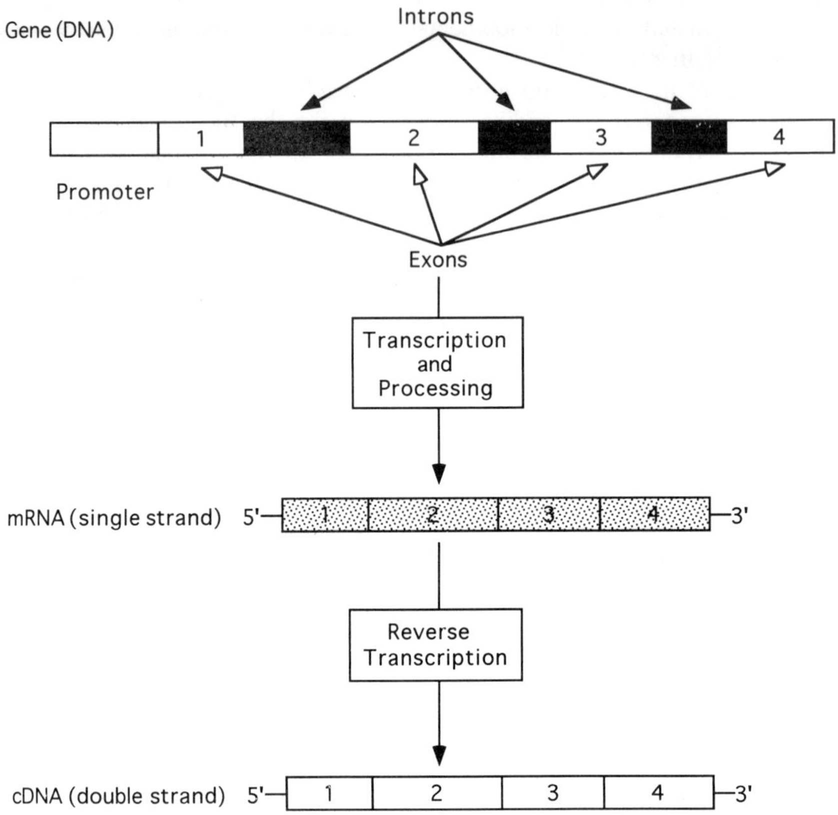

Fig. 2.10. Relation between a gene, its mRNA, and its cDNA.

DNA, if not corrected by the DNA repair systems of the cell, become incorporated into the genome and are passed on to the descendants of the mutated cell. The natural rate of mutations in DNA is maintained very low because of the high-fidelity replication mechanisms and efficient systems for surveillance and repair of DNA damage.

The consequence of sequence changes at the DNA level on the sequence of encoded protein is shown by the example in Table 2.3, where an AUG codon representing methionine in proteins is subjected to single base changes. The various types of mutations and their influence on information transfer are illustrated in Box 2.1.

Table 2.3. Consequence of mutations in DNA on protein sequence

Sequence in DNA	Codon in mRNA	Amino acid in protein
ATG	AUG	Met
GTG	GUG	Val
CTG	CUG	Leu
TTG	UUG	Leu
AGG	AGG	Arg
ACG	ACG	Thr
AAG	AAG	Lys
ATA	AUA	Ile
ATC	AUC	Ile
ATT	AUU	Ile

Mutations occur randomly and spontaneously in nature and are the cause of inherited diseases. The causes of heritable diseases such as sickle-cell anemia, beta-thalassemia, phenylketonuria, and others have been traced to single-base substitutions in the DNA encoding a single protein, and many of the complex diseases such as Alzheimer's disease and cancer have a genetic component as well. Mutations in the regulatory regions of the gene and in the intronic regions can also lead to disease. Such mutations are found in the hemoglobinopathy, beta-thalassemia.

Box 2.1. Nature of mutations

Base changes in the coding segment of DNA lead to changes in the protein, depending on the nature and position of the base changes. Single bases may be changed, deleted, or inserted. Single base changes alter the amino acid encoded by the triplet except where, due to the degeneracy of the genetic code, the altered triplet codes for the same amino. Insertions or deletions of single bases alter the reading frame, leading in most cases to an altered amino acid sequence of the protein beyond the point of insertion or deletion. Likewise stretches of bases can be deleted or inserted, offsetting the reading frame; in the cases of insertions or deletions of an integral number of triplets, the length of the encoded protein increases or decreases respectively, with attendant functional consequences. These concepts are illustrated below by using the coding sequence of a small protein containing tryptophan and leucine represented by a single codon and six degenerate codons respectively (Table 2.2). The synthesis of all proteins is initiated at an AUG codon, which encodes a methionine, and is terminated at one of the three nonsense triplets (TER) used to specify the end of a reading frame.

Correct DNA sequence and protein:

```
                |start----------------------stop|
AAT CCC ATG TTA TGG TGG TGG CTT TGG TAA AAA TTT
--- --- Met Leu Trp Trp Trp Leu Trp TER --- ---
```

Point mutations:

1. Amino acid change (''missense'' mutation)

```
                          *
*** *** *** *** *** TGT *** *** *** *** *** ***
--- --- +++ +++ +++ Cys +++ +++ +++ +++ --- ---
```

2. No change (due to degeneracy: ''DNA polymorphism'')

```
                              *
*** *** *** *** *** *** *** CTG *** *** *** ***
--- --- +++ +++ +++ +++ +++ Leu +++ +++ --- ---
```

3. Early termination (''nonsense'' mutation)

```
              *
*** *** *** TAA *** *** *** *** *** *** *** ***
--- --- +++ TER --- --- --- --- --- --- --- ---
```

Deletions and insertions:

1. Single base insertion:

```
                *
AAT CCC ATG TTA ATG GTG GTG GCT TTG GTA AAA ATT T??-
--- --- Met Leu Met Val Val Ala Leu Val Lys Ile ???-
```

2. Single base deletion:

```
                       *(G)
AAT CCC ATG TTA TGG TGT GGC TTT GGT AAA AAT TT?-
--- --- Met Leu Trp Cys Gly Phe Gly Lys Asn ???-
```

Deletion or insertion of a larger number of bases moves the reading frame as shown above, except that a number of amino acids will be removed or added respectively.

The undirected production of mutations in the laboratory using agents that damage DNA, followed by selection of mutated cells with desired traits, has been a widely used approach in areas such as antibiotics production. As discussed below, one of the potent advances in rDNA technology is the ability to alter chosen DNA sequences at will in a directed manner, by a technique called ''site-directed mutagenesis'' to produce proteins with desired amino acid replacements. Such altered proteins are useful for the study of protein function. This approach of changing DNA to create changes in proteins is termed ''reverse genetics'' in contrast to the conventional ''forward genetics'', which relies on identifying amino acid changes of consequence in proteins followed by the tracing of the changes to DNA (Berg, 1991).

Modification of proteins beyond the ribosome

Amino acid moieties of many proteins are enzymatically modified within the intracellular compartments following their incorporation into the polypeptide chains. For example, many asparagine residues in proteins of eukaryotic cells have carbohydrates attached to them, converting the protein into a glycoprotein. Several other "post-translational modifications" involving many of the 20 amino acids in proteins have been observed. Table 2.4 is a partial list of post-translational modifications found in mammalian proteins.

Table 2.4. Common post-translational modifications in mammalian proteins

Modification	Example	Function influenced
Disulfide bonds	Growth hormone	Bioactivity
Subunit assembly	Antibodies	Antigen binding
Proteolysis	Insulin	Bioactivity
Glycosylation	Gonadotropins Erythropoietin	Bioactivity Pharmacokinetics
Phosphorylation	Epidermal Growth Factor receptor	Signal transduction
Sulfation	Cholecystokinin Factor VIII	Bioactivity Circulating half-life
γ-Carboxylation	Clotting factor IX	Bioactivity
Amidation	Calcitonin	Bioactivity
Lipid addition	Oncogenes	Membrane localization

In many cases, the role of many post-translational modifications is not well understood, but in some cases they have been found to be required for the biological activity of the protein molecules. In some cases where the enzymatic or co-factor activity of a protein is unaffected by the lack of a specific post-translational modification, it has been found to impact properties such as stability and circulating half-life. Thus, while the lack of glycosylation of many proteins is without influence on their functionality, they become unstable and are cleared faster from circulation.

The ability to perform a specific post-translational modification is dependent on the organism, and within a multicellular organism on the cell type in which the protein is expressed. For example, while mammalian cells glycosylate proteins, bacterial cells lack the enzymes necessary for glycosylation. Cells of yeast, a unicellular, lower eukaryote, are capable of glycosylation, but the composition and structure of the carbohydrate complex is different from that obtained in a mammalian cell (Goochee *et al.,* 1991). Differences in protein modification capability are found even among mammalian cell types of different organs and tissues expressing the same protein.

Recombinant DNA technology has paved the way for the efficient production of many mammalian proteins of therapeutic interest in a wide range of cells derived from prokaryotic bacteria, fungi, insects, and animals. Considerations of the post-translational capability of the host cell have important consequences to the quality of the protein product. These aspects are elaborated further in the section below on protein expression, and in Chapter 3.

Secretion of proteins

All proteins are synthesized by the ribosomal machinery within the cytoplasm of cells. However, a number of proteins such as hormones and serum proteins are found in the extracellular space. All cell types, from bacteria to mammalian cells, have a mechanism for exporting proteins. The export is accomplished through a secretion signal sequence, which is a short stretch of 15 to 20 predominantly hydrophobic amino acids found at the amino terminus of the protein to be secreted. During protein synthesis by eukaryotic ribosomes, the amino terminus of the protein emerging from the ribosome is directed into a membrane vesicle by protein factors which bind to the signal sequence. The protein "threads" through the membrane into the luminal space of the vesicle where the signal sequence is removed by proteolysis. This process, depicted in Fig. 2.11, occurs as the protein emerges from the ribosome and, therefore, the export of proteins is co-translational. The membrane vesicles into which the proteins are deposited move to the cell surface and fuse with the cell membrane, releasing the protein into the extracellular space. Many post-translational modifications occur within the membrane vesicles as they move towards the cell surface via a membranous intracellular organelle called the Golgi apparatus (Kaufman *et al.,* 1991).

Proteins such as cell-surface receptors, destined to remain at the cell surface, contain additional signals along the polypeptide which halt its further transit or "threading" through the membrane, leaving the carboxyl terminus of the protein within the cytoplasm. Thus, the protein becomes embedded in the membrane with an extracellular domain, a transmembrane domain, and a cytoplasmic domain. Many cell-surface proteins span the membrane only once, but many others have multiple transmembrane domains. The mechanism of insertion of the multiple membrane-spanning proteins is not yet fully defined. Many of the receptors discussed in Chapter 4 span the membrane seven times, and other proteins are known that span it several more times.

Proteins are also transported across membranes after their complete synthesis and release from the ribosome. This form of protein export, known as post-translational secretion, occurs in bacteria, and in higher eukaryotic cells in the transport of proteins into cellular organelles such as the mitochondria. As in the case of the co-translational secretion, amino acid stretches serve as targeting signals which are removed after the protein reaches the destined compartment.

In producing proteins by rDNA technology, attachment of secretion signals to the protein of interest results in the appearance of the protein in the extracellular space. Such a strategy of production may be necessary for some proteins, permitting them to undergo the normal post-translational modifications by moving through the secretory pathway which includes the Golgi apparatus. The Golgi apparatus of the cell contains many of the enzymatic activities which perform the post-translational modifications. Furthermore, in being secreted, a protein is separated from the high concentration of proteins present in the cell cytoplasm, and is released into the relatively protein-deficient extracellular medium, facilitating its purification. The secretion capabilities of cells can be increased by over-producing the proteins involved in the secretory pathway (Edgington, 1992).

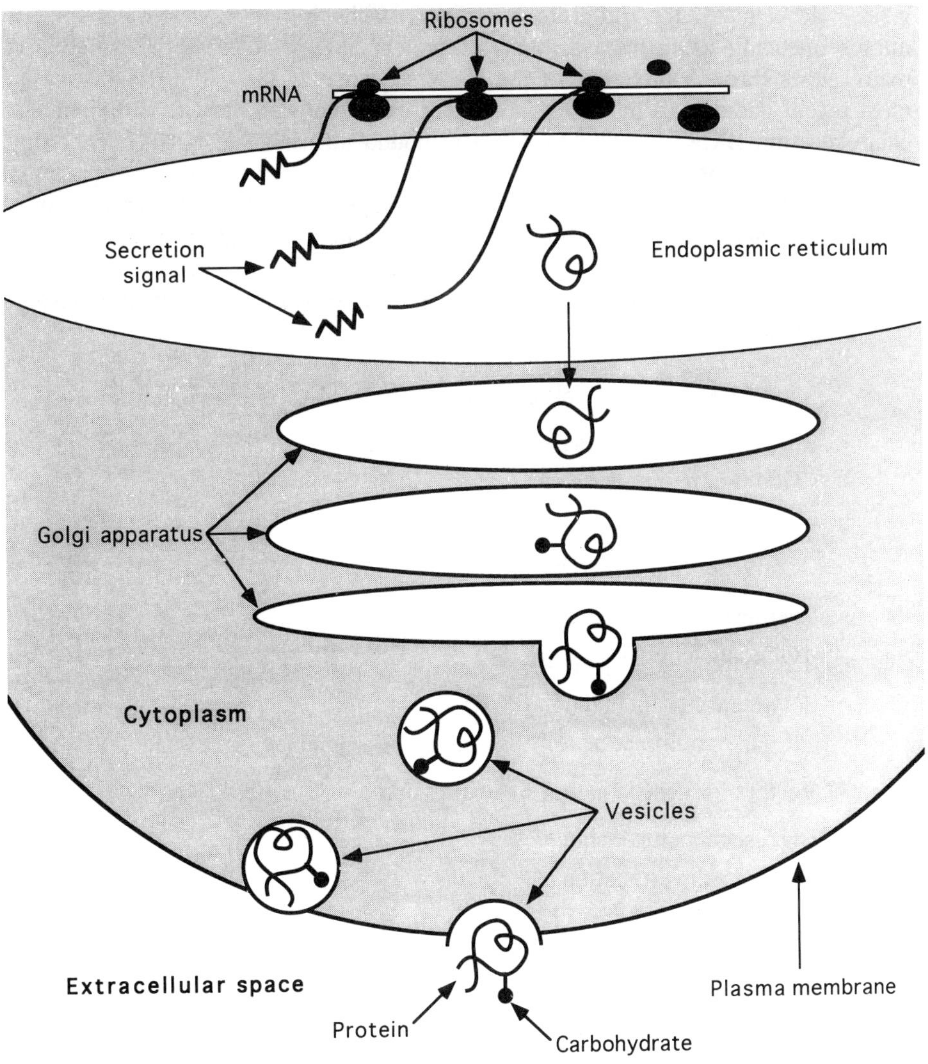

Fig. 2.11. Pathway of protein secretion in eukaryotic cells.

BASICS OF GENE MANIPULATION

Identification of DNA stretches of interest and their manipulation, be it to isolate and analyze a gene, or to overproduce a protein, or to diagnose a genetic disease, lies at the heart of rDNA technology. The tools used to manipulate DNA are the result of the confluence of distinct research pathways in bacterial and phage genetics, and bacterial physiology which were pursued for decades before the birth of rDNA technology. More recent developments in the chemical synthesis of DNA and the resultant use of synthetic oligonucleotides for isolation, sequencing and mutation of genes, and the ability to chemically synthesize entire genes, accelerated the progress of rDNA technology. Advances in protein microsequencing using trace amounts of protein have resulted in the isolation of many genes through inference of the DNA sequence of the coding segment. The most recent addition to the arsenal of molecular biology techniques is polymerase chain reaction (PCR), which has had a profound influence on rDNA technology. Concurrent developments in computer technology have led to the development of highly efficient and rapid algorithms for storage, analysis and comparison of nucleic acid and protein sequences. This organized accumulation of data has led to the formation of widely accessible data bases which are crucial for the conduct of rDNA technology. The major techniques and technologies currently used in rDNA applications are listed in Table 2.5 and are discussed below.

Table 2.5. Tools of recombinant DNA technology

- Restriction endonucleases and DNA ligase
  Cutting, rejoining DNA
- Reverse transcriptase
  Conversion of mRNA into cDNA
- Chemical DNA synthesis
  Oligonucleotides
- Polymerase chain reaction (PCR)
  Rapid amplification of specific DNA segments
- Vectors for gene isolation and expression
- DNA sequencing techniques
  Sequence verification
- Protein microsequencing, peptide synthesis
- Site-directed mutagenesis
  Creation of specific mutant proteins
- Protein overproduction
  Appropriate host/vector systems

Cutting and rejoining of DNA: restriction and ligation

The DNA content of the smallest genome such as that of the DNA virus SV40 is of the order of thousands of base pairs and the analysis of even such small genomes would be impossible if they could not be reproducibly fragmented into smaller pieces. The discovery of restriction endonucleases from several bacterial species provided the tool for the specific cleavage of DNA. Once cleaved, the fragments of different sizes could be separated electrophoretically, isolated, and analyzed.

Restriction enzymes are endonucleases which cleave specific sequences within double-stranded DNA stretches. The recognition and cleavage sequences of a routinely used group of endonucleases (called type II enzymes) may be four, five, six, or eight bases long and are symmetric across the two strands of DNA. Fig. 2.12 illustrates the cleavage specificity of a widely used six-base-motif-specific endonuclease, *Eco*R I.

By convention, the first three letters of the enzyme name refer to the bacterium which is the source of the enzyme, which, for *Eco*R I is *Escherichia coli*, and the subsequent letters denote the specific enzyme. In the cleavage sequence shown in Fig. 2.12, the two antiparallel strands of DNA are shown, where the numbers 5′ and 3′ denote the direction of the strands (see Fig. 2.5b). The recognition sequence of *Eco*R I, reading in the 5′ to 3′ direction, is GAATTC. The rules of complementarity of base pairing (A with T, and G with C) dictate the sequence of the complementary strand to have the same sequence when read in the 5′ to 3′ direction. This recognition sequence is therefore a "palindrome", which reads the same in either direction and has a two-fold axis of rotational symmetry. *Eco*R I cleaves at every location in the DNA where this sequence motif occurs. The phosphodiester bond between the G and the A on both strands is hydrolyzed by the enzyme, allowing the scission of the DNA strands at this sequence. Each end of the DNA fragment created in this cleavage event has a single-strand overhang which is capable of base-pairing with its partner generated in the cleavage event, or with other ends generated by *Eco*R I in any cleavage event. Such ends are known as "cohesive" or "sticky" ends. Thus, for example, it is possible for the *Eco*R I-generated ends of bacterial DNA and human DNA to associate by base-pairing. The cohesive ends involved in such an association can be sealed by another enzyme called the DNA ligase, which catalyzes the formation of the phosphodiester bonds on both strands, resulting in uninterrupted DNA as shown in Fig. 2.12. Note that such ligation points can be recleaved by *Eco*R I.

Over the course of the last two decades, over 700 restriction enzymes recognizing over a hundred unique sequence motifs in DNA have been isolated (some restriction enzymes from different sources recognize the same cleavage site). Table 2.6 lists a few commonly used restriction enzymes and their recognition sites. The overhangs produced by different enzymes vary and some restriction enzymes (*Eco*R V, *Sma* I) create blunt ends at the cleavage site. However, DNA ligase is also capable of joining blunt-ended DNA under specific reaction conditions.

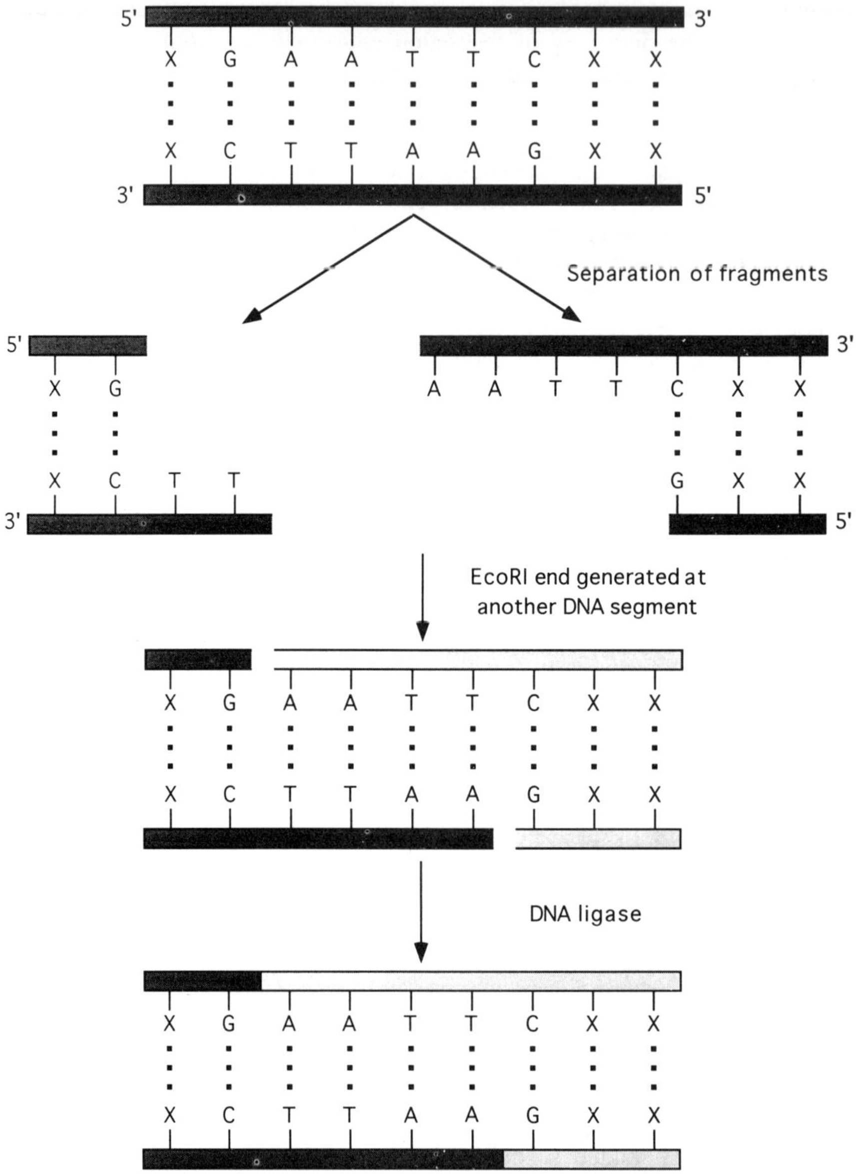

Fig. 2.12. Cleavage of DNA by restriction endonuclease *Eco*R I and joining by DNA ligase. The two shades of the DNA backbones represent DNA ends generated in different cleavage events.

Table 2.6. Recognition sequences of some commonly used six-base-specific restriction endonucleases

Endonuclease	Recognition sequence*
*Eco*R I	G^AATTC
*Eco*R V	GAT^ATC
*Bam*H I	G^GATCC
Hind III	A^AGCTT
Kpn I	GGTAC^C
Sal I	G^TCGAC
Nde I	CA^TATG
Xba I	T^CTAGA
Pvu I	CGAT^CG
Xho I	C^TCGAG
Sma I	CCC^GGG

*"^" denotes the cleavage point.

Cleavage sites for restriction enzymes occur randomly in the DNA. The frequency of a particular restriction site is dependent on the size of the DNA and the size of the recognition sequence. The probability of finding a particular four-base run in DNA is 1/256 (1/4 × 1/4 × 1/4 × 1/4) and that of a five-base run is 1/1024. The probability of occurrence reduces to 1/4096 for a specific six-base stretch and to 1/65536 for an eight-base stretch. The expectation and the occurrence of prototypic four-, six-, and eight-base-specific restriction sites in the 5243 base pair, circular genome of the simian virus SV40 is shown in Table 2.7.

Table 2.7. Frequency of restriction endonuclease sites in SV40 virus DNA (5243 base pairs)

Endonuclease	Recognition sequence	Frequency	
		Expected	Observed
Alu I	AGCT	20	34
*Sau*3A I	GATC	20	8
Taq I	TCGA	20	1
*Eco*R I	GAATTC	1	1
*Bam*H I	GGATCC	1	1
Hind III	AAGCTT	1	6
Not I	GCGGCCGC	<1	0
Pac I	TTAATTAA	<1	0

Although the general trend follows the expected probabilities, there are wide deviations from the expected numbers. Such deviations are common, and are attributable to the variations in the G–C content of the DNAs and the variable nearest-neighbor frequencies of the bases.

Every segment of DNA has a unique combination of restriction endonuclease sites and thus has a unique restriction map. Fig. 2.13 shows the restriction map of the region of the bovine genome containing the gene for the bovine growth hormone (Ramabhadran *et al.*, 1985). The entire growth hormone gene can be isolated on an *Eco*R I fragment of 4.3 kilobases and the coding region can be isolated on an *Bam*H I–*Hind* III fragment of 3.5 kilobases for further manipulation.

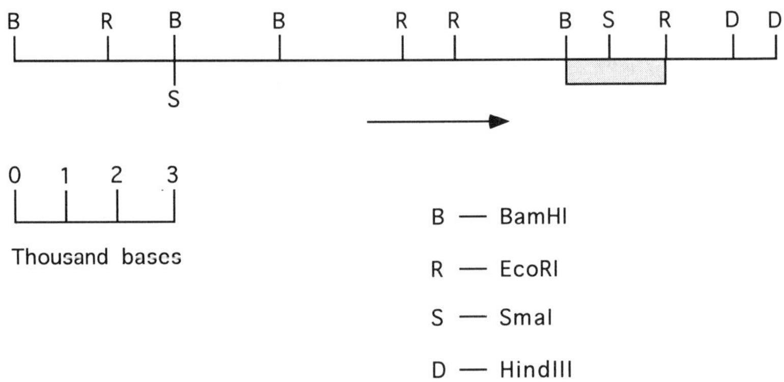

Fig. 2.13. Restriction map of the region of the bovine genome containing the gene for bovine growth hormone generated with selected restriction enzymes. The arrow denotes the promoter region and the box represents the protein coding sequence containing introns.

Chemical synthesis of DNA

A major advance which has been indispensable to progress in rDNA technology is the ability to synthesize oligonucleotides of a defined sequence. This is achieved by coupling the 5′ hydroxyl of the deoxyribose of the first nucleoside (a base linked to sugar) to a solid support such as controlled-pore-glass or polystyrene beads, and the chain is elongated by repeated cycles of addition of the next unit in the chain. The technique known as the phosphotriester method uses deoxyribonucleoside 3′-phosphoramides. Polymerization of nucleotides (phosphorylated sugar-linked base) into a strand of nucleic acids is complicated by the number of reactive groups in the nucleotide. Establishing the desired phosphodiester bond requires the "blocking" of all other reactive groups with protective groups which should be removable after synthesis of the polynucleotide chain. The progress made in the rapidity and yield of the polymerization reaction over the last two decades has been astounding and the technology has been fully automated (Fox, 1991). Thus, oligonucleotides of nearly 150 bases can be synthesized with a per-cycle time of under ten minutes (Vu *et al.,* 1990).

Synthetic oligonucleotides are indispensable for the detection of genes by hybridization, for the sequencing, total synthesis, and amplification of genes using the recently developed technique of polymerase chain reaction. These applications are discussed below. Oligonucleotides are also being developed as the therapeutics for highly specific inhibition of expression of selected genes (such as viral genes) as discussed in Chapter 6.

Nucleic acid hybridization

As discussed in the preceding section on DNA, the two strands of a double-stranded DNA molecule are held together by hydrogen bonds between the bases. Agents which disrupt the hydrogen bonding interaction between the strands cause the strands to separate, resulting in ''denaturation''. Heat and extremes of pH cause denaturation of DNA. Upon removal of the denaturing agent, the two strands of DNA can reform the hydrogen bonds. Under the right renaturation conditions, it is possible for the strands to assume the original, native form with uninterrupted hydrogen bonding along the length of the molecule. This phenomenon is known as reassociation or reannealing. Strands of DNA from different organisms can also anneal with each other in regions having sequence homology, to form hybrid molecules. Oligonucleotides also interact specifically with denatured DNA at locations corresponding to their complementary sequence. For a sufficiently long (12–15 bases) oligonucleotide, the specificity and the energy of interaction is high enough for the hybrid molecule to be stable. Thus, an oligonucleotide complementary to the sequence of a given gene would bind only to the gene even in situations where the DNA corresponding to the gene is a minor fraction of the total DNA. If the oligonucleotide carries a radioactive phosphorus (^{32}P) or other detectable label, its binding can be monitored and the presence of the gene confirmed. This is the principle involved in the Southern blotting procedure (named after its inventor, Southern) used to detect genes as shown in Fig. 2.14. Fragments generated by the restriction-enzyme digestion of DNA are separated on a gel, transferred and bound to filter paper (nylon membrane), and denatured to separate strands. This is followed by hybridization with a labeled oligonucleotide complementary to a gene segment; the region of the membrane containing the gene retains the label. The Southern blotting technique is employed routinely in gene isolation.

RNA molecules are also able to anneal with complementary sequences within themselves, within other DNA or RNA molecules, or with oligonucleotides. Thus, the RNA product of a gene can be detected by probing the RNA preparation separated on a gel with labeled oligonucleotides. This procedure was (facetiously) named ''Northern'' blotting.

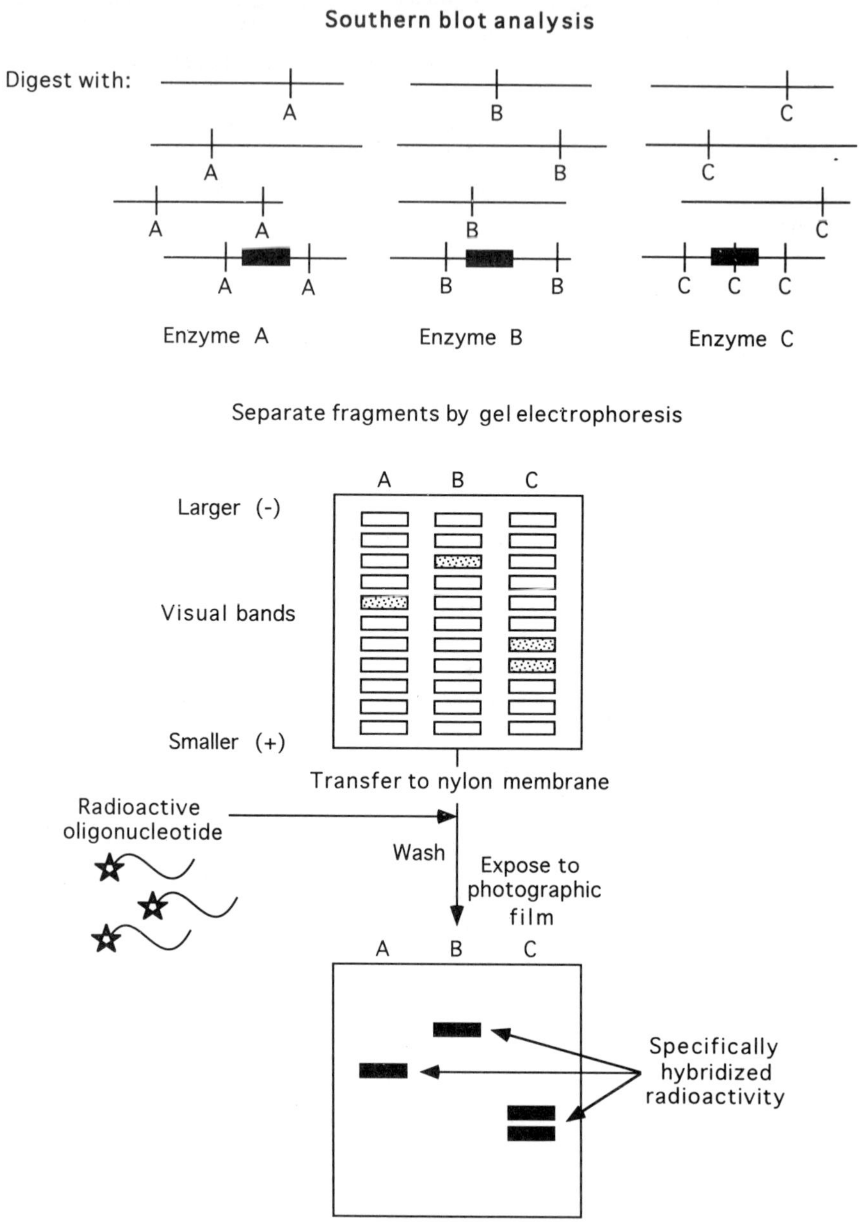

Fig. 2.14. Detection of specific DNA fragments by Southern blot hybridization.

DNA sequencing

Another seminal advance of the seventies was the development of techniques for the sequencing of DNA. The availability of restriction enzymes was critical for the development of DNA sequencing because they enabled reproducible fragmentation of DNA into small pieces required for sequencing. The widely used method of DNA sequencing also uses sequence-specific synthetic oligonucleotides. The technique involves preparation of radioactively labeled copies of the DNA region being sequenced, with a defined start but random terminations at one of the four bases (A, G, C, or T). Four individual labeling and chain elongation reactions, with random terminations at each of the four bases, are run. Size-based separation of the termination fragments from the four reactions on gels and visualization of the fragments using the incorporated radioactive label allow the sequence of the DNA segment to be read as shown in Fig. 2.15.

A single set of four reactions permits the reading of the sequence of about 500 bases from the start point defined by the oligonucleotide primer. Sequencing can be extended further by continuing the process with a new oligonucleotide primer complementary to the newly determined sequence and, thus, longer sequences can be determined. Although most of the sequence determinations are performed manually at this time, automation of this procedure using fluorescent labels for the fragments is well under way and is expected to facilitate sequencing of large stretches of DNA (Hunkapillar *et al.,* 1991; Fox, 1991). Recent initiatives aimed at sequencing the human genome of nearly 3 billion base pairs rely heavily on the speed and automation of DNA sequence determination. Other strategies of sequencing such as the one using computerized approaches and hybridization methods are also in early stages of development (Barinaga, 1991).

Protein microsequencing and peptide synthesis

Developments in the methods for the sequencing of proteins obtainable only in small amounts have been invaluable for the development of recombinant DNA. A sequence of about ten to twenty amino acids from the amino terminus of full-length proteins, or of defined fragments of the protein produced by chemical or protease cleavage, can be obtained from 30 to 100 picomoles of a protein (Yuksel *et al.,* 1991). (A picomole translates to 10 nanograms of a protein of about 100 amino acids.) Knowing the sequence of a stretch of amino acids permits inference of the DNA sequence which encoded it. This DNA sequence information can be used to synthesize oligonucleotide probes which, in turn, can be used to detect the gene for the protein by hybridization with DNA as discussed in the section below on gene isolation. However, because of the degeneracy of the genetic code discussed earlier, an amino acid may predict more than one DNA triplet sequence (Table 2.2). Methionine and tryptophan predict unique triplets in DNA because they are specified by single codons. Leucine, serine and arginine, which are specified by six codons each, predict any of the multiple triplets in DNA. Thus, given the amino acid sequence, it is possible to predict a set of possible coding DNA sequences. The number of possible DNA sequences corresponding to a protein sequence is determined by the number of codons used to specify each amino acid in the

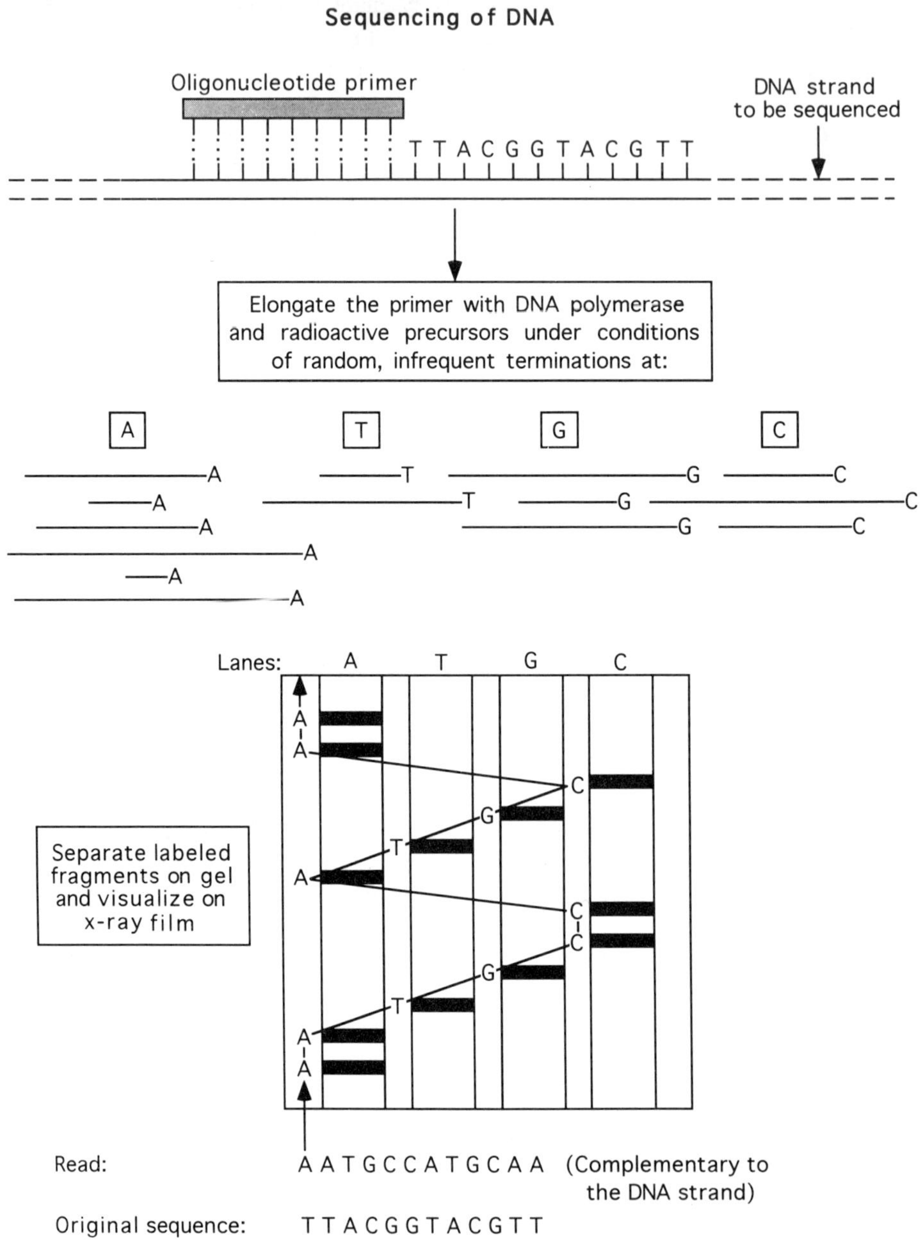

Fig. 2.15. Sequencing of DNA by chain termination method.

sequence. For example, the sequence of three contiguous tryptophans predicts a unique sequence TGG–TGG–TGG in DNA, but a stretch of three leucines would predict $6 \times 6 \times 6 = 216$ different possible sequences. Nonetheless, by judicious choice of the stretch of amino acids it is possible to minimize the number of inferred coding sequences. This approach of using the protein sequence to "guess" the gene sequence is used routinely in gene isolation.

Protein sequence determination uses the standard sequential Edman-degradation procedure to cleave of the N-terminal amino acid of the protein followed by the characterization of the released amino acid in each degradation cycle on chromatographic columns (Wittman-Liebold and Kimura, 1984; Klemm, 1984). The procedure is fully automated, and protein sequencers, along with DNA synthesizers, are an integral part of every biotechnology research effort.

In addition to protein sequencing, the capability to chemically synthesize small proteins and peptides of defined sequence has played a vital role in the development of biotechnology (Kent, 1988; Kent and Parker, 1988; Atherton, 1991). Peptide synthesis is accomplished on solid-phase matrices to which the starting amino acid is coupled. The subsequent amino acids are added sequentially to elongate the peptide chain. Upon completion, the chain is released from the matrix, and the protecting groups used to mask other reactive side-chain groups are removed. The resultant peptide of interest is purified away from abnormal shorter peptides resulting from early terminations and unsuccessful cycles, and the authenticity of the peptide is confirmed by sequencing.

Using this method, peptides of up to a hundred amino acids can be synthesized, but the yields of full-length peptides decrease rapidly as synthesis of peptides longer than about 50 amino acids is attempted. In addition, the yield of a peptide is also dependent on the amino acid composition and on the sequence of the peptide. In a typical example, TGF-α, a 50 amino acid peptide was synthesized at an average coupling efficiency of 99.65% at each step (Kent, 1988).

Some small peptides have biological activities of therapeutic interest, and in these cases chemically synthesized peptides are used as drugs. The primary use of defined peptides in the laboratory is in the production of highly specific antibody reagents for the detection of proteins. Peptides chemically coupled to larger proteins are used as antigens to immunize animals. In addition, suspected biological activities of small peptides predicted by gene sequence can be verified by using synthetic peptides. Synthesis of small peptides using the cellular ribosomal machinery, while feasible, is complicated, and further purification and generation of bioactivity can be laborious. Therefore, for short peptides, the high yields of synthesis and the ease of purification make chemical synthesis a cost-effective alternative to ribosomal synthesis.

Isolation and amplification of genes: cloning

Individual mammalian genes comprise a tiny fraction of the total DNA of a mammalian cell. For example, a gene occupying 10,000 base pairs comprises a mere 3×10^{-5} fraction of the human genome. Therefore, if human genomic DNA

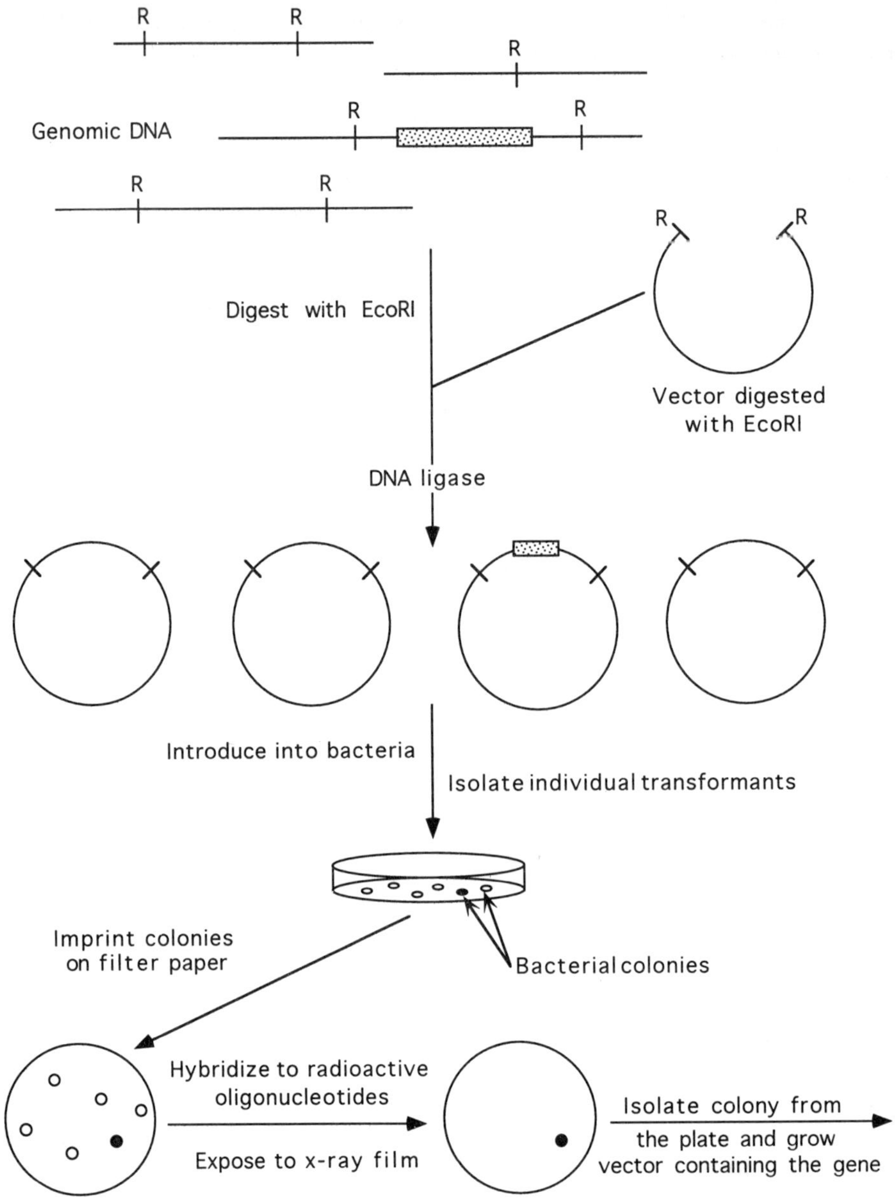

Fig. 2.16. Isolation of a single gene from a large genome.

were fragmented into 10,000 base-pair fragments, only one fragment in 300,000 would contain the gene of interest. Thus, the study and use of gene sequences require techniques for their identification and amplification.

Fig. 2.16 shows the process of cloning a hypothetical mammalian gene which is contained on an *Eco*R I fragment. DNA is digested with *Eco*R I and the resulting fragments are ligated to the DNA of a "cloning vector" producing recombinant DNA molecules. Vectors are DNA molecules which are capable of replication to very high copy numbers when a single copy is introduced into their host cell. They are either autonomously replicating circular DNA molecules known as plasmids or are DNAs of bacterial viruses (bacteriophages) which replicate to high numbers. Segments of foreign DNA ligated to the vectors are amplified along with the vector sequences when introduced into their host which, in most cases, is *E. coli.* Bacteria harboring the vector containing the foreign gene of interest are identified using labeled oligonucleotide complementary to the gene. In the case of genes whose DNA sequence is unknown, oligonucleotides are designed based on inference from the known sequence of the protein encoded by the gene. The amino acid sequence can predict the nucleic acid sequence, but because of the degeneracy of the genetic code discussed earlier (preceding section), multiple oligonucleotides are required to identify the gene.

As discussed earlier, eukaryotic genes contain introns which interrupt the coding sequences. It is possible to make a copy of the coding sequence without the introns by making a cDNA copy of the messenger RNA. This is accomplished by using the enzyme reverse transcriptase. The resultant DNA is called the complementary DNA or cDNA of the gene from which the messenger RNA was transcribed. A cDNA of interest can be isolated from the pool of cDNAs generated by reverse transcription of a messenger RNA pool using plasmid or bacteriophage vectors as described above. The pool of vector molecules containing the assortment of gene fragments from an organism, or cDNAs from an organ where a particular gene is transcribed, is known as a "library". The process of searching for the specific gene sequences in the library is called "screening" or "probing" the library.

Once identified, bacteria harboring the desired vector are grown and large quantities of vector containing the foreign DNA (recombinant DNA) are isolated for further characterization.

Polymerase chain reaction

A recent powerful addition to the arsenal of rDNA techniques is the method of polymerase chain reaction, commonly known as PCR (Erlich *et al.,* 1991; Erlich, 1989), which permits rapid and high-level amplification of DNA as shown in Fig. 2.17. A pair of synthetic oligonucleotides known as "primers", flanking the gene or the DNA segment to be amplified, are annealed to the heat-denatured total DNA mixture in which the gene to be amplified is present in very low concentration. Primers hybridize to the gene of interest at the ends of both strands as shown in Fig. 2.17. DNA-bound primers are elongated using the enzyme DNA polymerase, which extends the primer on both strands, creating two

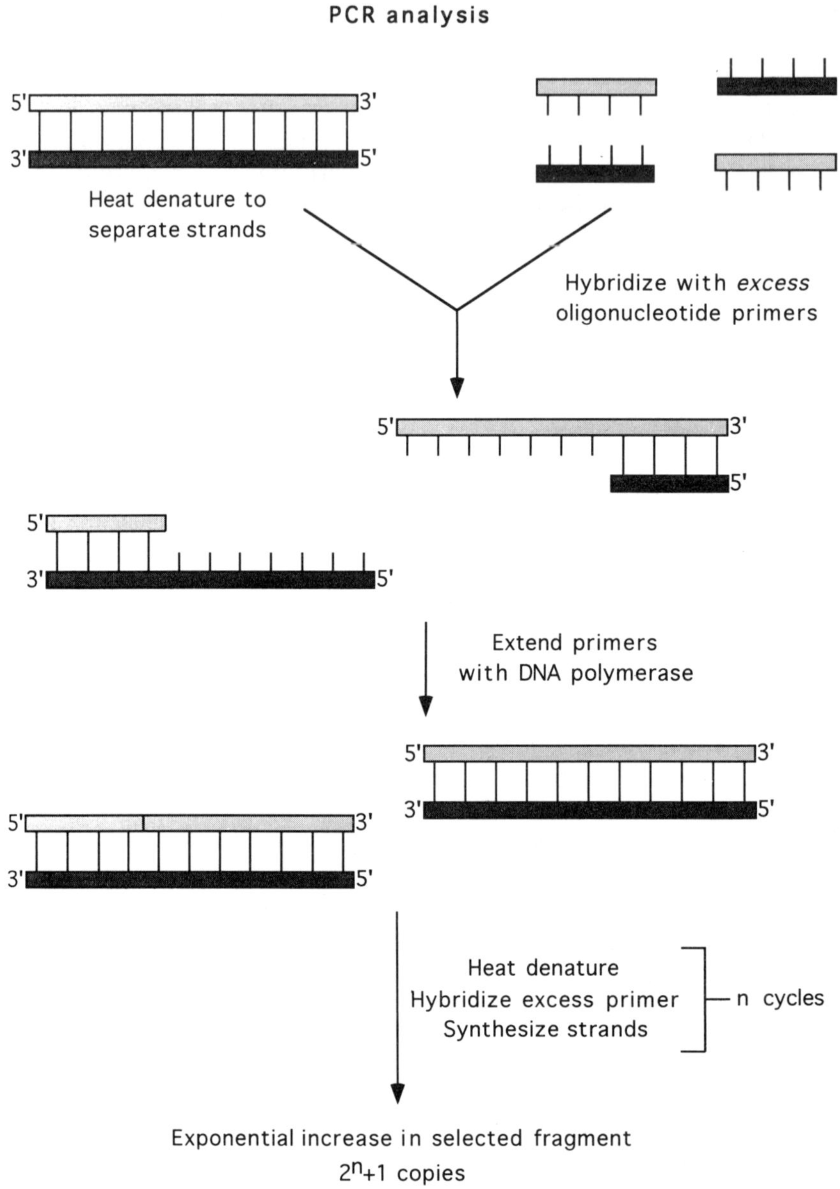

Fig. 2.17. Amplification of DNA segments by polymerase chain reaction (PCR).

double-stranded DNA copies of the gene of interest. The same series of steps of heat denaturation, primer annealing, and chain extension in the second cycle results in four copies of the DNA segment. Every repeat of the cycle results in a two-fold amplification of the copy number of the gene, and 10 cycles of heating, cooling and DNA synthesis can result in a 1024-fold amplification of the selected gene. The cycle times are short enough for several cycles to be accommodated into a period of a few hours. Use of a heat-stable *Taq* DNA polymerase from thermophilic bacterium obviates the need for adding polymerase at every synthesis step preceded by heating. The PCR procedure has been fully automated and is used routinely in almost every molecular biology laboratory. Many sophisticated variations of the technique have been developed for a variety of applications. A major drawback of the technique is its relatively high error rate resulting in misincorporation of 1 in 10^5 nucleotides per cycle compared to the error rate of 1 in 10^9 incorrect bases per cycle for cellular DNA polymerases. This high error rate necessitates the confirmation of the sequence of amplified PCR products, especially in applications such as protein production where the correct sequence is of utmost importance.

The design of oligonucleotide primers for PCR requires the knowledge of sequences flanking the DNA region to be amplified. Thus, this technique is useful only for the rapid manipulation of DNA segments of known sequence. This is often the case in applications such as the detection of the low-level presence of HIV viral genomes in biopsies, or the search for mutations in the cystic fibrosis gene among families with disease prevalence. PCR has also been applied successfully to examine specific regions of DNA from centuries-old archeological specimens (Cherfas, 1991). Although PCR has many applications in gene manipulation (Paabo, 1991), its major impact on the pharmaceutical industry is expected to be in the diagnostic applications (Eisenstein, 1990) described in Chapter 8. A related technique known as ligase chain reaction (LCR) is also emerging as a powerful technique for use in diagnostic applications, either independently or in combination with PCR (Weiss, 1991). This technique and its applications are also discussed in Chapter 8.

Directed mutation of DNA: site-directd mutagenesis

Change or deletion of codons at the DNA level results in replacement or deletion respectively of the corresponding amino acids, producing altered proteins. These alterations permit the determination of the contribution of single amino acids or that of defined regions composed of a few amino acids to the function of proteins. For example, determination of the key residues which are involved in the action of a protease like that of the HIV virus is useful in the design of drugs to inhibit the protease. In addition, proteins with novel activities can also be created by deleting or mutating existing proteins, or by splicing together segments of different proteins. This approach to the analysis of the function of proteins by creating changes in coding sequence has been dubbed ''reverse genetics'' in contrast to the classical or ''forward'' genetics, which traces the nature of genetic and structural changes associated with a given mutant phenotype (Berg, 1991).

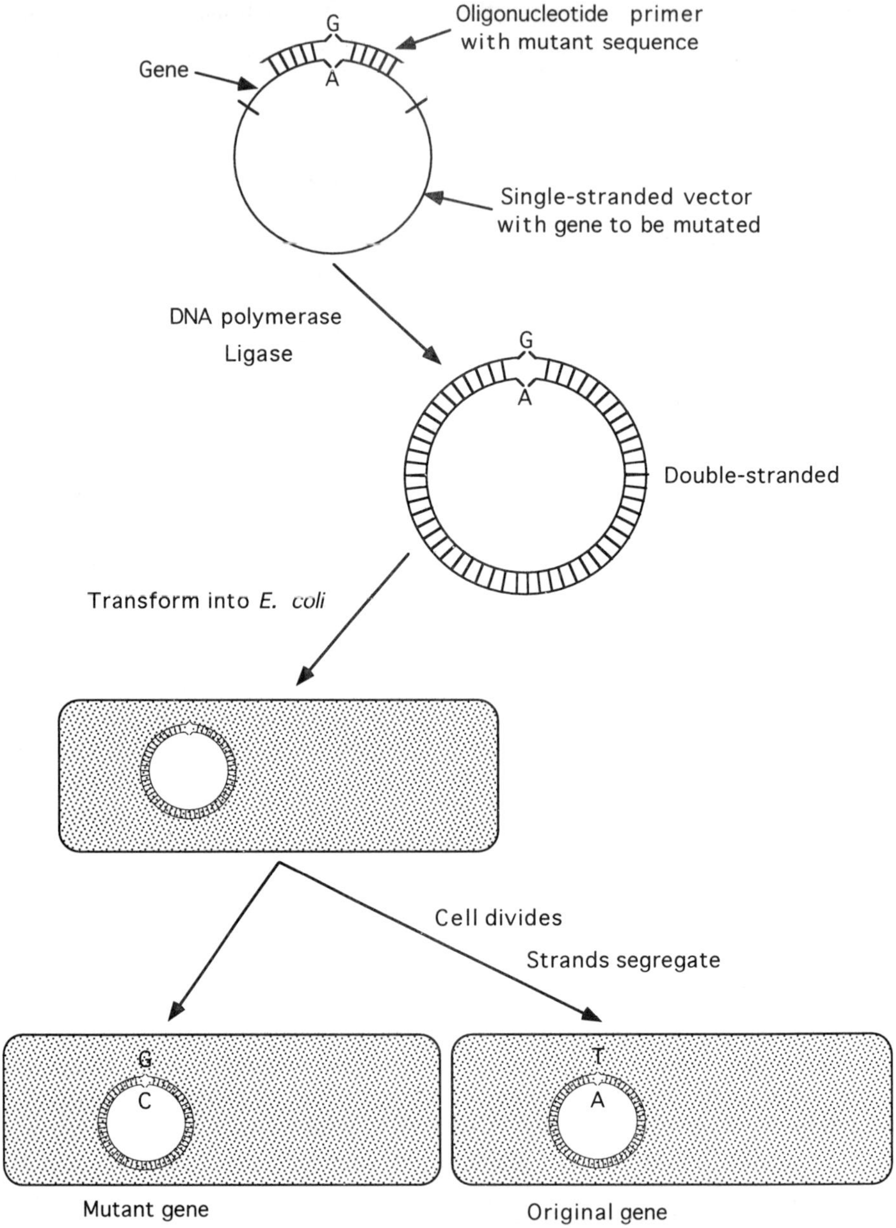

Fig. 2.18. Principle of site-directed mutagenesis of DNA using an oligonucleotide primer.

Deletion of a segment within a gene is easily achieved by digestion with restriction enzymes followed by ligation, thereby deleting a section of the coding information. Single amino acid changes are introduced by using synthetic oligonucleotides which contain the desired codon change. The oligonucleotide is annealed with the complementary strand from the unmutated gene, resulting in a base mismatch as shown in Fig. 2.18. A new strand is synthesized by elongating the annealed oligonucleotide primer. Introduction of the hybrid DNA molecule into the *E. coli* bacterium results in progeny vectors derived from the parental and the mutant strands. Mutants are identified by their preferential hybridization to the labeled mutagenesis primer, and the mutation is confirmed by DNA sequencing.

Computer analysis of sequence and information bases

Progress in biotechnology has been accelerated by the astounding developments in computer technology over the last decade, in both the capability and the accessibility. This is most evident in the specialized applications of computers to the analysis of protein structure discussed in Chapter 5. However, the use of smaller computers for analysis and comparison of sequence data is a routine activity in all molecular biology laboratories. Sequences determined in the laboratory can be fed into computers for storage, compilation, and analysis. Powerful programs are available for the rapid analysis of DNA sequences to determine all the restriction sites contained within the sequence. This information is indispensable to the experimental manipulation of DNA sequences. Other programs are available for translating a given DNA sequence into its amino acid sequence, for determining the possible hydrogen-bonding interactions and folding of RNA molecules, and the possible secondary structures of protein molecules. It is also possible to make rapid comparisons of DNA or protein sequences from different sources and species, using varying degrees of stringency of similarity (for example, being identical vs. belonging to the same chemical class of amino acids), to detect structural relationships which may indicate functional similarities (Gribskov and Devereux, 1991).

Over the last two decades, thousands of sequences of genes, cDNAs, and proteins have been published. Universally accessible data banks containing the published sequences have been established, and new sequences are being added as they are determined. At this time, more than 65 million bases of DNA and RNA sequences from 3000 species, 30,000 protein sequences covering 8 million amino acid residues, and the complete atomic coordinates of 655 proteins are in various data banks (Courteau, 1991; Pearson *et al.,* 1991). These data bases permit the analysis of any published sequence by any researcher tied into the computer network. It is a routine procedure now to compare a newly derived DNA or protein sequence against all known sequences in the data bank to ascertain if the gene or protein has already been isolated in another context. The search for relatedness to genes from the same species or from other species is many times quite useful in assigning a possible function to the newly discovered sequence. Database searches have led to astounding and serendipitous discoveries on many occasions. For example, scientists studying the cell-surface receptor for the human rhinovirus, a cause of common colds, discovered that the sequence of the protein matched the sequence of a protein known as the immune-cell adhesion molecule, or I-CAM, which was discovered by immunologists as a cell-surface molecule regulating cell–cell interactions. Database searches and computerized similarity searches have been valuable also in the analysis of many other cell-surface receptor families, ion channels, prohormone-processing proteases, etc.

Gene expression and protein overproduction

The final goal of all the techniques described in the preceding sections is to produce the protein products of the isolated genes for analysis and clinical applications. The production of a protein from its gene is termed ''expression'', and the DNA components used for expression are termed expression vectors. Production of the protein of interest occurs in a host cell which is compatible for the maintenance and/or replication of the expression vector. Together, the host cell and the expression vector are called an expression system.

As discussed earlier, the genetic code is universal for all cells from simple bacteria to plants and humans. Therefore, any cell is capable of translating the message transcribed from a human gene or cDNA, provided the appropriate regulatory signals recognized by the particular cell type are attached to the message. This underlying unity of biological systems allows for the production of a human protein in any cell type for which vector systems are available. The choice of a particular expression system is determined by factors such as the application for which the protein is expressed, properties of the protein, and the economics of production in cases where large quantities are desired.

Expression vectors

Protein production by the rDNA approach is accomplished through the use of expression vectors which are an assembly of covalently linked segments of DNA, each performing a specific function. The three basic components of most expression vectors are shown in Fig. 2.19. These are: (1) DNA regions which permit the replication of the vector in the bacterial host cell used in vector assembly, and also allow the selection of the host cells containing the vector. (The host cell here is generally *E. coli*, in which most vectors are assembled); (2) DNA regions which confer selectability and maintenance in the host cell chosen for expression, if it is different from the bacterial host wherein the vector was assembled; (3) the gene or cDNA to be expressed, linked to appropriate transcription and translational control elements capable of functioning in the expression host.

Most of the expression vectors currently in use are constructed and propagated in *E. coli* bacterium. Large amounts of the vector DNAs are extracted from *E. coli* cultures and introduced into the chosen host cell. (A notable exception to this generalization are vectors derived from mammalian and insect viruses, but even in these cases at least some of the components of the expression vector are assembled in *E. coli.*) Thus, vectors assembled by the manipulation of DNA by restriction nucleases and ligase are introduced in the naked-DNA form into *E. coli* rendered competent to accept extraneous DNA. This process is termed "transformation". Once the vector enters the *E. coli* cell, it has to be replicated and maintained in order to avoid its loss due to the dilution that accompanies rounds of cell division. The presence of a DNA sequence on the vector which functions as the origin of replication permits the vector to replicate in the host cell.

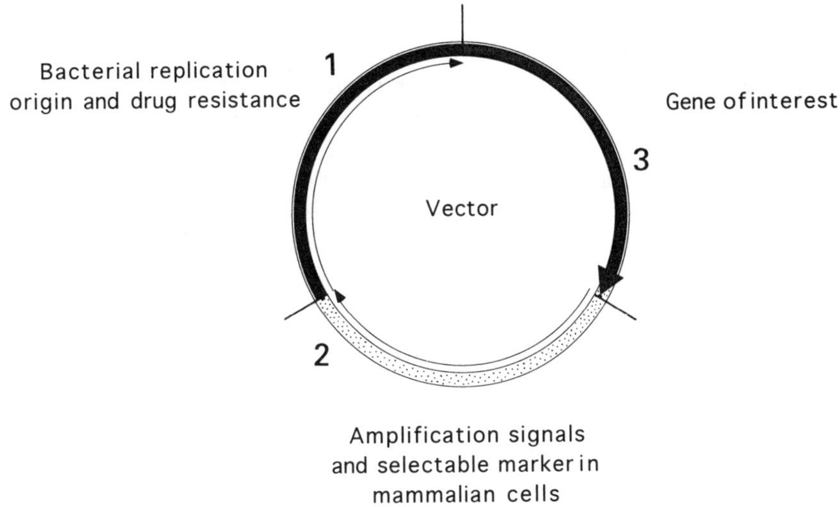

Fig. 2.19. Components of a typical expression vector.

When cells are transformed with naked vector DNA (as opposed to packaged, protein associated DNA in viruses) only a fraction of the cells, ~10% under the best conditions, take up the DNA. Therefore, the cells receiving the DNA or the "transformants" have to be isolated from among the non-receiving "untransformed" cells. This is accomplished by using the selectable property encoded by the vector, such as resistance to antibiotics (ampicillin, tetracycline, etc.). Exposure of the mixed population of transformed and untransformed cells to the antibiotic results in the elimination of untransformed cells. Transformed bacterial cells can be isolated, grown, and vector DNA prepared from them for introduction into the expression host cell of choice.

The second component of an expression vector comprises DNA sequences required for the selection, maintenance and copy-number amplification of the vector in the host cell wherein protein expression is desired. Obviously, this region is not needed for expression in *E. coli*. The selectable markers used in other host cells may be an enzyme conferring the ability to produce a nutrient essential for growth of the host cell, or transformation of cell morphology, or resistance to antibiotics (such as hygromycin or geneticin). Sequences for the maintenance of the vector DNA are required for the autonomous replication of the plasmid in these host cells except in cases where the vector sequences "integrate" into chromosomes of the host cells and are then replicated with the chromosome. The maintenance sequences are usually composed of a replication origin and coding sequences for accessory protein(s) which act on the replication origin. Both the origin and the coding information for the accessory proteins are usually derived from viruses that normally replicate in the particular expression host cells.

The third component of an expression vector is the expression cassette comprising the DNA (either cDNA or gene) encoding the protein to be produced and the sequences required to direct the transcription, RNA processing, and translation of the RNA. The coding sequence is preceded by a promoter sequence which is capable of directing transcription in the chosen host cell and is followed by sequences involved in RNA processing and termination of transcription. Transcription and RNA processing involve RNA polymerase and other proteins specific to the class of host cells, and therefore promoters and regulatory elements are not usually interchangeable between host cell systems. In cases where the goal is to obtain large quantities of a protein (as is the case of proteins for drug use), the promoter and other regulatory elements are chosen to produce maximum transcription. In addition, specific sequences which are known to prolong the half-life of the mRNA and increase the frequency of its translation by ribosomes are transcribed into mRNA along with the coding sequences. Table 2.8 lists the factors which influence the production level of a protein. In optimizing the yields of expressed genes, the final level of expression obtained is the sum of the efficiencies of all these steps. Some of the factors, such as gene copy number and promoter efficiency, are parameters that are easier to manipulate and to quantify, while others such as translational efficiency and mRNA stability are less easily controlled because their molecular mechanisms are not well understood.

Table 2.8. Factors affecting protein production levels

- Vector/gene copy number
- Transcription efficiency of promoter
- Efficiency of mRNA maturation and transport
- Translational efficiency
- mRNA stability
- Protein stability

Expression hosts

As discussed earlier, because of the universality of the genetic code, it is possible to produce a protein in any cell type whose biology is understood, and for which vectors and the method for transformation exist. Currently in the biotechnology industry, proteins of biological interest are expressed in bacteria, yeast and other fungi, insect cells, and mammalian cells. Intact oocytes derived from the frog *Xenopus* are also amenable for use in the expression of mRNAs or genes introduced into them by microinjection. This system is mainly used for the characterization of protein products of an mRNA, and is not very useful for the large-scale production of proteins. Recent advances in the use of transgenic animals for secreting therapeutic proteins in milk are an exciting extension of the expression in mammalian cells, and circumvent the need to culture engineered mammalian cells (see below).

Two factors which dictate the choice of a host/vector system are the ability to produce the protein in a form acceptable for the particular application, and the economics of production. While biological activity of the protein is the criterion for acceptability in most cases, in some applications such as vaccines, the protein is useful irrespective of its biological activity. Evaluation of the economics should include not only the cost of growing the engineered cell, but also the downstream purification techniques necessitated by the characteristics of the production system. Table 2.9 is a list of the expression systems currently in use, and their advantages and disadvantages.

Table 2.9. Expression systems and characteristics

Expression system	Prototype	Advantages	Limitations
Bacterial	*E. coli*	Inexpensive media	No post-translational modifications
		rapid high-density growth	endotoxins
		high protein yield	insolubility
		secretion	
Fungal	*S. cerevisiae*	Inexpensive media	Limited post-translational modifications
		high-density growth	different post-translational modifications
		some post-translational modifications	lower protein yield
		secretion	
Insect	SF9 cells baculovirus	High protein yields	Different post-translational modifications
		many post-translational modifications	expensive media and growth
			lytic, not continuous
Mammalian	Chinese hamster ovary cells	Correct post-translational modifications	Expensive media and growth
		secretion	slow growth
		authenticity of product	mammalian pathogens

Among the host/vector systems listed in Table 2.9, bacteria offer the greatest economy of growth. Media used for their growth are inexpensive and their growth rate is rapid. This is one of the earliest and best-characterized expression systems owing to both its simplicity and the history of the developments in the field. Many vectors for foreign gene expression in bacteria, predominantly *E. coli*, have been developed and optimized (Morales and Bagdasarian, 1991; Bogosian *et al.*, 1991; Rodriguez and Denhardt, 1988). Thus, bacterial systems are the first choice if a protein can be produced in an active form, or if the protein is needed as antigenic material where activity is not an issue. One of the major problems encountered in the production of proteins in bacterial hosts is the aggregation of these proteins into an amorphous entity called an "inclusion body" (Georgiou and Bowden, 1991; Bowden *et al.*, 1991). Disulfide bonds present in many proteins of interest do not form in the bacterial cytoplasm. Therefore it is necessary to extract the protein present in a denatured form and refold it into an active form. The conditions for the refolding process varies with each protein and is often laborious. The refolding process also becomes more difficult as the size of the protein and the number of disulfide bonds in it increase. Many of the folding problems can be overcome by inducing the bacterial host to secrete the protein into the extracellular space or the bacterial periplasm (Morales and Bagdasarian, 1991; Masui *et al.*, 1983; Rodriguez and Denhardt, 1988). This is achieved by attaching the secretion signal from a normally secreted bacterial protein to the amino terminus of the protein to be secreted. The signal sequence is cleaved in the secretion process, but the accuracy of cleavage of the signal in the chimeras cannot be assumed, and must be verified. Furthermore, the efficiency of secretion is variable with each protein.

Another limitation of bacterial expression systems is the inability of bacteria to preform many of the post-translational modifications which are normally present in mammalian proteins. Further, the assembly of proteins composed of multiple subunits (e.g. antibodies) does not occur in a bacterial cell. There are many examples where the protein is biologically active without the particular modification, and may be usable in the clinic. However, the roles of many of the modifications are not fully understood. While without effect on the bioactivity in test systems, they can have an influence on functions such as immunogenicity and circulating half-life. Humulin, human growth hormone, and interferons are some of the proteins produced in *E. coli* cells which are currently in use in the clinic. Among these, some of the interferons are glycosylated in nature. But interferons without glycosylation, produced in *E. coli,* are in clinical use (Pestka and Langer, 1987).

Yeast and other fungi are unicellular eukaryotes, and, like bacteria, they can be grown to very high cell densities in short times using inexpensive media. Vast experience in fermenting yeast has been accrued through their use in fermentation in the food and beverage industries, and other industrial applications. As in the case of bacterial expression, proteins can be produced in the cytoplasm of the engineered cell, or their secretion into the medium can be engineered. Fungal cells have post-translational modification capabilities not found in bacteria, but these may differ from those found in mammalian cells. For example, even though yeast cells are able to glycosylate human proteins, the nature of the sugars and the length of the sugar chains differ significantly from those added by mammalian cells. Differences in the nature of the oligosaccharides added are observed even among different yeasts (Marino, 1991; Buckholz and Gleeson *et al.* 1991; Goochee, 1991). Recombivax HB and Energix-B are two currently approved hepatitis B vaccines produced in the baker's yeast *Saccharomyces cerevisiae* (PMA Survey Report, 1991).

Cells of multicellular organisms can be grown in the laboratory by cell culture methods. These cells can be engineered for the production and secretion of recombinant proteins by using a variety of vectors. Among the expression hosts, animal cells are the most expensive to cultivate. Cell culture media used for their growth are complex and have to be supplemented with animal sera or purified growth factors. Because of the nutritional richness of the media, they can be easily contaminated with fungi and bacteria. Thus, a high degree of sterility is a must for routine cell culture, and is of utmost importance for pharmaceutical production. Cells derived from mammalian species are possible hosts for viral agents that may be pathogenic to man, necessitating routine testing of the cells and the protein product for adventitious agents. Therefore cell culture production is an expensive proposition, and is the last resort if less-expensive alternative systems are found unsuitable. One of the chief advantages of the higher eukaryotic and mammalian cell systems is their ability to affect many of the important post-translational modifications, and to secrete proteins efficiently (Kaufman *et al.,* 1991). Secreted proteins are easier to purify because of the relatively lower concentration of proteins in the medium, especially when serum-free media are used for culturing the cells (Thilly, 1986; Spier and Griffiths, 1985a,b).

The expression system for proteins in insect cells using an insect virus known as baculovirus is a new addition to the choice of available host/vector systems (Luckow, 1991). In this system, the gene or cDNA to be expressed is incorporated into the DNA genome of the baculoviral vector replacing a highly expressed but non-essential gene. Infection of insect cells in culture with the recombinant baculovirus results in the replication of the virus and the concomitant production of the foreign protein to very high levels. Being higher on the evolutionary scale in relation to bacteria and fungi, insect cells are able to affect many post-translational modifications of increased complexity. However, the detailed chemical structures of many of these modifications are not yet well understood (Goochee *et al.,* 1991; see also Appendix (chapter 2) for an update).

The greatest advantage of the higher eukaryotic cell expression systems is their ability to produce proteins in a form much closer to the naturally occurring material. Because therapeutic proteins are generally products of mammalian or human tissues, it is not surprising that the expression system best suited for their production is mammalian cells. All mammalian cells are capable of performing most of the simple post-translational modifications and secretion of proteins. However, the different mammalian cell lines currently in use are established from different tissues which differ in their ability to affect specific post-translational modifications. For example, the antithrombotic, protein C, a member of the blood coagulation system, requires for activity gamma carboxylation of specific glutamic acid residues. This post-translational modification occurs efficiently when protein C is expressed in a human kidney cell line, 293, but not as efficiently in other established cell lines (Grinnell *et al.*, 1987). Similarly, two preparations of erythropoietin, a highly glycosylated protein, produced in two different engineered mammalian cell lines, while showing similar bioactivities *in vitro*, differ strikingly in their *in vivo* activities. This difference has been attributed to the difference in the circulating half-lives of the two preparations, resulting from the differences in the sialic acid content of the carbohydrate chains attached to the proteins by the two cell lines (Goto *et al.*, 1991; Goochee *et al.*, 1991). Upon the establishment of cells in culture, some of the specific modification capabilities found in the tissue of origin are maintained, but many are lost during establishment and continuous culturing. Thus, even among mammalian cells, it may be necessary to identify the appropriate cell line for the production of proteins which require complex post-translational modifications for biological activity. Tissue plasminogen activator (tPA) marketed as Activase, erythropoietin marketed as Epogen, coagulation factor VIII, and humanized monoclonal antibodies are some of the protein drugs expressed in mammalian cells.

A recent exciting development in the expression of proteins is the production of therapeutic proteins in the milk of transgenic farm animals (Moffat, 1991a; Bialy, 1991; Spalding, 1992). Fertilized farm animal embryos are injected with an expression vector containing the gene or cDNA for the gene of interest linked to a promoter for a milk protein gene. The resultant transgenic animals express the protein in the mammary glands (and in no other organs), and secrete the protein into milk. Alternatively, animals can be engineered for the production of the therapeutic protein in other cells such as erythrocytes, as in the case of human hemoglobin synthesis in the red blood cells of transgenic pigs (Spalding, 1992). The transgenic animal method utilizes the advanced protein production capabilities of mammalian cells without having to resort to the use of expensive media and laborious techniques required for cell cultivation. Transgenic animals can be bred to produce herds of drug-producing cattle. Optimistic predictions have been made for the economics of this approach; for example, it is projected that a single transgenic cow will produce sufficient Factor VIII to satisfy the need of the US patient population of 120 grams per year (Paleyanda *et al.*, 1991). However, this technology is relatively new, and the economics of production and the safety issues are only beginning to be addressed.

The attempts at ''biopharming'' are not restricted to transgenic cattle. Methods for the expression of pharmaceutically important proteins in plant cell cultures and in intact plants are showing promise (Moffat, 1991b). For example, tobacco and alfalfa plants have been shown to secrete antibodies, and human serum albumin has been produced in transgenic potatoes and tobacco. However, structural differences have been observed in the proteins produced in plants. Here again, issues of protein yields, and regulatory and safety concerns remain to be addressed.

Table 2.10 lists the characteristics of an ideal expression system. High production rates per cell increase the economy of production. Maintenance of vectors, especially at high copy-numbers, in several expression systems requires the use of antibiotics such as ampicillin and tetracycline, or toxic antimetabolites such as methotrexate which pose problems of worker exposure, disposal, and product safety. Thus, systems which avoid the use of such compounds are preferable. In many recombinant expression systems, the vector can be lost from the transfected cell, and the cells without the vector may overgrow the culture because of higher growth rate. Production in the absence of cell growth permits the maintenance of the bioreactor at a fixed cell density and harvesting of the product over extended periods of time, of the order of weeks to months. The ability to cultivate cells from higher eukaryotes which are serum-dependent in serum-free media reduces the medium cost and facilitates downstream purification of the product. Finally, safety issues relating to the expression system determine their utility and also the costs of safety testing of the product. These issues may be the immunogenicity of the protein product, or contamination by carcinogenic or infectious components of the expression system such as mammalian DNA or animal viruses. These issues relating to protein drugs are discussed in further detail in Chapter 3.

Table 2.10. Characteristics of an ideal expression system

- Rapid growth rate, high cell densities
  High biomass production
- Low-cost medium
  Little or no expensive nutrients such as animal sera
- High production rates per cell
- Low vector copy number/high production
  No selection for high copy number
- Stable under cultivation
  No vector loss
- Production in the absence of cell growth
  Long-term harvesting
- No toxic substances for maintenance of the vector
- Safety
  Lack of immunogenicity, carcinogenic components or viruses

MONOCLONAL ANTIBODIES

Monoclonal antibody technology is the second of the two major components of the revolution that is biotechnology. The emergence of this technology during the 1970s concurrent with the emergence of rDNA technology is a fortunate coincidence which has led to their synergistic interaction, making biotechnology more than the sum of the two technologes. The development of monoclonal antibodies is the culmination of many years of earlier research in immunology and in cell-culture methodologies. Their highly defined specificity and availability in unlimited quantities have made monoclonal antibodies valuable in many diagnostic and therapeutic applications. Further, the ability to manipulate genes encoding the antibodies using rDNA techniques has facilitated their engineering to make monoclonal antibodies better suited for clinical applications as described in Chapter 3.

Antibodies

Antibodies are protein molecules present in high abundance in the immunoglobulin fraction of the sera of vertebrates, and also in other body fluids. They are secreted by a class of blood cells known as B lymphocytes. Their production is stimulated by substances known as ''antigens'', which are foreign to the organism. Antibodies protect the organism by sequestering and eliminating foreign antigens entering the organism. Most antigens are themselves simple proteins or proteins with other substances such as carbohydrates attached to them. They may be components of invading organisms such as bacteria or viruses, or environmental agents which accidentally enter the organism. Antibodies elicited by an antigen react specifically with that antigen by binding non-covalently through complementarity of the surfaces between the antibody and the antigen, in a manner analogous to a ''lock-and-key'' or ''glove-and-hand'' fit. The region of the antigen which is involved in binding to its antibody is called the ''epitope''. An epitope is usually composed of a small stretch of amino acids within the entire protein antigen. Because of their large size, most antigens contain many distinct epitopes against which the immunized organism produces distinct antibodies. Thus, exposure of an organism to an antigen results in the production of a set of distinct antibodies, each reacting with different parts of the antigen. Depending on the extent of the surface complementarity with the epitope, antibodies may bind with different affinities to the antigen.

Structure of antibodies

Antibodies (Abs) or immunoglobulins (Igs) are glycosylated proteins composed of four subunits held together by disulfide bridges. They are made of two identical ''heavy chains'' (*heavy* signifying their larger size compared to the other subunit) and two identical ''light chains'', which are assembled as shown in Fig. 2.20. An antibody molecule is symmetric around its long axis and is composed of an antigen binding site in each segment. Thus, antibody molecules are bivalent in their antigen binding capacity.

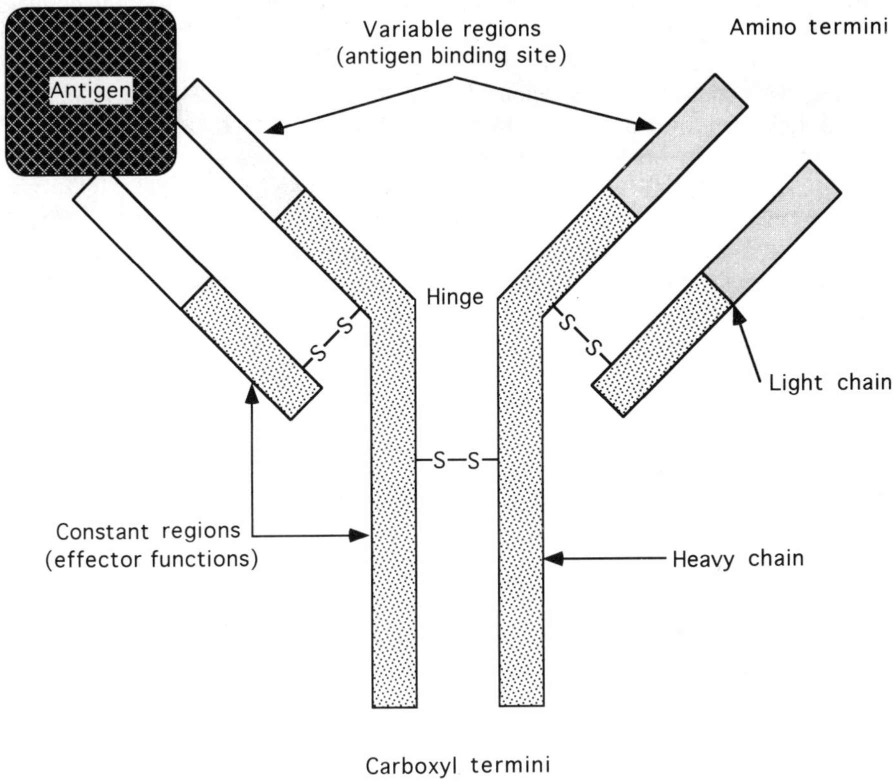

Fig. 2.20. Structure of an antibody molecule showing the heavy and light chains, and the constant and variable regions of each chain.

Antibodies are divided into two functional domains known as "the constant" and "the variable" regions. Both the light and the heavy chains contribute to each of the domains. The variable region contains the antigen binding site. Because different antibodies bind their respective antigens by surface complementarity, the structure of the variable region is different among antibodies with different antigen specificities. This variability of structure is accomplished by varying the amino acid sequence within the variable region. The immune system is capable of mounting an immune response against an infinite number of antigens. Therefore, the potential for the production of a wide variety of variable regions is inherent in the immune system. The segment of an antibody containing the variable region and the constant region, up to the hinge region shown in Fig. 2.20, is known as the "Fab" region, and the remaining constant region is called the "Fc" region. Digestion of antibodies with the protease papain, which cleave at the hinge region, generates an Fc fragment and two monovalent Fab fragments capable of binding antigen. The Fab fragments are useful or may be preferable in some diagnostic and therapeutic applications.

The constant regions are members of a limited set of distinct amino acid chains, and determine the class or "isotype" of the antibodies. In human antibodies, the constant regions belong to one of the five classes, IgG, IgM, IgA, IgD, and IgE, determined by the structure of the constant region of the heavy chain. Antibodies in some classes are further divided into subclasses. Thus, human IgG is divided further into four distinct subclasses, IgG_1, IgG_2, IgG_3, and IgG_4. The constant regions of the antibodies confer upon them "effector functions", which involve the interaction of the antibodies with a variety of other molecules. These functions include neutralization of infectious agents such as viruses, complement fixation reactions which result in the lysis of invading foreign cells, opsonization which facilitates the uptake and digestion of foreign materials by phagocytic cells, antibody-dependent cell-mediated cytotoxicity resulting in the destruction of virus-infected cells by other cells of the immune system (T lymphocytes), and mast cell degranulation which results in the release of the contents of the mast cell granules as in hypersensitivity. The different antibody classes differ in their ability to perform these reactions. In addition, the constant regions determine properties such as the circulating half-life, distribution of the antibody in the different body compartments, and the transfer across the placenta. These properties of the different classes of human antibodies are listed in Table 2.11. Most of the antibodies currently used in diagnostic and therapeutic applications belong to the IgG class.

Generation of antibody diversity

Despite their structural similarities, antibodies are distinct macromolecules largely because of the unique sequence of each variable region, and because of the limited differences in the constant region. One of the exciting challenges in immunology has been the elucidation of the mechanisms responsible for generating antibody diversity. A detailed discussion of the mechanism is beyond the scope and the goal of this chapter. However, some understanding of the basic mechanism is essential for the discussion of chimeric antibodies in Chapter 3. The mechanism is described below in simplified terms. One of the references should be consulted for a detailed discussion.

Genes encoding the heavy and the light chains of an antibody are assembled by the reorganization of DNA sequences encoding antibodies. This rearrangement occurs only in immunoglobulin-producing cells. In all cells in a vertebrate organism, including those that differentiate into antibody-producing B-lymphocytes, the coding sequences of the antibody genes are maintained discontinuously, separated by many thousand bases of DNA, as shown in Fig. 2.21. Each copy of the genome contains one copy each (two copies each in the diploid genome) of the sequences coding for the limited set of constant regions. As shown in Table 2.11, the set of heavy chain constant regions in humans consists of nine members, IgG1, IgG2, IgG3, IgG4, IgA1, IgA2, IgD, IgE, IgM. The set of light chain constant regions consists of two members, lambda and

Table 2.11. Properties conferred on human antibodies by constant regions

Property	IgG1	IgG2	IgG3	IgG4	IgM	IgA1	IgA2	IgD	IgE
Molecular wt (kDa)	146	146	170	146	970	160	160	184	188
Carbohydrate (%)	2–3	2–3	2–3	2–3	12	7–11	7–11	9–14	12
Serum concentration (mg/ml)	9	3	1	0.5	1.5	3	0.5	0.03	0.00005
Complement fixation (classical pathway)	+	+	+++	–	+++	–	–	–	–
Placental transfer	+	+	+	+	–	–	–	–	–
Binding to mast cells	–	–	–	–	–	–	–	–	+++
Half-life (days)	21	20	7	21	10	6	6	3	2
Synthetic rate (mg/kg body weight/day)	33	33	33	33	33	24	24	0.4	0.002

Source: Table 1, p. 95, *Immunology* (2nd edition), Golub and Green, 1991.

kappa. Variable regions are encoded by two large sets of DNA regions, one set for heavy chains and the other for light chains. In the unrearranged configuration, the set of sequences encoding the constant regions is separated from the set encoding the variable regions by many thousands of bases. During the maturation of an antibody-producing B cell, one of the variable region sequences for the heavy chain is combined at the DNA level with one of the heavy chain constant regions, resulting in a complete heavy chain gene. Likewise, the combination of a light chain variable region with a constant region of the light chain results in a productive light chain gene. Each B cell is restricted to produce only one complete heavy chain gene, and one complete light chain gene, thus producing only one characteristic antibody. It is estimated that in a human genome, there are about 2.7×10^4 heavy chain variable sequences and 4.7×10^2 light chain variable sequences. A random combination of the heavy and light chains is capable of yielding up to 1.27×10^7 unique antibody molecules. In addition, somatic mutations and inexactness in the joining mechanism at the DNA level introduce further diversity. Thus, the immune system is capable of producing antibodies in response to a large number of antigenic epitopes (Golub and Green, 1991).

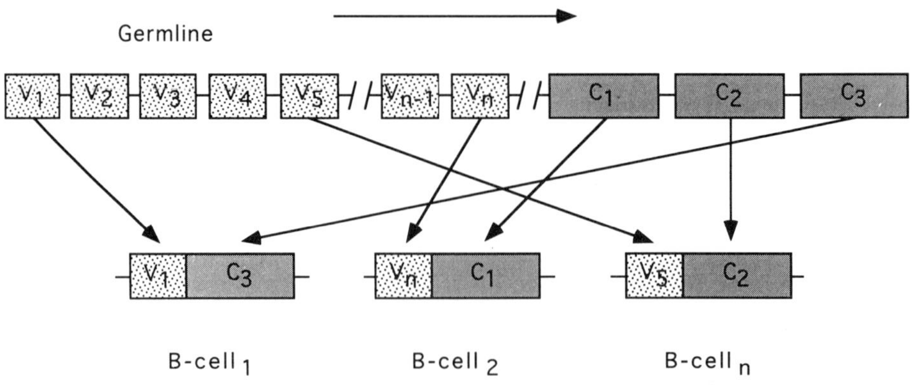

Fig. 2.21. Generation of antibody diversity by random assortment and joining of constant and variable region DNA segments.

Each developing B cell undergoes random combinatorial assembly of heavy and light chains and displays the assembled immunoglobulin on its surface. Thus, the immune system consists of a wide repertoire of cells of different antigen binding capabilities. Upon contacting an antigen or an epitope that is capable of binding the antibody displayed on the cell surface, the particular B cell divides to produce a large population of daughter cells or ''clones'' secreting the antibody characteristic of the parent B cell, as shown in Fig. 2.22. Thus, in eliciting an immune response, an antigen merely induces the amplification of a B cell lineage whose antibody product is capable of binding the antigen.

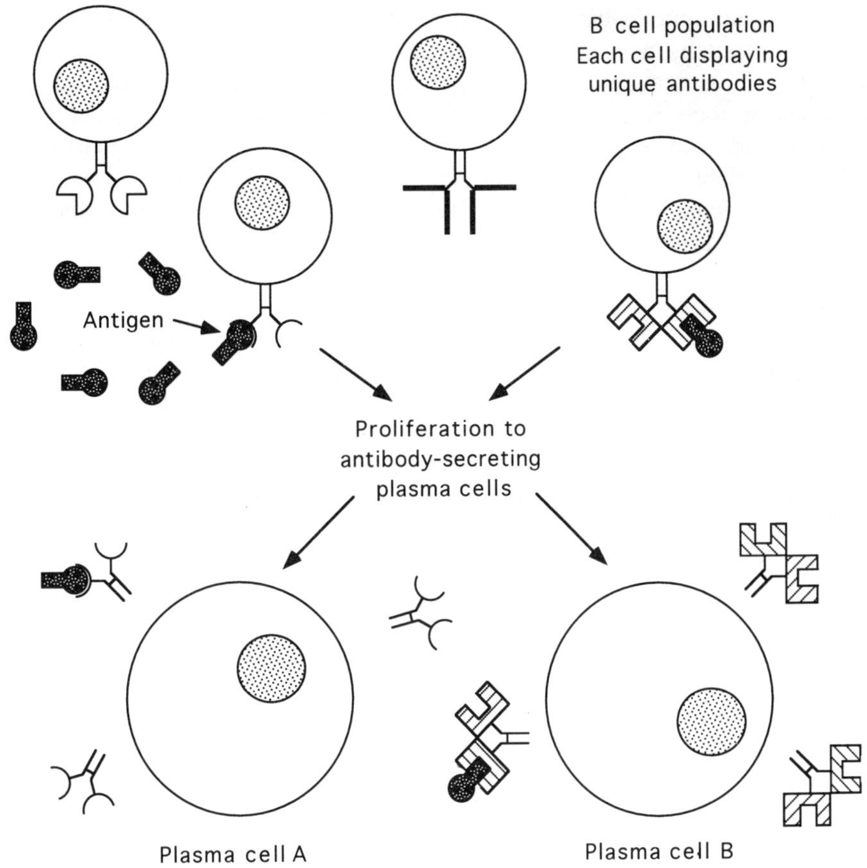

Fig. 2.22. Antibody response to an antigen and the production of polyclonal antibodies. Among the four B cells shown, antibodies produced by two bind different regions of the antigen, and are stimulated to multiply.

Polyclonal antibodies

Exposure to a specific antigen causes clonal expansion of all B cells capable of reacting with the multiple epitopes present on the antigen. Thus, the immune response to the entire antigen results in the production of antibodies by several clones of B cells. The resultant mixture of antibodies present in the serum is called a polyclonal antibody. In addition, because an animal is naturally exposed to a host of other antigens in its environment, its serum also contains antibodies produced by clones specific for each of these antigens. Therefore a polyclonal antibody preparation obtained from an animal is a mixture of many distinct antibody classes, only some of which are specific for the antigen used in experimental immunization.

The immunoglobulin fraction derived from the polyclonal hyperimmune serum of humans and animals has been used clinically in combating conditions such as bacterial infections and maternal immunization by Rh-positive cells from the fetus. Polyclonal sera raised against proteins have also been valuable diagnostic and research tools. However, the undefined composition of polyclonal antisera results in wide and unpredictable cross-reactivities. Furthermore, the quantities of antibody available are limited to the amount of serum an immunized animal can yield. Monoclonal antibodies described below circumvent these problems of definition and quantity associated with polyclonal sera.

Monoclonal antibodies

A polyclonal serum against a protein is composed of several antibodies directed against the different epitopes present in the protein. As discussed earlier, each antibody in the mixture is produced by a clonal line of B cells which are the progeny of a single B cell which responded to the antigen. If it were possible to isolate one of the B cells producing the desired antibody and to propagate it in culture indefinitely, and collect the secreted antibody, a homogeneous and defined antibody preparation directed at a single epitope in the protein would be obtained. Such an antibody derived from a clonal population of B cells is called a ''monoclonal'' antibody.

Generation of cell lines secreting monoclonal antibodies

Normal B cells are incapable of extended growth outside the animal. The production of monoclonal antibodies, however, involves establishment of a B cell clone producing the antibody in long-term culture. This is accomplished by immortalizing the B cell using a transforming virus such as the Epstein-Barr virus (EBV), or by fusing it with another immortalized cell. The latter approach is called hybridoma technology because it involves fusion of two cells to produce a hybrid cell. This is the approach used most widely for the production of mouse monoclonal antibodies.

The basic principle of hybridoma technology is shown in Fig. 2.23. B cells obtained from the spleens of mice immunized with the antigen of interest are fused with established mouse myeloma cells. Myeloma cells are transformed cancerous cells of the B lymphocyte lineage with infinite growth capacity. While many myeloma cell lines continue to secrete their antibody, others lose the ability to produce antibodies. Spleen cells from immunized animals are fused with non-antibody-producing myeloma cells, resulting in a hybrid cell which inherits the properties of both the fusion partners. Thus the hybrids are capable of continued growth in culture like the myeloma cell and also maintain the antibody production of the spleen B cell.

Fusion of the population of B cells present in the spleen of an immunized animal results in the production of large numbers of hybrid clones. Identification of clones producing antibodies of interest requires screening of the supernatants of the individual clones for antigen binding. Rapid and sensitive assays with large throughputs have been developed for such screening. Once identified and established in culture, the hybrid cells can be grown in cell culture or in the peritoneal cavity of mice, and the secreted antibody can be obtained in unlimited quantities.

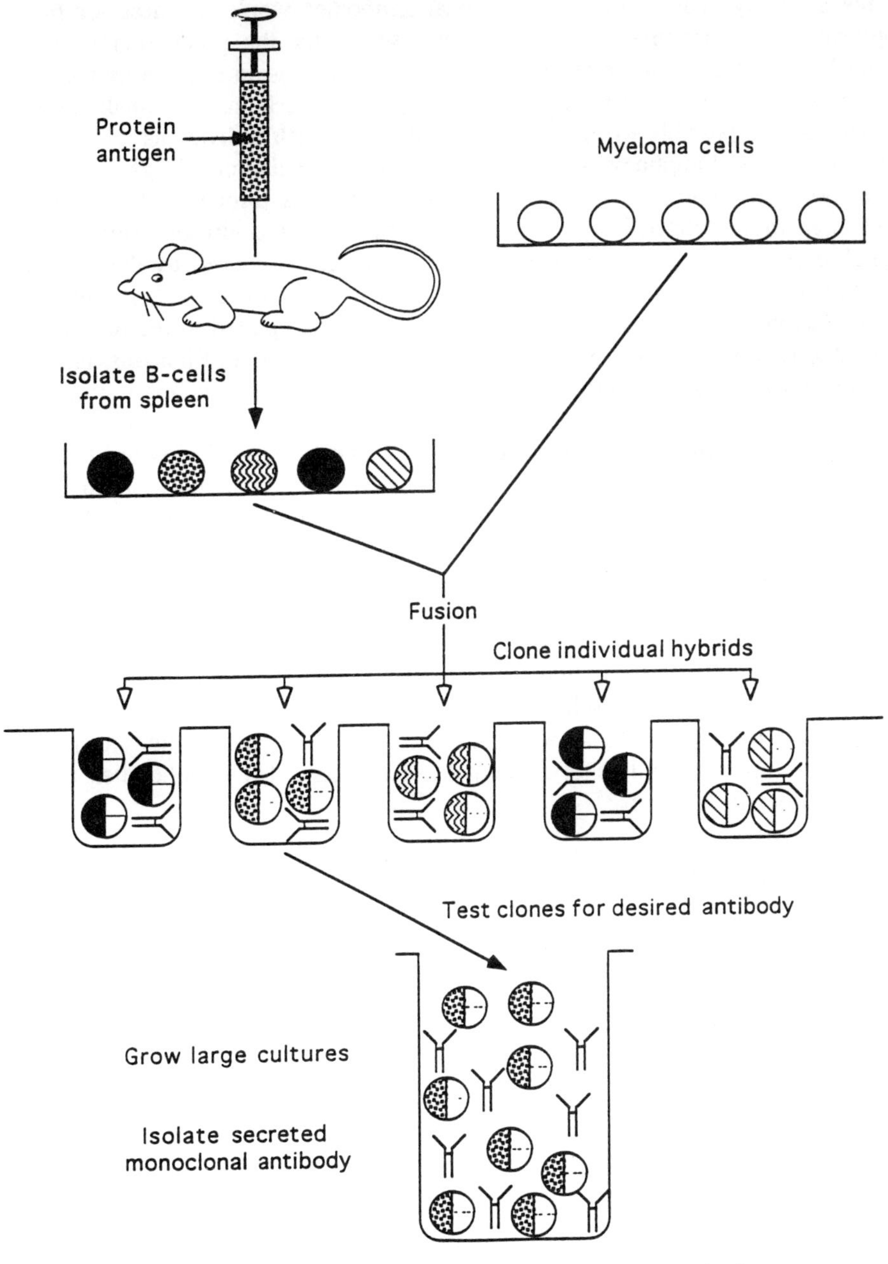

Fig. 2.23. Production of monoclonal antibodies by hybridoma technology.

The hybridoma technology has been very successful with rodent cells. The mouse or rat antibodies generated are valuable in *in vitro* diagnostic applications and as laboratory reagents. However, their use in therapeutic and *in vivo* imaging applications is hampered by immune reactions against the mouse-specific domains of the antibody. Thus, human monoclonal antibodies would be ideal for *in vivo* applications. Hybridoma technology is not suited for the production of human monoclonals because of the technical limitation of the fusion technology and, more importantly, because it is neither possible to immunize humans with the antigens of interest nor possible to obtain spleen cells from such individuals. However, in some instances, lymphocytes from the peripheral circulation of individuals who have mounted an immune response to certain antigens through natural exposure have been immortalized by transformation with oncogenic viruses. Human monoclonal antibodies to gram negative bacteria have been produced by this approach. In addition, techniques for the immunization of isolated spleen cell in culture, for use in fusions, have shown some success, and may be applied to the development of human monoclonals as a way to circumvent immunization of humans. However, this method is technically difficult and has not found widespread application (Scott and Fleischman, 1991).

The paucity of methods for the production of human monoclonals has led to the development of methods for the ''humanizing'' of mouse monoclonal antibodies of therapeutic value. DNA encoding the antigen-binding variable region of a mouse antibody is combined by using standard rDNA techniques, with the DNA sequences for the constant region of a human antibody, producing chimeric mouse–human hybrid heavy and light chain genes. Coexpression of the two chains in mammalian cells results in the secretion of the ''humanized'' antibody. Further refinements of the technique to increase the humanization of the mouse antibodies are also under development (Scott and Fleischman, 1991). Chimeric and other engineered antibodies represent the fusion of rDNA technology and monoclonal antibody technology which form the two pillars of modern biotechnology. These antibodies are discussed further in Chapter 3.

Table 2.12. Characteristics and uses of monoclonal antibodies

- Defined specificity
  - Single epitope
  - Single class
- Unlimited supply
  - Cell culture production
  - Production in ascites fluid
- Diagnostic applications
  - Immunoassays
  - Imaging
- Therapeutic applications
  - Antibodies and toxin conjugates
  - Chimeric antibodies

The characteristics and uses of monoclonal antibodies are listed in Table 2.12, and their applications are discussed in greater detail in the following chapters.

RECOMMENDED READING

Alberts, B., Bray, D., Lewis, J., Raff, M., Roberts, K., and Watson, J.D. (1989). *Molecular Biology of the Cell* (New York: Garland Publishing).

Baulieu, E-E. and Kelly, P.A. (eds) (1990). *Hormones: From Molecules to Disease* (New York: Chapman and Hall).

Branden, C. and Tooze, J. (1991). *Introduction to Protein Structure* (New York: Garland Publishing).

Darnell, J.E., Jr. (1985). RNA. *Sci. Am.* **253,** 68–78.

Doolittle, R.F. (1985). Proteins. *Sci. Am.* **253,** 88–99.

Felsenfeld, G. (1985). DNA. *Sci. Am.* **253,** 58–67.

Golub, E.S. and Green, D.R. (1991). *Immunology: A Synthesis* (Sunderland, Massachusetts: Sinauer Associates Inc.).

Griffiths, E. (1991). Polypeptide production by recombinant DNA technology. In *Polypeptide and Protein Drugs: Production, Characterization and Formulation.* R.C. Hider and D. Barlow, eds. (Chichester: Ellis Horwood), pp. 82–102.

Harlow, E. and Lane, D. (1988). *Antibodies: A Laboratory Manual* (New York: Cold Spring Harbor Laboratory).

Hood, L.E., Weissman, I.L., Wood, W.B., and Wilson, J.H. (1984). *Immunology* (Reading, Massachusetts: Benjamin/Cummings Co.).

Judson, H.F. (1992). A history of the science and the technology behind gene mapping and sequencing. In *The Code of Codes: Scientific and Social Issues in the Human Genome Project.* D.J. Kevles and L. Hood, eds. (Cambridge, MA: Harvard University Press), pp. 37–80.

Richards, F.M. (1991). The protein folding problem. *Sci. Am.* **264,** 54–63.

Stryer, L. (1988). *Biochemistry* (New York: W.H. Freeman & Co.).

Thornton, J.M. and Barlow, D.J. (1991). Peptide and protein structure. In *Polypeptide and Protein Drugs: Production, Characterization and Formulation.* R.C. Hider and D. Barlow, eds. (Chichester: Ellis Horwood), pp. 9–30.

Watson, J.D., Tooze, J., and Kurtz, D.T. (1983). *Recombinant DNA: A Short Course* (New York: Scientific American Books/W.H. Freeman & Co.).

Weatherall, M. (1990). *In Search of a Cure* (Oxford: Oxford University Press).

Weinberg, R.A. (1985). The molecules of life. *Sci. Am.* **253,** 48–57.

REFERENCES

Atherton, E. (1991). Current chemical strategies in peptide synthesis. In *Polypeptide and Protein Drugs: Production, Characterization and Formulation.* R.C. Hider and D. Barlow, eds. (Chichester: Ellis Horwood), pp. 70–81.

Barinaga, M. (1991). Will ''DNA chip'' speed genome initiative? *Science* **253,** 1489.

Berg, P. (1991). Reverse genetics: its origins and prospects. *Bio/Technology* **9,** 342–344.

Bialy, H. (1991). Transgenic pharming comes of age. *Bio/Technology* **9,** 786–788.

Bogosian, G., Kane, J.F., Obukowicz, M.G., and Olins, P.O. (1991). Optimizing protein production in recombinant strains of *Escherichia coli.* In *Recombinant DNA Technology and Applications.* A. Prokop, R.K. Bajpai, and C. Ho, eds. (New York: McGraw-Hill), pp. 285–315.

Bowden, G.A., Paredes, A.M., and Georgiou, G. (1991). Structure and morphology of protein inclusion bodies in *Escherichia coli. Bio/Technology* **9,** 725–730.

Buckholz, R.G. and Gleeson, M.A. (1991). Yeast systems for commercial production of heterologous proteins. *Bio/Technology* **9,** 1067–1072.

Cherfas, J. (1991). Ancient DNA: still busy after death. *Science* **253,** 1354–1356.

Courteau, J. (1991). Genome databases. *Science* **254,** 201–207.

Edgington, S.M. (1992). Rites of passage: moving biotech proteins through the ER. *Bio/Technology* **10,** 1413–1420.

Eisenstein, B.I. (1990). The polymerase chain reaction: a new method of using molecular genetics for medical diagnosis. *New England J. Med.* **322,** 178–183.

Erlich, H.A., Gelfand, D., and Sninsky, J.J. (1991). Recent advances in the polymerase chain reaction. *Science* **252,** 1643–1650.

Erlich, H.A. (Ed.) (1989). *PCR Technology: Principles and Applications for DNA Amplification* (New York: Stockton Press).

Fox, S. (1991). Applications for synthesizing and sequencing DNA beyond the genome project. *Genetic Engineering News* June, 6–8.

Georgiou, G. and Bowden, G.A. (1991). Inclusion body formation and the recovery of aggregated recombinant proteins. In *Recombinant DNA Technology and Applications.* A. Prokop, R.K. Bajpai, and C. Ho, eds. (New York: McGraw-Hill), pp. 333–356.

Gitschier, J., Wood, W.I., Goralka, T.M., Wion, K.L., Chen, E.Y., Eaton, D.H., Vehar, G.A., Capon, D.J., and Lawn, R.M. (1984). Characterization of the human factor VIII gene. *Nature* **312,** 326–330.

Golub, E.S. and Green, D.R. (1991). *Immunology: A Synthesis* (Sunderland, Massachusetts: Sinauer Associates Inc.).

Goochee, C.F., Gramer, M.J., Andersen, D.C., Bahr, B.J., and Rasmussen, J.R. (1991). The oligosaccharides of glycoproteins: bioprocess factors affecting oligosaccharide structure and their effect on glycoprotein properties. *Bio/Technology* **9,** 1347–1355.

Goto, C., Akai, K., Murakami, A., Hashimoto, C., Tsuda, E., Ueda, M., Kawanishi, G., Takahashi, N., Ishimoto, A., Chiba, H., and Sasaki, R. (1988). Production of recombinant human erythropoietin in mammalian cells: host-cell dependency of biological activity of the cloned glycoprotein. *Bio/Technology* **6,** 67–71.

Gribskov, M. and Devereux, J. (Eds) (1991). *Sequence Analysis Primer* (New York: Stockton Press).

Grinnell, B.W., Berg, D.T., Walls, J., and Yan, S.B. (1987). Trans-activated expression of fully gamma-carboxylated recombinant human protein C, an anti thrombotic factor. *Bio/Technology* **5,** 1189–1192.

Hunkapillar, T., Kaiser, R.J., Koop, B.F., and Hood, L. (1991). Large-scale and automated DNA sequence determination. *Science* **254,** 59–67.

Kaufman, R.J., Wise, R.J., Wasley, L.C., and Droner, A.J. (1991). Factors limiting expression of secreted proteins in mammalian cells. In *Recombinant Technology in Hemostasis and Thrombosis.* L.W. Hoyer and W.N. Drohan, eds. (New York: Plenum Press), pp. 171–195.

Kent, S.B.H. (1988). Chemical synthesis of peptides and proteins. *Ann. Rev. Biochem.* **57,** 957–989.

Kent, S.B.H. and Parker, K.F. (1988). The chemical synthesis of peptides and proteins. In *Therapeutic Peptides and Proteins: Assessing the New Technologies.* D.R. Marshak and D.T. Liu, eds. (New York: Cold Spring Harbor Laboratory), pp. 3–20.

Klemm, P. (1984). Manual Edman degradation of proteins and peptides. In *Methods in Molecular Biology, Volume 1: Proteins.* J.M. Walker, ed. (Clifton, New Jersey: Human Press), pp. 243–254.

Luckow, V.A. (1991). Cloning and expression of heterologous genes in insect cells with baculovirus vectors. In *Recombinant DNA Technology and Applications.* A. Prokop, R.K. Bajpai, and C. Ho, eds. (New York: McGraw-Hill), pp. 97–152.

Maniatis, T. (1991). Mechanisms of alternate pre-mRNA splicing. *Science* **251,** 33–34.

Marino, M.H. (1991). Expression of heterologous proteins in yeast. In *Recombinant DNA Technology and Applications.* A. Prokop, R.K. Bajpai, and C. Ho, eds. (New York: McGraw-Hill), pp. 29–65.

Masui, M., Coleman, J., and Inouye, M. (1983). Multipurpose expression cloning vehicles in *Escherichia coli.* In *Experimental Manipulation of Gene Expression.* M. Inouye, ed. (New York: Academic Press), pp. 15–32.

McKnight, S.L. (1991). Molecular zippers in gene regulation. *Sci. Am.* **264,** April, 54–64.

Miller, H.I. (1991). Regulation. In *The Genetic Revolution: Scientific Prospects and Public Perceptions.* B.D. Davis, ed. (Baltimore: The Johns Hopkins University Press), pp. 196–211.

Moffat, A.M. (1991a). Transgenic animals may be down the pharm. *Science* **254,** 35–36.

Moffat, A.S. (1991b). "Plant pharmers" transform tobacco to produce proteins. *Genetic Engineering News* November/December, 1–55.

Morales, V.M. and Bagdasarian, M. (1991). Cloning in bacteria: vectors and techniques. In *Recombinant DNA Technology and Applications.* A. Prokop, R.K. Bajpai, and C. Ho, eds. (New York: McGraw-Hill), pp. 3–28.

Mudge, A.W. (1989). Neuropeptides find a role? *Nature* **339,** 663.

Nadal-Ginard, B. (1990). Muscle differentiation and alternate splicing. *Curr. Opinion in Cell Biol.* **2,** 1058–1064.

Paabo, S. (1991). Amplifying DNA from archeological remains: a meeting report. *PCR Methods and Applications* **1,** 107–110.

Paleyanda, R., Young, J., and Velander, W. (1991). The expression of therapeutic proteins in transgenic animals. In *Recombinant Technology in Hemostasis and Thrombosis.* L.W. Hoyer and W.N. Drohan, eds. (New York: Plenum Press), pp. 197–209.

Pearson, P.L., Maidak, B., Chipperfield, M., and Robbins, R. (1991). The human genome project initiative — do databases reflect current progress? *Science* **254,** 214–215.

Pestka, S. and Langer, J.A. (1987). Interferons and their actions. *Ann. Rev. Biochem.* **56,** 727–777.

PMA Survey Report (1991). Biotechnology Medicines in Development (Washington, DC: Pharmaceutical Manufacturers Association).

Ramabhadran, T.V., Reitz, B.A., and Shah, D.M. (1985). High-level expression of bovine growth hormone gene in heterologous mammalian cells. *Gene* **38,** 111–118.

Rodriguez, R.L. and Denhardt, D.T. (Eds) (1988). *Vectors: A Survey of Molecular Cloning Vectors and Their Uses* (Boston: Butterworths).

Royer, P. and Kemper, B. (1990). Calcium regulatory hormones. In *Hormones: from Molecules to Disease.* E-E. Baulieu and P.A. Kelly, eds. (New York: Chapman and Hall), pp. 637–669.

Scott, M.G. and Fleischman, J.B. (1991). Monoclonal antibodies in diagnostic medicine. In *Recombinant DNA Technology and Applications.* A. Prokop, R.K. Bajpai, and C. Ho, eds. (New York: McGraw-Hill), pp. 255–282.

Spalding, B.J. (1992). Transgenic pharming advances. *Bio/Technology* **10,** 498–499.

Spier, R.E. and Griffiths, J.B. (Eds) (1985a). *Animal Cell Biotechnology,* Volume 1 (New York: Academic Press).

Spier, R.E. and Griffiths, J.B. (Eds) (1985b). *Animal Cell Biotechnology,* Volume 2 (New York: Academic Press).

Thilly, W.G. (Ed.) (1986). *Mammalian Cell Technology* (Boston: Butterworths).

Vu, H., McCollum, C., Lotys, C., and Andrus, A. (1990). New reagents and solid support for automated oligonucleotide synthesis. *Nucleic Acids Res.* Symposium Series **22,** 63–64.

Weiss, R. (1991). Hot prospect for new gene amplifier. *Science* **254,** 1292–1293.

Wittman-Liebold, B. and Kimura, M. (1984). Microsequencing of peptides and proteins with 4-*N,N*-diethylaminobenzene-4-isothiocyanate. In *Methods in Molecular Biology, Volume 1: Proteins.* J.M. Walker, ed. (Clifton, New Jersey: Humana Press), pp. 221–242.

Yuksel, K.U., Grant, G.A., Mende-Mueller, L., Niece, R.L., Williams, K.R., and Speicher, D.W. (1991). Protein sequencing from polyvinylidenedifluoride membranes: design and characterization of a test sample (ABRF-90SEQ) and evaluation of results. In *Techniques in Protein Chemistry II.* J.J. Villafranca, ed. (New York: Academic Press), pp. 151–162.

3

Biological drugs

Biological drugs are macromolecular components of living systems used as drugs usually to treat natural deficiency states or in prophylaxis. Because of their macromolecular nature they are not amenable to synthesis in the laboratory and are obtained from extracts of cells, tissues, and organs. Almost all of the "biological drugs" currently in use are proteins and therefore the term "biological drugs" is used interchangeably with the term "protein drugs". The greatest impact of biotechnology to date has been on the production of pharmaceutical proteins. This is because the earliest benefit to accrue from biotechnology was the capacity to produce proteins in large quantities. This chapter explores the advances in the production and use of protein therapeutics resulting from the application of biotechnology. Following a discussion of general principles, a few specific examples are considered. The production of chimeric proteins with novel activities, using gene splicing techniques, is also described.

BIOLOGICAL DRUGS OF THE PRE-BIOTECHNOLOGY ERA

The use of components of biological systems for therapeutic purposes predates the advent of biotechnology by nearly two centuries. Historically, vaccines were among the first documented biological drugs, whose use began in the late eighteenth century with the successful vaccination against smallpox by Jenner (Behbehani, 1991). This was followed in the nineteenth century by the discovery of antitoxins derived from the blood of immunized animals (Weatherall, 1990). In both these cases, the preparations were crude and the active ingredient of the drug was not defined. It is now well established that the active components of both vaccines and antitoxins were proteins which formed the antigens and antibodies respectively. Recognition of the protein nature of biological drugs began with the emergence of endocrinology and the use of glandular extracts for the successful treatment of deficiency states. The discovery and commercialization of extracts of endocrine glands for the treatment of diabetes and growth deficiency occurred in the early part of this century. Advances in analytical and protein purification techniques led to the identification of the active principles of the extracts to be proteins (Weatherall, 1990). Development of plasma fractionation techniques during World War II extended the list of available protein therapeutics to include blood products such as human coagulation factors and human immunoglobulins (Dwyer, 1987; Snape, 1991; DMD, 1991). Developments in cell culture methodology were facilitated by the introduction of antibiotics, which made possible the long-term culturing of mammalian cells without microbial contamination. Large-scale growth of mammalian cells under laboratory conditions in bioreactors permitted their use as substrates for the development of protein therapeutics, notably several viral vaccines currently in clinical use, and also a few growth factors and enzymes (Griffiths, 1985). The first vaccine derived from cell culture, for polio, was introduced in 1954, and several more have been produced by this method since. Thus, methods of production, and the therapeutic regimen for these proteins, were well established before the emergence of rDNA technology. Many of the products developed in the pre-biotechnology era are presently in use; Table 3.1 is a list of the key protein drugs developed during this era.

Table 3.1. Protein drugs of the pre-rDNA era

Protein	Source
Insulin	Bovine, porcine
Growth hormone	Human cadavers
Factor VIII	Human plasma
Immunoglobulins	Human and animal sera
Plasma proteins	Human plasma
Vaccines	Cultured cells
	Human plasma
	Whole animals

The development of proteins as therapeutics prior to the 1980s suffered from some major limitations. In some instances, concentration of the desired protein in the source material was low, rendering its isolation and purification laborious and expensive. In other cases, the ability to produce sufficient quantities of some proteins was limited by the availability of starting material, resulting in insufficient production to meet the needs of the patient population. Aside from the quantitative limitations, the presence of infectious agents, mainly viruses, in the tissues and biological fluids of humans and animals posed the risk of infection to the patients. All protein drugs suffered from one or all of these drawbacks (Snape, 1991).

The following examples illustrate the magnitude of the problem associated with the production and use of protein therapeutics in the pre-biotechnology era. Production of a one-year supply of the coagulation factors needed to treat a single hemophiliac required the fractionation of approximately 8000 pints of human blood; insulin for the treatment of one diabetic for a year was obtained from 7 to 10 pounds of pancreas from approximately 70 pigs or 14 cows; a one-year supply of the human growth hormone for one patient had to be obtained by extracting the human pituitary glands from about 80 human cadavers because animal growth hormones, unlike animal insulins, are not effective in man (Micklos and Freyer, 1990). Whereas a single pituitary contains only 5 to 10 milligrams of human growth hormone (Kelly, 1990), the therapeutic dosage is between 0.06 and 0.1 milligram/kilogram bodyweight, thrice weekly (Kuret and Murad, 1990).

The starting source materials used for the production of therapeutic proteins were heterogeneous mixtures obtained from several humans or animals, requiring the pooling of source material from a large number of individuals to eliminate individual and batch to batch variation of post-translational modifications in the final product. Thus, starting plasma lots used in fractionation are made from pools of plasma derived from 10,000 to 12,000 individuals (Snape, 1991).

Mammalian sources of proteins, especially those of human origin, were often contaminated with adventitious infectious agents such as microorganisms and viruses. In many cases, these agents are viruses that cause devastating diseases in the recipient of the drug (Osborn, 1988). Viral agents most significant in products from human plasma are hepatitis B, hepatitis C, HIV-1 and HIV-2 (Snape, 1991). The consequences of contamination of human factor VIII by HIV-1 on the hemophiliac population have been devastating, resulting in HIV infection of not only over two-thirds of the patients but also of their spouses and sexual partners (Booth, 1988). Similarly, administration of cadaver-derived human growth hormone to short-statured children has been traced to be the cause of the slow, neurodegenerative Creutzfeldt–Jakob disease which resulted in the discontinuation of its use (Brown *et al.*, 1985; Aldhous, 1992). Early batches of polio vaccine preparations produced in monkey cells in culture were contaminated with the simian virus SV40, which is capable of replicating in human cells. Fortunately, inoculations with these vaccine lots seem not to have produced adverse consequences in the subjects (Osborn, 1988; Geissler, 1990). The incidence of contamination by many, if not all, infectious agents is detectable by the testing of the starting materials and the final products, but such tests increase production costs. Risks are also greatly reduced where possible by the viral inactivation steps which are incorporated into the purification protocol. However, the diagnostic tests and inactivation procedures are not useful against new, heretofore unknown infectious agents which enter the donor population before they are well characterized. This is illustrated by the case of the HIV virus contamination of factor VIII preparations derived from plasma which was being routinely tested for other known infectious agents.

In addition to the established drug proteins discussed above, several proteins with interesting biological activities and clinical potential were identified in the pre-biotechnology era by using cell culture and protein purification methods. The development of these proteins as drugs was limited by their low concentrations in body fluids and tissues. Plasminogen activators, erythropoietin, and insulin-like growth factors (IGFs) are examples of proteins which were believed to have clinical potential but were difficult to commercialize because of the technical difficulties and economic considerations resulting from lack of suitable sources (Griffiths, 1985; Kadouri and Bohak, 1985; Neta *et al.*, 1990).

PROTEIN THERAPEUTICS THROUGH THE BIOTECHNOLOGY ROUTE

The first obvious application and the greatest impact to date of rDNA and hybridoma technologies has been on the production of many desired human proteins in unlimited quantities. The cloning of genes and their high-level expression in defined host cells capable of continuous and infinite growth has lifted the restrictions on the development of biological drugs imposed heretofore by availability, protein abundance, and contamination of starting materials used. These advances are discussed below under three categories, namely (a) protein therapeutics derived through rDNA, (b) vaccines which are derived through rDNA, and (c) monoclonal antibody therapeutics produced through hybridoma technology.

Protein therapeutics

The earliest development efforts were focused on scarce proteins whose therapeutic utility and regimen were well established. Thus, human insulin was the first rDNA product to appear on the market, followed by the human growth hormone. Human insulin was produced in *E. coli* at high yields and is marketed under the trade name Humulin, as a replacement for bovine and porcine insulins. Similarly, the human growth hormone was produced in high abundance in *E. coli*, and has been brought to the market under the trade names of Protropin and Humatrope. Production through biotechnology has eliminated both the safety issues and the shortage of this protein. For example, a typical human pituitary obtained from a cadaver contains 5 to 10 milligrams of growth hormone (Kelly, 1990), whereas one liter of *E. coli* culture yields 20 milligrams or more of the hormone (Ross, 1981). Furthermore, the availability of the growth hormone in unlimited amounts has stimulated research into ''investigational use'' applications of the protein to wound healing, AIDS, and ageing (PMA Survey Report, 1991; Kuret and Murad, 1990). Other established protein drugs, such as factor VIII, have been recently approved by the FDA (Table 1.3) and yet others such as factor IX are rapidly approaching the approval stage (Hoyer and Drohan, 1991). Thus, while many of the drugs produced by non-rDNA methods continue to be on the market, the current trends suggest that they will be replaced by equally effective, but safer versions produced through rDNA technology. Other components of blood such as albumin and hemoglobin are also being developed using rDNA methods (Potera, 1992). A novel approach in this area is to produce human hemoglobin in the erythrocytes of transgenic pigs created using human hemoglobin genes (Hodgson, 1991d; Swanson *et al.*, 1992).

Interferons, tissue plasminogen activator (t-PA), erythropoietin, and other cytokines and lymphokines were already known, and attempts to commercialize these proteins by using cell-culture production methods were in the initial stages at the time when rDNA-based production became feasible. Thus, for example, the early batches of interferon used in clinical trials were produced by stimulating isolated human leukocytes and from an established lymphoblastoid cell line (Petricciani, 1985). The advent of cloning and expression technologies accelerated the appearance of these proteins in the clinic. Natural interferon alpha, which was shown to be a mixture of very similar proteins derived from several closely related genes, is now available in a single component form with controlled specificity and potency in comparison to the natural mixture of variable composition. t-PA and erythropoietin, both glycoproteins requiring the use of mammalian cells as production hosts, have also currently reached the clinic. Other cytokines such as the granulocyte-macrophage colony stimulating factor (GM-CSF) and granulocyte colony stimulating factor (G-CSF) have also undergone commercial development and have been approved. Development of other natural cytokines and novel engineered versions is in progress (Geller, 1993). Well over a hundred FDA investigational new drug applications, involving new protein drugs, and different uses of already approved proteins, are awaiting approval. Among these are growth factors such as epidermal growth factor (EGF), fibroblast growth factors (FGFs), platelet-derived growth factor (PDGF), and insulin-like growth factors (IGFs) putatively useful in wound healing and diabetes. Interleukins, members of a family of proteins which modulate predominantly the cells of the immune system, are in clinical trials as therapeutics, and as adjuvants in cancer chemotherapy; recently, recombinant interleukin-2 has received approval for use in metastatic kidney cancer (Table 1.3; Drake, 1990; PMA Survey Report, 1991; Fradd, 1992a). Of the nineteen FDA-approved protein therapeutics in early 1993 (Table 1.3), fifteen are in the therapeutic protein category. Several more are in clinical trials, and an equal or greater number are in the development stage as evidenced by the reports in the popular press and research literature.

Vaccines

The production of safe and effective vaccines against bacterial and viral agents has been impacted greatly by rDNA techniques. Many of the viral vaccines currently in use are produced in whole animals, eggs, or cell cultures by infecting with the virus strain. The safety of these preparations is assured by using an attenuated, and hence non-pathogenic, virus strain in the case of live vaccines, or by subsequent inactivation of the virus in the cases of killed vaccines (Melnick, 1985). However the degree of safety of vaccine preparations depended on the probability of reversion of the attenuated vaccine strain to virulence in the case of live vaccines, and on the degree of inactivation of the virus in the case of killed vaccines. rDNA technology has provided new methodologies for the production of both live viral vaccines and safer equivalents to killed vaccines.

Vaccines against a wide range of infectious agents are in development in a large number of pharmaceutical companies (Edgington, 1992a).

The active ingredients of most vaccines are protein or glycoprotein components of bacteria and viruses. Once the vaccinating antigen is identified, the administration of this component devoid of other components of the infectious pathogen is sufficient to raise a protective immune response against natural infection. Thus, for instance, the surface protein of the hepatitis B virus (HBV), known as the surface antigen or HBsAg, was identified as being sufficient for conferring resistance to viral infection, but specific conformation and association of the antigen was essential for immunoprotective antigenicity. The conventional, pre-biotechnology HBV vaccines consisted of purified aggregates of the surface antigen which occur as particles of 22-nanometer diameter in the blood of healthy, HBV-positive human donors. Such vaccines, which use only parts of an infectious agent, are termed "subunit vaccines". Such protein subunits, depending on their size, are amenable either to chemical synthesis or to synthesis via rDNA methods, or to both (Dreesman *et al.,* 1985; Ellis and Conley, 1991; Yoneyama, 1990).

The determination of the sequence of the HBV genome provided the genetic information required for the expression of HBsAg in heterologous systems. Thus, rDNA production of the HBsAg was the obvious route to an effective and safe HBV vaccine; indeed, this was the first rDNA-derived vaccine to be approved in the US. This vaccine, produced by the expression of HBsAg in yeast, is available under the trade names Recombivax HB, Engerix-B, and Bimugen. Other more potent vaccines using amino terminally extended versions of HBsAg, known as pre-S, are also under development because of their higher efficacy (Ellis and Kniskern, 1991).

One of the major thrusts in vaccine research is the development of subunit vaccines against HIV (Spalding, 1992; Emini and Putney, 1992; Edgington, 1992b). Although the prospects of a useful HIV vaccine are not clear, many candidates are in phase I clinical trials. The benefit of a virus-free, subunit vaccine as opposed to killed whole virus vaccine is easy to appreciate in this case because of the social and medical consequences of vaccine failure. Nonetheless, vaccines using killed, stripped HIV are also under development in the hope of stimulating antibody-mediated humoral immunity and cell-mediated immunity (Kurnick and McCluskey, 1990). Two classes of HIV vaccines are under development — therapeutic and preventive. Because of the long incubation period required for the progression of a latent HIV infection into full-blown AIDS, therapeutic vaccines are aimed at delaying or preventing the development of AIDS in infected individuals who are seropositive but otherwise healthy. These vaccines are expected to augment the immune response to HIV already mounted by the infected individual. Preventive vaccines are intended for use in the uninfected population.

HIV is a well-characterized virus. Like all retroviruses, it has a membrane envelope studded with a glycoprotein. This glycoprotein of 160 kilodaltons, gp160, is responsible for the interaction of the virus with the cell-surface receptors on T lymphocytes. Entire genomes of several HIV strains have been sequenced, providing coding information of all the components of the virus, including gp160. The gp160 glycoprotein is composed of two segments, a transmembrane segment of 41 kilodaltons, and an extracellular, glycosylated domain of 120 kilodaltons, gp120, which contains the regions required for interaction with the T-cell receptor. The interior of the HIV virus contains proteins p17 and p24. A major proportion of the HIV subunit vaccine development effort is directed at gp160, gp120, and their segments, expressed in yeast, insect, and mammalian cells. However, the high rate of mutation in HIV, causing constant change in its proteins, presents a serious problem for vaccine development where constancy of the immunoprotective antigen is a prerequisite for success. HIV vaccines developed to date have not lived up to the expectations raised by the success with rDNA-based vaccine development in general (Edgington, 1992a, 1992b).

Subunit vaccines against other viral, parasitic and bacterial agents are under development (Ellis, 1992). These agents include herpes viruses, the Epstein-Barr virus, the cytomegalovirus (Ellis and Conley, 1991), malarial and other such parasites, and bacteria such as *Bordetella pertussis*, the causative agent of whooping cough (Burnette, 1990; Brennan *et al.*, 1992). In the last case, the toxin is a hexameric protein, and one of the component subunits, S_1, contains the toxic enzymatic activity (ADP-ribosylase), which has to be inactivated in whole-bacterial vaccine preparations without destroying the immunoprotective antigenicity of the toxin. Site-directed mutagenesis has been used to create a version of the S_1 subunit which lacks the toxic enzymatic activity but retains the ability to combine with other subunits of the toxin to produce immunoprotective antigen. This development should lead to pertussis vaccines without side-effects such as acute encephalopathy, irreversible brain damage, and death associated with the whole bacterial component currently used in the diphtheria–tetanus–pertussis (DPT) vaccines. Novel vaccines composed of chimeric proteins combining the immunoprotective antigens of two or more infectious agents are also under development (Ellis and Conley, 1991).

Live attenuated vaccines

The replication competent cowpox virus was the first vaccine to be used in prophylaxis against smallpox (Behbehani, 1991), and this was followed by other live vaccines such as the more recent Sabin vaccine against polio (Melnick, 1985). By virtue of replication of the virus in the vaccinated host, live vaccines offer advantages over killed or subunit vaccines in terms of lower dosage required, and the degree and duration of immunity. Live vaccines also produce broader immunity involving both humoral antibodies and cell-mediated immunity (Kurnick and McCluskey, 1990). Furthermore, immunity at the portal of entry and the site of virus multiplication is induced by eliciting the production of appropriate antibody isotypes (Ogra and Garofalo, 1990). The main drawbacks of such vaccines are limited shelf-life, carryover of unrecognized adventitious agents from the substrates used in their production, and, most importantly, the reversion of the attenuated virus strain to virulence and pathogenesis.

Using rDNA technology it is possible to introduce the genes coding for the vaccinating antigens of many unrelated agents into an established, attenuated virus strain in a ''piggyback'' fashion. This approach is not limited to viruses; attempts are also in progress to engineer bacteria belonging to *Salmonella, Escherichia,* and other genera as vectors to deliver foreign immunoprotective antigens. The most advanced among these vectors is the recombinant live-virus vaccines using the vaccinia virus (Moss, 1991; Moss, 1992), the agent used for the world-wide eradication of smallpox (Behbehani, 1991). The vaccinia virus is a member of the pox virus family whose genome consists of DNA of ~190 kilobases, and encodes about 200 proteins. Many of these proteins, and hence the DNA segments which encode them, are not essential for virus replication. Therefore, these segments can be replaced with coding sequences of antigens of interest, to produce recombinant vaccine strains.

The method used for construction of the recombinant vaccinia virus vectors is shown in Fig. 3.1. The simple approach of using restriction endonucleases and ligase to recombine foreign genes into the vaccinia genome is impractical because of the large size of the genome. Digestion with almost any restriction endonuclease results in fragmentation of the genome, and, furthermore, the restriction enzyme sites are not always conveniently located. Therefore, an alternative strategy of using DNA recombination enzymes of the host cell to integrate the foreign DNA of interest into the virus is used in the construction of a recombinant vaccinia virus. Restriction and ligation operations are performed on a vector of smaller size known as the ''transfer vector''. The transfer vector contains segments of the viral sequences between which the antigen coding sequence of interest and the required control elements are inserted.

The transfer vector engineered with the foreign antigen is transfected into a mammalian cell infected by the vaccinia virus. During the replication process of the wild-type virus, a small fraction of recombinant viruses incorporating the foreign gene into the virus, at the location of the flanking viral sequences in the transfer vector, are generated by cellular enzymes that recombine DNA precisely (by homologous recombination; see Chapter 7). Vectors are designed so that the recombinant viruses are identified by using biochemical or genetic selections. Infection of mammalian cells with the recombinant virus results in the expression of the foreign immunoprotective antigen in the infected cells.

Using this approach, several antigens have been introduced into the vaccinia virus. Antigens from HBV, herpes virus, influenza virus, and HIV have been expressed successfully and have been shown to elicit humoral and cell-mediated immune responses. The large size of the vaccinia genome, and the dispensability of a high proportion of it, permit the incorporation of the genes for several foreign antigens into a single recombinant virus, to obtain polyvalent vaccines. The utility and efficacy of the recombinant vaccinia viral vaccines is under investigation. The main obstacles anticipated are the low frequency complications associated with the use of vaccinia virus, and the questions regarding the efficacy

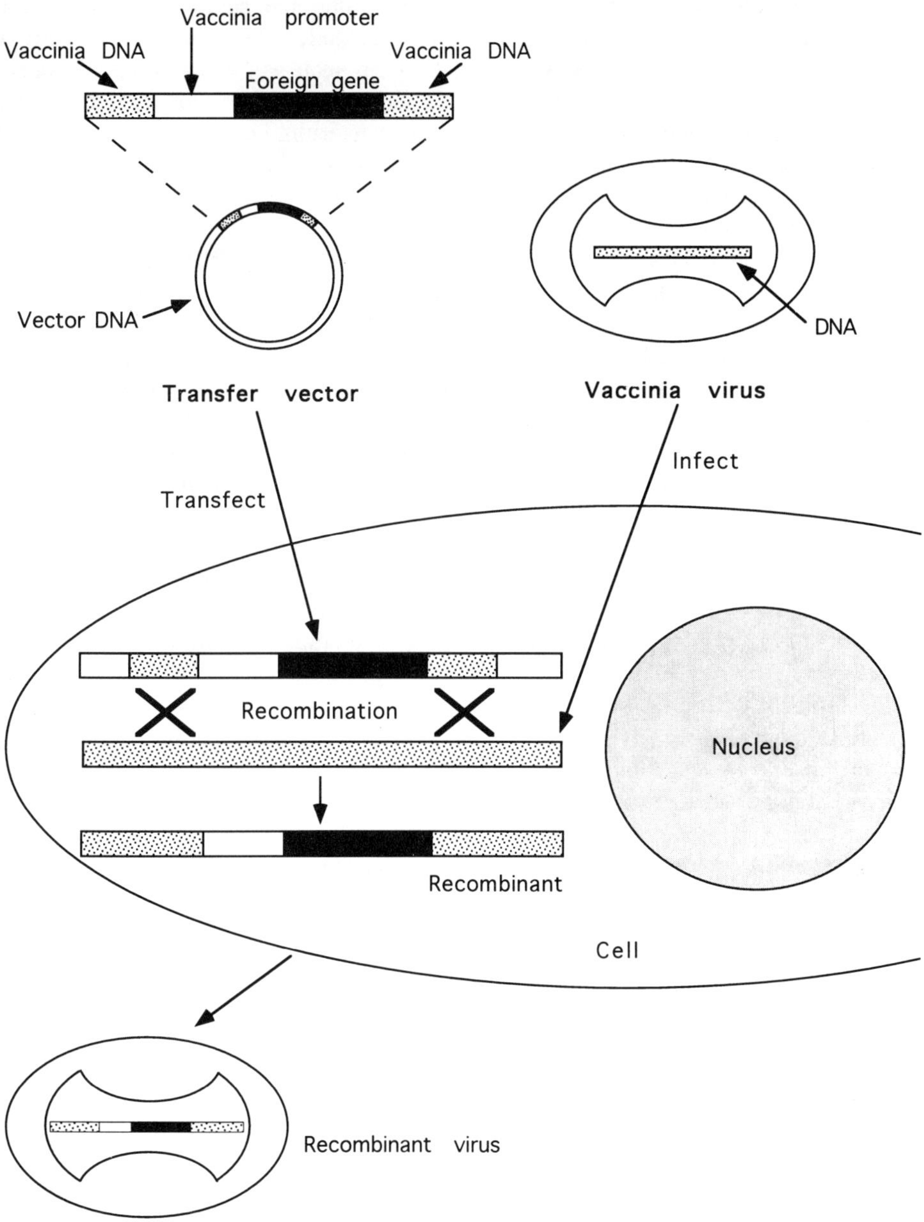

Fig. 3.1. Construction of recombinant vaccinia virus vectors.

of recombinant vaccinia vectors in provoking an immune response in a population previously vaccinated in the context of the global smallpox eradication program (Ellis and Conley, 1991; Behbehani, 1991). Recombinant herpes viral and adenoviral vectors are being developed along the same principles but lag behind the vaccinia system (Whitley and Meignier, 1992; Graham and Prevec, 1992). In addition, attenuated strains of bacteria such as *Salmonella typhimuirium* and *Escherichia coli* are being genetically engineered to present foreign antigens. Live attenuated tubercle *Bacillus* (a bovine bacterium, bacille Calmette-Guerin), the widely used BCG vaccine against tuberculosis, is also being developed to express foreign antigens as the technologies and vectors for expressing foreign proteins in this bacterium are becoming available (Stover *et al.,* 1991). gp120, gp41, and other HIV proteins have been expressed in BCG for use as live attenuated HIV vaccines (Spalding, 1992).

Monoclonal antibodies

The use of immunoglobulins in the therapy of infections via passive immunization has a long history since the nineteenth century, even before the nature and chemical structure of antibodies were recognized (Weatherall, 1990). However, the use of antibody-containing sera and their subfractions has been complicated by the large doses required because of the low concentrations of specific antibodies in the preparations, and by reactions such as serum sickness and anaphylaxis induced by other components of the crude preparations (Dwyer, 1987). Thus, while many potential applications of antibodies were recognized (Dwyer, 1992; Lally, 1991), their actual use in therapy was limited by the lack of methods for producing pure antibody preparations. The discovery and development of monoclonal antibody (Mab) technology now provides avenues for the use of pure antibody preparations as therapeutics and imaging agents, and for their use in novel applications such as immunotoxins, receptor mimetics, and antiidiotypic vaccines as discussed below (Waldmann, 1991; Campbell, 1991; Mernaugh *et al.,* 1992; Abrams, 1993).

Applications of Mabs use two distinct approaches. In the first, intact antibodies seek out target molecules or cells, and initiate actions against them by stimulating the resident immune mechanism through the effector regions of the Mab (constant regions; Chapter 2). In the second, antibodies act merely as vehicles for the delivery of poisons to cells or tumor sites. In such cases only the antigen specificity of the antibody is required, and protein toxins or radioisotopes linked to the variable region of the antibody are responsible for the cell killing.

The first Mab preparation approved for therapeutic use was the OKT3 antibody, as an immunosuppressive agent for the reversal of acute kidney transplant rejection (PMA Survey Report, 1991). OKT3 is a mouse monoclonal antibody directed against the CD3 cell-surface marker present on T cells. T cells are central to many of the systemic immunological phenomena, and different subsets of the T-cell population are distinguishable by their unique and shared surface markers (Waldmann, 1991; Campbell, 1991). The CD3 marker is common to all T cells. Administration of OKT3 interferes with the function of T cells including the subsets involved in rejection of transplants. The exact mechanism of action of this antibody is not known. OKT3 Mab has now been used successfully in thousands of patients since its approval by the FDA. However, an increase in occurrence of lymphomas in patients receiving higher doses of OKT3 has been reported (Leff, 1991). This may be a side-effect caused by the broad-spectrum action of OKT3 against *all* T cells. Mabs directed against a selected subset of T cells might be more efficacious because of their restricted targets. Antibodies directed at other T cell-surface molecules, such as the CD5 marker, are under development (Waldmann, 1991; Dutton, 1991a; PMA Survey Report, 1991). More recently, a Mab under the trade name Oncoscint has been approved for imaging applications for the detection of ovarian and colorectal cancers (Table 1.3; News Briefs, *Bio/Technology,* 1993).

One of the major problems encountered with the use of mouse antibodies is the development of antibodies by the patient against the mouse determinants. This is known as the human anti-mouse antibody (HAMA) response. The HAMA reduces the effectiveness of a mouse antibody in applications where repeated doses of the antibody are used, which is likely to be the case in therapeutic applications (LoBuglio *et al.,* 1989; Dutton, 1991b). In addition, the constant regions of mouse antibodies may be inappropriate for eliciting the appropriate effector functions in humans. The development of human Mabs by techniques used in the production of mouse monoclonals or by other methods has been marred by technological limitations and by the ethical considerations described in Chapter 2 (Scott and Fleischman, 1991; Masuho, 1992). This has led to the development of "humanized" antibodies, which are created by combining the variable region of a mouse monoclonal antibody with selected constant regions of human antibodies, at the gene level. Both the heavy and light chain genes are recombined in this fashion. The co-expression of such "chimeric" genes by transfection of mammalian cells results in the production of "chimeric" antibodies as shown in Fig. 3.2 (Seabrook and Atkinson, 1991; Winter and Milstein, 1991). In addition, the chimerization procedure permits changing of the isotype of the antibody defined by the constant region. For example, the human immunoglobulin gamma 1 isotype is more effective in triggering cell killing and thus would be appropriate in cancer therapy, while the immunoglobulin gamma 4 isotype, which is relatively inactive in cell killing, may be more appropriate for imaging applications (Winter and Milstein, 1991). In one clinical trial, human–mouse chimeric antibodies directed against antigens on colorectal cancer cells had longer circulating half-lives in patients. Therefore, unlike mouse antibodies, chimeric antibodies require less frequent administration to maintain antibody levels, thereby reducing the overall therapeutic dose. Patients' antibody reactions to the therapeutic antibody were significantly decreased and, when present on rare occasions, were directed against the epitopes in the variable region deriving from the mouse component (LoBuglio *et al.,* 1989; Dutton, 1991b).

Centoxin, a Mab developed for use in gram-negative bacterial sepsis, was one of the first chimeric antibodies to undergo extensive clinical trials and came close to FDA approval. However, Centoxin and other such antibodies targeted at gram-negative sepsis have failed to show efficacy so far (Diller, 1992; Sterling,

1993). Other chimeric antibodies directed against the CD4 marker of T cells for use in rheumatoid arthritis, and against the tumor necrosis factor (TNF; Beutler and Cerami, 1990) for the treatment of bacterial infections, are also under development (PMA Survey Report, 1991).

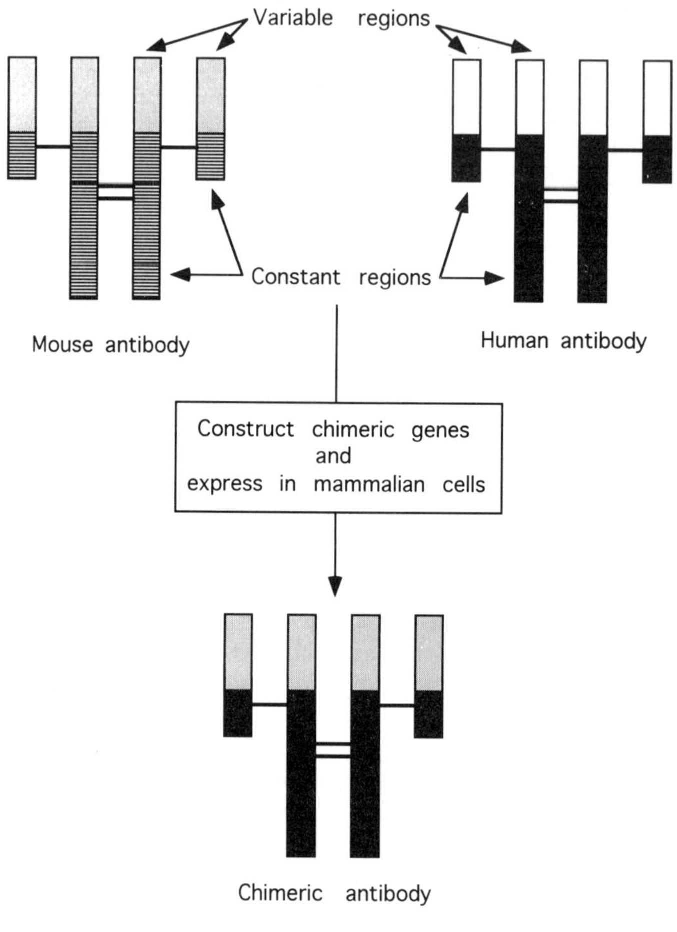

Fig. 3.2. Structure of mouse–human chimeric antibody.

Immunoconjugates

OKT3, Centoxin, and other such antibody drugs use the effector function of their constant regions in their biological action. However, the variable regions of antibodies alone may also be used as targeting vehicles for the delivery of toxins and radioisotopes to tumors. In these applications, presence of the constant region is not essential but this protein stretch can be used to couple to the toxin or isotope. Oligosaccharide chains found in the constant region can serve as convenient attachment points for coupling.

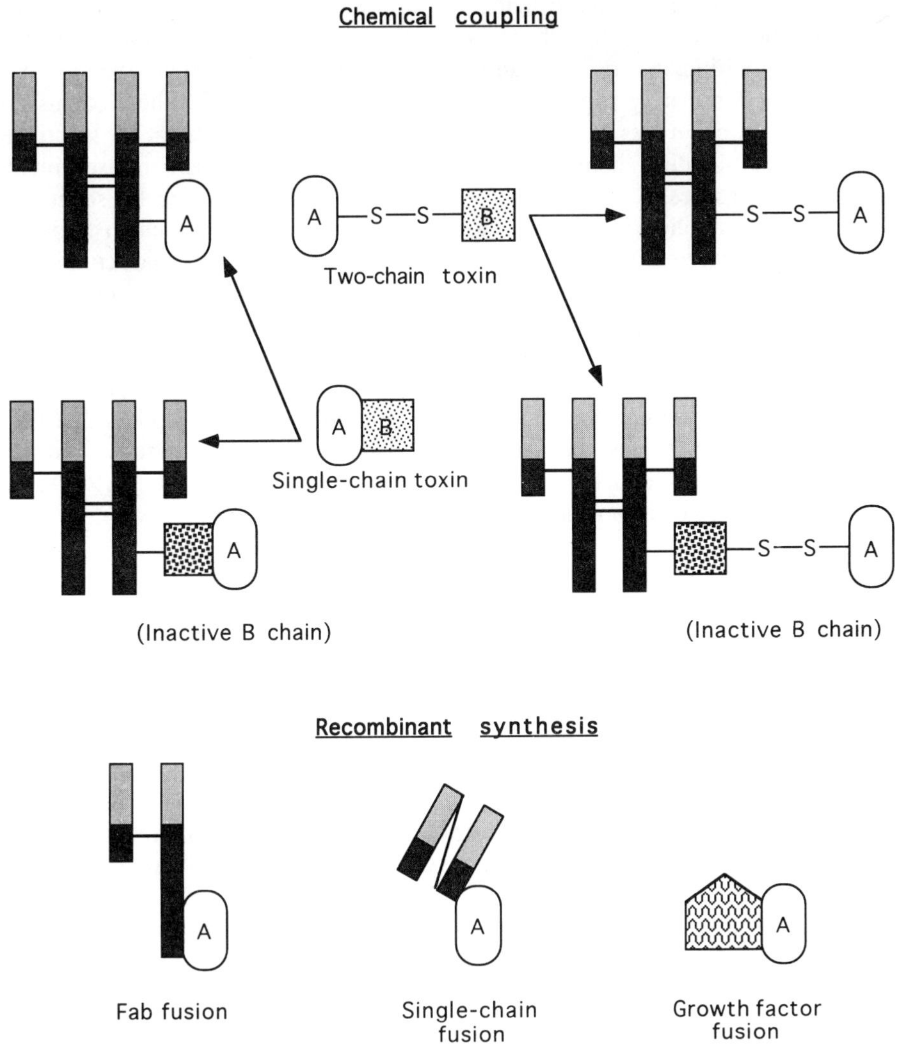

Fig. 3.3. Principle of design of immunotoxin conjugates by chemical coupling of toxins, or through their recombinant synthesis as fusion proteins. The antibody components which are parts of the Fab fusion and single-chain fusion are shown in Fig. 3.4.

Fig. 3.3 shows the principle behind the design of immunotoxins. A number of protein toxins of bacterial and plant origin are useful for the production of immunotoxins. These include the diphtheria toxin and pseudomonas exotoxin from bacteria, and ricin, arbin, pokeweed antiviral proteins, saporin, and gelonin from plants (Pastan *et al.,* 1986; Pastan and FitzGerald, 1991). All of these toxins kill cells by entering the cells, and enzymatically inactivating the translational machinery of the cells. Some, such as diphtheria toxin, arbin, and ricin, are composed of two protein chains, A and B. The B chains bind to the cell-surface receptors and allow the toxins to enter the cell and express the cytotoxic activity present in the A chains. In other cases, such as the pseudomonas toxin and saporin, the cell-binding domain and the toxic enzymatic activity reside in a single protein, fortunately as two separate domains. Receptors for these toxins are found on many cell types in the body, and therefore it is essential to inactivate the natural cell-binding domain of the toxins to prevent their indiscriminate cytotoxicity. In the case of two-chain toxins this is easily achieved by separating the chains, and coupling the A chain to the antibody. With single-chain toxins, it is possible to preferentially inactivate the cell-binding activity and couple the toxin to the antibody. Once the inactivation of the cell-binding domain is achieved, the binding specificity of the antibody determines the target of the immunotoxin. Chemical methods are used to couple the antibody to the toxin. Protein fusions (Box 3.1) between the antibody and relevant portions of the toxin can also be produced by constructing fusion genes (Pastan and FitzGerald, 1991). In addition, immunotoxins can be created by fusing onto antibody constant regions other enzymatic activities such as RNA-degrading enzymes (RNAses), which are toxic to cells upon internalization (Rybak *et al.,* 1992).

Box 3.1. Fusion proteins

Different proteins or their segments can be synthesized as a single fusion protein by manipulating the respective genes to generate a contiguous translational reading frame devoid of intervening termination codons. Translation of the mRNA derived from this fused gene initiates at an appropriated methionine codon at the 5′ end of the message representing the amino terminus of one of the proteins which will form the amino terminal region of the fusion protein. Translation terminates at the "stop" codon at the 3′ end of the message, past the coding sequence of the entire fusion protein. Thus, the second member of the fusion protein forms its carboxyl terminus. In the event that the segments of two proteins in the fusion fold correctly and maintain their biological functions, the fusion protein will possess both biological activities, resulting in proteins with novel functions. Expression in the form of fusion proteins is also useful in the recombinant production of small proteins and peptides. Small peptides (generally below 80 to 100 amino acids), when expressed in some host cells such as *E. coli*, are susceptible to rapid degradation. In such cases, they are expressed as fusions with larger proteins which stabilize the peptide against proteolysis. In other cases, specific peptide segments are fused to proteins of interest to aid their purification by affinity methods.

In most cases, the activity of the immunotoxin is lower than that of an equivalent amount of native toxin. Antibodies chosen are ones that react with cell-surface marker proteins expressed by cancer cells, although markers restricted specifically to cancer cells have been difficult to identify. If the immunotoxin bound to the cell surface is internalized, a small fraction of the internalized toxin component enters the cytoplasm, causing cell death. Toxin conjugates can also be created with other ligands that bind cells with specificity. Some cancer cells express receptors for specific growth factors in high numbers. For example, the receptor for the epidermal growth factor is present in large amounts in squamous cell and epidermoid carcinomas, glioblastomas, and some metastatic ovarian and bladder cancers. Similarly, the interleukin-2 receptor is present on the malignant cells of patients with adult T-cell leukemias. In such cases, the corresponding growth factor can be used as a vehicle for toxins as shown in Fig. 3.3 (Pastan and FitzGerald, 1991); several such growth factor–toxin conjugates are in clinical development (Hodgson, 1993).

Currently, an antibody directed against the CD5 marker of T cells coupled to the ricin A chain for use in rheumatoid arthritis is being tested. Several anti-cancer immunoconjugates use blocked ricin, where both the A and B chains are present, but the cell-binding site of the B chain is chemically blocked. This prevents the indiscriminate action of ricin while maintaining its internalization properties (PMA Survey Report, 1991; Pastan and FitzGerald, 1991). Such immunoconjugates are reported to be 1000 times more potent than chemotherapeutics like methotrexate and adriamycin (Spalding, 1991a). Several toxic immunoconjugates using antibodies or growth factors are in various stages of development (Hodgson, 1993).

De novo immunogenicity of the toxin component and the presence of antibodies to these toxins due to previous natural exposure to pseudomonas bacteria or due to diphtheria vaccination are some of the factors limiting the use of immunoconjugates, especially in therapeutic regimens involving repeated administration (Pastan and FitzGerald, 1991). Cytotoxic proteins derived from humans, such as RNAase, in the immunoconjugates can be used to reduce the immune reaction which occurs when immunoconjugates contain toxins derived from foreign sources (Rybak *et al.*, 1992).

Antibodies can also be conjugated to appropriate radioisotopes for local irradiation of a tumor against which the antibody is directed. In contrast to the immunotoxin molecule being capable of killing only the cells it enters, the radioconjugates cause the inactivation of inaccessible cells in the tumor by virtue of the penetrating power of the radiation. This "cross-fire" killing range is determined by the properties of the linked isotope and can extend from 5 to 10 mm. The radiation dose to the tumor is determined also by the decay half-life of the radioisotope. Technetium-99, yttrium-90, rhenium-186 and iodine-131 are some of the radioisotopes used in therapeutic immunoconjugates (Waldmann, 1991). The conjugation of isotopes to the antibody is achieved by chelation, and the utility of a particular radioisotope is determined by the availability of methods for its conjugation. Different methods for coupling of isotopes to antibodies have been developed (Spalding, 1991a).

Radioconjugates can also be used as imaging agents if the emission from the isotope is capable of reaching an external radiation detector. Several such conjugates, useful in the detection of cancer metastases, are under development, and one conjugate, Oncoscint CR/OV recently approved by the FDA for the detection of colorectal and ovarian cancers, uses the externally detectable, gamma-ray-emitting isotope, indium-111. The same antibody coupled to yttrium-90, which emits radiations of a shorter range, is in phase II trials for the treatment of ovarian and colorectal cancers (Waldmann, 1991; PMA Survey Report, 1991; Hodgson, 1993).

On another front, antibody–enzyme conjugates can be used to achieve localized activation of prodrugs at selected locations in the body. Prodrugs are inactive precursors which are converted to active drugs by enzymatic mechanisms within the organism. In this application of antibodies, an enzyme capable of activating a prodrug is coupled to an antibody reactive with the antigenic determinants of a specific tissue type or a tumor. Administration of the enzyme conjugate followed by administration of the prodrug results in the activation of the prodrug at locations to which the antibody–enzyme conjugate is targeted (Hiller, 1991).

The use of antibody conjugates in the applications described above is limited by the several major problems, some of which have already been mentioned above. First, antibodies that show reactivity strictly specific for cancer cells have not been identified. The receptors on cancer cells are also found on normal cells, albeit at lower levels, and this results in the killing of normal cells as well. Second, owing to their large size, antibodies do not penetrate tumors well, and therefore the uptake into the tumor is limited to a small fraction of the total injected (0.01% to 0.001% per gram of tumor). The low uptake combined with cross-reactivity at sites other than the tumor increases the possibility of undesirable side-effects. Third, conjugation of toxins or radioisotopes to the antibody may alter its distribution and clearance. Lastly, as described earlier, mouse antibodies produce a HAMA reaction in humans (Waldmann, 1991; Dutton, 1991b; Hodgson, 1993).

Genetic engineering methods have been useful in addressing the HAMA reaction and the limitation of uptake imposed by the large size of the antibody molecules. The creation of chimeric mouse–human antibodies (discussed above) has been used to reduce the HAMA, although epitopes in the mouse variable region in the chimeras can contribute to some HAMA reaction. It is possible to further "humanize" antibodies by incorporating the minimal antigen binding regions and to eliminate most, if not all, of the mouse epitopes. The rationale and techniques used in humanization are discussed in a section below.

The uptake of an antibody can be increased by reducing the size of the antibody molecule to its minimum essential binding region. The variable region of an antibody alone is sufficient for targeting the conjugated isotope or toxin. The variable region can be obtained as the Fab fragment (Fab contains a portion of the constant region; Fig. 2.20) by digestion of the antibody with proteases.

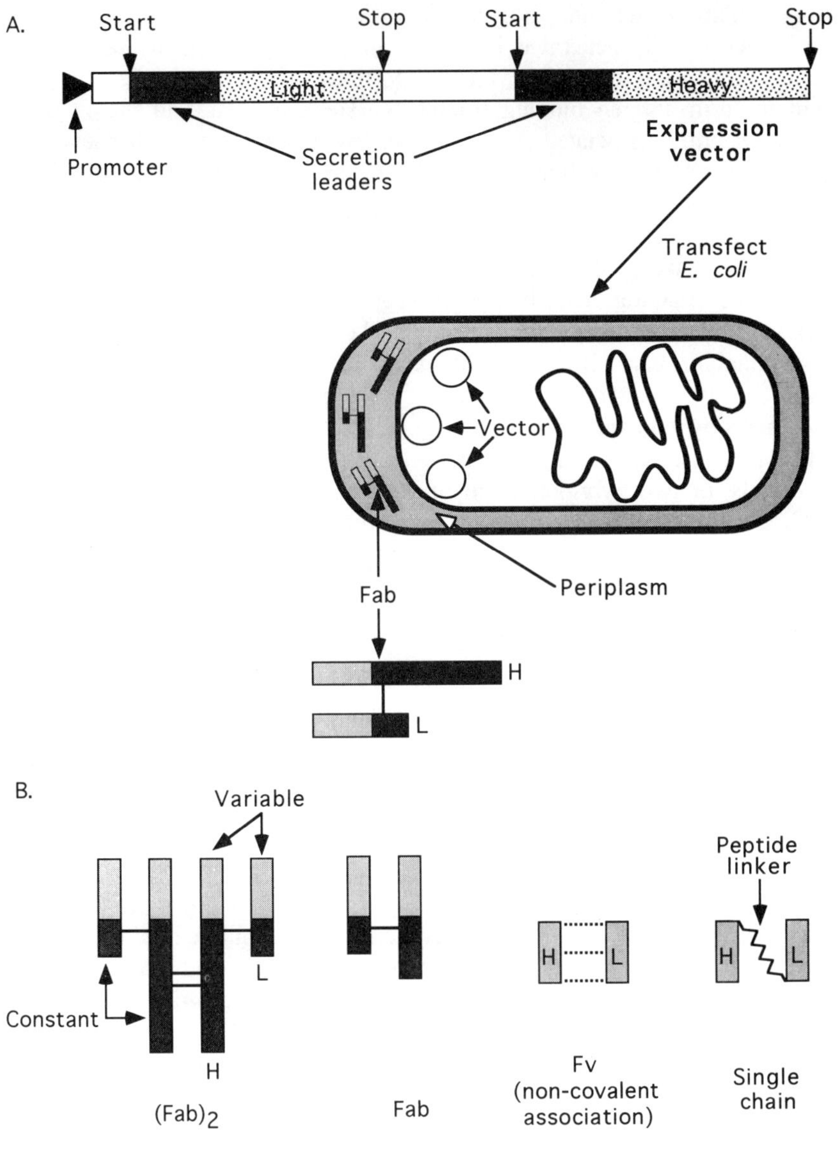

Fig. 3.4. A. Recombinant synthesis of Fab fragment in bacteria by secretion. B. Structures of Fab, Fv and single-chain antibodies.

However, recently Fab fragments have been produced by secreting the Fab segments of the heavy and light chains into the periplasmic space of *E. coli* bacterium, or into the medium by eukaryotes as shown in Fig. 3.4A (Pluckthun, 1991; Hodgson, 1991a; Davis *et al.,* 1991). The secretory process results in the folding, disulfide bond formation, and association of the heavy and light chains resulting in Fab chains with antigen affinity similar to that of the native antibody and its proteolytically generated Fab fragment. Further, using the same approach, segments comprising only the variable portions of the antibodies, Fv, can be secreted to form antigen binding fragments. The two chains in the Fv fragment are not covalently associated and therefore are susceptible to dissociation (Fig. 3.4B). Stability of the Fv fragment can be further increased by linking the heavy and light chain segments via an extraneous peptide linker, producing single-chain Fv, ScFv, also known as a single-chain antibody shown in Fig. 3.4B. The relatively small size of the Fab and the Fv fragment is expected to increase their uptake in the imaging and therapeutic applications described above, but their antigenicity and pharmacokinetics remain to be determined.

Bifunctional or bispecific antibody molecules capable of binding two distinct antigens can be created by chemically coupling the halves of two different antibodies or by co-expression of the genes for the two antibodies in the same cell. The four genes (two light chains and two heavy chains) can be introduced into the cells, or two hybridoma cell lines expressing the two different antibodies may be fused to produce hybrid hybridomas or "quadromas" (Scott and Fleishman, 1991; Waldmann, 1991). Such antibodies are useful in specific targeting of toxins, enzymes and cytotoxic cells to selected cell types and tumors. In such cases one variable region binds to the target cells while the other binds the toxin or the drug.

Another novel application of Mabs is the development of antiidiotypic antibodies as vaccines and receptor mimetics (Netzer, 1988; Thanavala, 1989; Campbell, 1991; Mernaugh *et al.,* 1992). The principle of the antiidiotype antibody is described in Box 3.2.

Box 3.2. Antiidiotypic antibodies

The variable region of antibody containing the antigen binding site is known as the idiotype of the antibody. An antigen and the antibody directed against it interact through surface complementarity that is often compared to a "lock and key" or "glove and hand" fit. In such a situation, it is possible to create the image of the "key" or the "hand" using the "lock" or "glove" respectively as molds, and vice versa. Thus, the shape of the antigen binding region of the antibody reflects the contour of the epitope it is directed against. The binding region of a new, second antibody raised against the binding pocket of this (first) antibody often has a shape similar to the epitope of the first antibody, as shown in Fig. 3.5. The natural occurrence of antiidiotypic antibodies has been demonstrated in several cases.

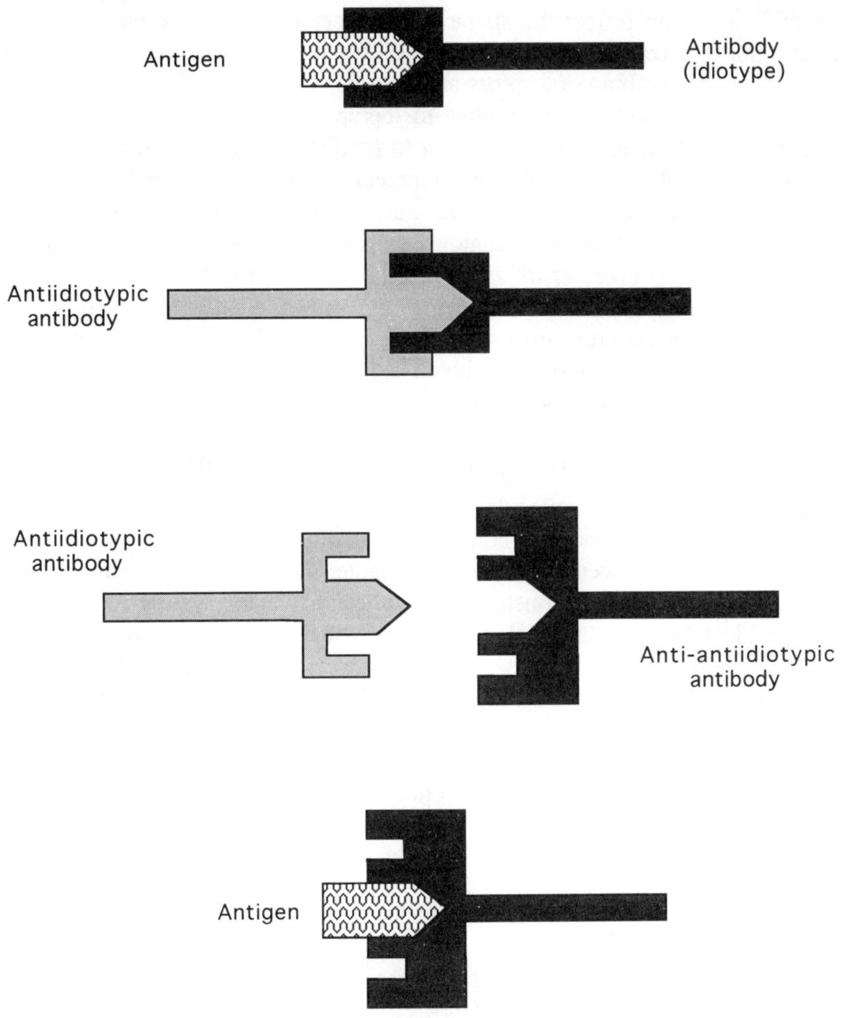

Fig. 3.5. Antiidiotypic antibodies.

Antiidiotypic antibodies raised against antibodies to pathogens can be used as vaccines because of the structural similarity of the idiotype of the antiidiotypic antibody to the antigenic component of the pathogen. This approach is useful in situations where vaccination with the pathogen or its subunits poses risks (Thanavala, 1989). For example, antiidiotypic antibodies raised against anti-HIV gp120 antibodies induced broadly neutralizing anti-HIV antibodies (Kang *et al.*, 1992). Alternatively, antigen binding regions of antiidiotypic antibodies raised against anti-receptor antibodies show binding properties of the receptor, and may be useful in screening assays. Conversely, the antibodies directed against the receptor-binding-region of ligands can reflect the shape of the receptor and hence be useful for the structural characterization of the receptor in situations where the isolation and/or crystallization of membrane receptors are difficult (Netzer, 1988). The concepts and applications of antiidiotypic antibodies in therapy are in early stages of development, and their ultimate utility is difficult to predict. Another exciting development in the antibody technology is the development of antibodies that behave like enzymes in catalyzing chemical reactions. Such catalytic antibodies, also known as "abzymes", are raised against analogs of the transition state intermediates in chemical reactions (Lerner *et al.,* 1991; Lerner and Tramontano, 1988). Abzymes may be useful in specifically identifying and enzymatically inactivating foreign agents such as bacteria and viruses, or in seeking out blood clots and proteolyzing them. These possibilities and other novel applications will doubtless be explored during the next decade of biotechnology.

COMMERCIAL DEVELOPMENT OF BIOLOGICAL DRUGS

The basic techniques of molecular biology and hybridoma technology for the production of proteins, and the considerations of choosing a host/vector system for protein production, were described in Chapter 2. Once a therapeutic protein is isolated and its potential demonstrated, and the host/vector system required for its production identified, commercial development of the protein begins. The steps in the pathway leading from the research laboratory to the clinic are listed in Table 3.2, and are discussed below. The choice of the host/vector systems influences the production economics of a biological drug from the fermentation plant, through purification and formulation, all the way to the clinical testing. A recent case study comparing the process economics of mammalian-cell and bacterial production of t-PA, a thrombolytic glycoprotein, explores these points in great detail (Datar *et al.,* 1993).

Table 3.2. Pathway to a biological drug

RESEARCH:
Identification of activity and assay
Isolation of gene or cDNA
Appropriate expression and characterization
DEVELOPMENT:
Optimization of expression system
Development of high-throughput assays
Adaptation of expression system to scale-up process
Large-scale harvest and purification
Quality definition and control
Formulation and delivery
Preclinical studies
Human clinical trials
Regulatory approval
Market launch

Optimization of expression systems

The crucial decision in the choice of an expression host is its adequateness to produce a biologically active product. Activity includes not only the biological efficacy *in vitro*, but also the pharmacokinetic and immunological properties which influence the dose and side-reactions in animals and man. While some of these properties are not predictable *a priori*, accrued experience and the extent of knowledge regarding the particular protein can aid in the choice of the appropriate expression system. It is therefore routine at the research level to investigate bacterial and eukaryotic expression systems. Given two or more expression hosts that produce active protein, at the development stage the consideration shifts to the economy of the system. While the intrinsic production efficiency of the host/vector system is a key factor, other factors such as medium cost, and the cost of process validation and assurance of safety of the product become important. By these criteria, bacterial systems are the first choice for protein production, and mammalian cell systems a last resort. A detailed discussion of the variety of host/vector systems has already been presented in Chapter 2, and the discussion here is focused on systems currently in use for production. A recent case study in process development using interleukin-3, a glycosylated protein, as the test candidate illustrates the process of determining the suitability of expression systems (van Leen *et al.*, 1991).

Once an expression system is chosen, it is beneficial to optimize the variables of the system to maximize production. If a bacterial system is sufficient, a choice has to be made between vectors for intracellular production and secretion. This choice is made on considerations of downstream purification and generation of bioactivity. Intracellular expression results in high yields, but often leads to the protein's aggregation into inclusion bodies (Georgiou and Bowden, 1991; Papoutsakis, 1991).

If a mammalian expression system is necessary, the specific host cell/vector combination has to be decided upon. This is because there are a variety of possible mammalian vectors, and the utility of many of these vectors is restricted to particular host cell types (Wilson, 1984). For example, bovine papilloma-virus-derived vectors are high copy-number vectors but their replication to high copy numbers, and therefore their utility, is restricted to a few mouse cell lines. The choice of the particular mammalian cell type is also determined by its ability to perform the post-translational modifications essential for efficacy of the product. While glycosylation is a universal modification carried out by all mammalian cells, its fine detail varies among cell types, resulting sometimes in differences in the pharmacokinetic properties of the protein. This is the case with erythropoietin, which is discussed in greater detail below (Goto *et al.*, 1988). Likewise, some cell types are more efficient than others in gamma-carboxylating the glutamic acids of some coagulation factors such as protein C (Grinnell *et al.*, 1987). Finally, characteristics of the engineered cell line, such as requirement for attachment (substrate attachment versus suspension growth), growth rate, serum requirement, and ease of handling (fragility), influence the economy and the choice of the fermentation process from among the variety of systems and modes available (Kearns, 1990). These choices may also influence the structure and the pharmacokinetics of the final protein product as has been exemplified by the recent study on the production of monoclonal antibodies (Maiorella *et al.,* 1993).

Extensive past experience in antibiotic production and in fermenting bacteria and yeast for food uses, and to a lesser extent in growing mammalian cell cultures for vaccine production, has generated technologies and techniques that have been useful in the fermentation of engineered cells. However there are several additional factors to be considered when engineered organisms are grown on a large scale. Therefore, choices based on past fermentation experience were not easily possible in the decade of the 1980s. However, recent experience accrued through the production of the first few recombinant proteins now in the clinic and in clinical trials, has made possible the inclusion of fermentation and downstream processing considerations in the current production schemes (Spalding, 1991b; Kearns, 1990). Thus for example, from past success, the Chinese hamster ovary (CHO) cell system has emerged as the cell line of choice for the production of several proteins requiring mammalian cells. However, there is a view that familiarity and early success with a few systems of cell culture production has made protein drug manufacturers reluctant to consider newer and more efficient methods being developed for culturing mammalian cells (Griffiths, 1992).

Once a host/vector system is selected, expression levels can be further optimized by manipulating the control elements in the expression vector. The factors which influence the expression level of a protein are listed in Table 2.8. Genetic elements in the vectors (such as promoters, and RNA processing signals) are tested for increasing the yield of the protein (Prokop and Bajpai, 1991; Bogosian *et al.,* 1991). For example, level of transcription and inducibility are properties of a promoter which are easily characterized. Inducible promoters are useful in cases where the constitutive production of proteins is detrimental to the growth of the host cell. The transcriptional activities of inducible promoters, which are normally repressed, are enhanced several-fold in the presence of their inducers, which could be specific chemicals or environmental agents like heat. This strategy is routinely used with bacterial and yeast expression systems, where the cultures are grown to high densities in the absence of the inducer, and the production of the protein is turned on by the addition of the inducer. In addition to efficiency and inducibility, the cost of the inducing agent also determines the choice of an inducible promoter.

While there are some general observations based on past experience, the appropriateness of each genetic element for the expression of each protein has to be determined independently. In addition, stability of the vector in the host cell assumes greater importance at the production stage as many generations of growth of the engineered cell are required for production in fermentors with capacities of thousands of liters. Vectors are stabilized by maintaining a selection pressure on the vector. For example, *E. coli* vectors contain genes which confer resistance to antibiotics such as ampicillin or tetracycline, which are useful in the selection of transformants (Chapter 2). The inclusion of antibiotics in the culture medium can be used to eliminate cells which lose the vector (and also prevent contamination of the culture with exogenous organisms). However, the cost of large amounts of antibiotics, the need for their elimination from the final product, and the consequence of worker exposure are also important factors to be considered in the overall production cost. Vectors can also be stabilized by incorporating into them coding sequences for enzymes required for the *de novo* synthesis of amino acids or precursors for DNA, and using them in host cells which have lost these enzymes by mutation. This approach has been employed successfully in yeast and mammalian expression systems. In such cases the host cell without the vector is incapable of growth if the required amino acids or precursors for DNA synthesis are not provided exogenously. Other genetic "tricks" to improve plasmid stability are also available (Margaritis and Bassi, 1991).

Within each host cell system, several independent isolates and laboratory variant strains are available, and the efficiency of expression can vary between them for reasons that are not always understood. For example, there are several independently isolated strains of *E. coli*, which vary in their ability to express the same protein using the same vector. Thus, it is routine to test several strains for optimal production, and this is usually achieved by screening a bank of available strains. In addition, notably in the *E. coli* system, there are several mutant strains which may be used to increase product yield and improve fermentation characteristics. Such mutants may have deficiencies in proteases, resulting in increased stability of the expressed protein (Kresze, 1991), cell-wall mutations permitting better secretion characteristics (Le and Trotta, 1991), or resistance to bacteriophages which can lyse bacteria leading to losses and delays in large-scale fermentation.

Independent clones isolated by transfection of a given host strain by the same vector can differ in their expression capabilities. Such "clonal variation" has been observed in most expression systems currently in use, and therefore examination of several independent clones for the desired expression and fermentation characteristics is a routine part of protein yield optimization. However, clonal variation is an ongoing process in all cultures that are propagated and is therefore not eliminated once a pure strain has been isolated. Thus, the properties and genetic background of the production strains have to be monitored constantly. Master cell banks (MCBs) and master working cell banks (MWCBs) are prepared to ensure consistency between different production runs (Kearns, 1990; Pramik, 1991; Langer, 1993). MCBs and MWCBs should be prepared with the anticipation of the quantity of the product to be manufactured, which, in turn, depends on factors such as the therapeutic dose, and the number of doses needed. Cell banks are tested for contamination by all possible adventitious agents such as bacteria and viruses. During the preparation of cell banks it is advisable not to handle more than one cell line at any given time so as to avoid the possibility of cross-contamination (Nelson, 1991). These precautions are essential because regulatory agencies require demonstration of equivalence if new cell banks are established to replace the ones already validated. All operations in the production are performed under good manufacturing practices mandated by the regulatory agencies.

Assays

High-throughput assays are vital to the efficient purification of proteins on a large scale. Immunoassays, such as radioimmunoassay and "Western" immunoblotting, detect the presence of the protein regardless of biological activity. These assays are simpler to establish and execute, and can be designed to have very high throughputs. Receptor-based assays such as radioreceptor assays go a step further in establishing maintenance of receptor-active conformation of the protein, but are usually more cumbersome than immunoassays because of the requirement for preparations of active receptors. Biological activity assays, using intact cells or whole animals, are ultimately essential to monitor the maintenance of biological activity of the protein through the purification steps. Compared to immuno- and receptor-based assays, the cell-based *in vitro* assays are often complicated and lengthy, but they are almost always less laborious and inexpensive compared to whole animal assays, and are therefore preferable. However, cell-based *in vitro* assays may be incapable of determining subtle differences that may contribute to differences in *in vivo* activity. Some proteins (human growth hormone, for example) may not have suitable *in vitro* biological assays, and testing in whole animals may be the only available method. All of the above assays are useful at various points in the purification process. Therefore their establishment and validation form the cornerstone of biological drug production effort (Langer, 1993).

Fermentation

Once the expression of the protein is optimized and seed stocks are made, the next step in production is their growth on a large scale to generate sufficient product. The scale of fermentation is determined by the therapeutic dose of the product, the total number of doses required, and the shelf-life of the product. The ideal characteristics of a bioreactor or a fermentor are listed in Table 3.3.

Fermentations involving microorganisms are performed in stirred-tank bioreactors, which are generally of one thousand to ten thousand liter capacity, in a batch mode. These include bioreactors in smaller pilot plants used for optimization, and those in the production plants. Fermentors or bioreactors are stirred either mechanically or pneumatically. As discussed before, the fermentation of recombinant yeast or bacteria in general has benefitted from past experience with these organisms in the pharmaceutical and food industries. However, the properties and requirements for the growth of recombinant organisms are different as is the goal of fermentation (which here is the production of proteins). The need to avoid vector loss, harvesting of cells to purify proteins, and assuring authenticity of the protein product are considerations that are specific to rDNA-based fermentation operations. Both vector stability and the authenticity of the protein product are sensitive to oxygen supply and nutrient limitation. Limitations of amino acids can result in incorporation of incorrect amino acids into the protein product (Prokop and Bajpai, 1991).

Table 3.3. Characteristics of an ideal bioreactor

Contain the culture completely
Exclude contamination
Minimize mechanical damage to cells
(mixing operations and air–liquid interfaces)
Provide control of environment
(pH, dissolved oxygen, temperature, etc.)
Ensure uniform nutrient availability
Provide sampling access with no contamination
Be reliable and robust in operation
Be easy to clean, sterilize, and maintain
Have reasonable capital cost

(Adapted from Nelson, 1991.)

Large-scale growth of animal cells is a later development, and the requirements for growing them differ in many aspects from microbial fermentation due to factors such as their size, fragility, sensitivity at the gas–liquid interface, and the requirement for attachment to solid substrates in the case of some mammalian cells. In addition, nutritive-richness of the growth media together with the slow growth rate of animal cells makes these fermentation operations highly susceptible to contamination by rapidly growing bacteria. Further, the undefined composition of animal sera used in the growth of animal cells, especially when required in large volumes, adds a variable that is particularly difficult to control, both because of inherent variability of sera from different animals, and also due to deliberate adulteration and mislabeling by serum by suppliers (Hodgson, 1991b). Fortunately, several media formulations using little to no serum have been developed recently. The use of serum-free media is facilitated if cells previously adapted to the media are used as hosts in the engineering of expression. The use of cells adapted to growth in serum-free media as expression hosts is an example of how the fermentation considerations can influence the early development decisions in the choice of host cells and vectors. Further, the use of serum-free media in combination with host/vector systems which allow regulated secretion of the product into the serum-free medium in the absence of cell growth permits the production of starting material highly enriched in the therapeutic protein (Danheiser, 1993).

Past experience with stirred-tank fermentation with microorganisms has made stirred tanks the logical first choice for use with animal cells, and they are currently in use in fermentations involving engineered mammalian cells and hybridomas. This system can be adapted to the growth of cells requiring substrate attachment by using microcarrier beads to which the cells attach. The microcarriers are then used in a stirred tank. With this adaptation the stirred-tank reactors can be accommodated to the growth of virtually any cell type. Several types of impellers for stirring the tanks have been designed to increase the efficiency of stirring while reducing the effects of mechanical stress on cells (Oldshue and Bajpai, 1991). Because stirred-tank bioreactors are best suited for the growth of microorganisms, a variety of bioreactors addressing the special needs of animal cells have been developed during the 1980s (Spalding, 1991c; Griffiths, 1992). These include hollow fiber perfusion reactors, static maintenance reactors, and the fluidized bed reactors. At present, these novel reactors are primarily used by their inventors in contract manufacturing. However, they are making inroads into the fermentation operations of pharmaceutical companies as the use of hybridomas and engineered animal cells attains prominence. The appropriateness of a bioreactor type for a given cell/vector system and the economics of protein production have to be determined by laborious, case-by-case comparative studies (McKillip *et al.,* 1991; Maiorella *et al.,* 1993; Datar *et al.,* 1993).

In addition to permitting high yield fermentation, the production plants have to address safety issues involved in the use of engineered organisms. These include containment and the prevention of environmental release of live organisms, in compliance with regulations which are formulated by governmental agencies. This concern applies not only to fermentor operations, but also to solid and liquid wastes produced in the operation. Thus, depending on the associated risks, the fermentation plant itself is contained and, if necessary, is operated under negative pressure to prevent the release of live organisms into the environment. The effluent air is filtered to remove recombinant organisms. Kill tanks are used for the steam sterilization of effluent wastes. In addition to the environmental aspects, containment restrictions arising from concerns related to worker exposure are also to be considered. This is dependent on the type of organism being grown. In the US, rDNA guidelines issued by the National Institutes of Health (NIH), and guidelines for working with pathogenic organisms issued by Centers for Disease Control (CDC) have set containment levels based on the risk factors encountered with each organism. In addition, worker exposure at the time of sampling during the fermentation run and during the final harvesting procedure should be minimized. For example, the production of aerosols represents one of the common avenues for worker exposure (Nelson, 1991).

Purification of biological drugs

The basic techniques used in the purification of protein drugs have been developed in biochemical laboratories over the past several decades. However, the objectives of protein purification as applied to rDNA products differ from those encountered in the basic research laboratory. Purity of the final product is one of the objectives that is shared by protein purification processes in both situations.

An objective critical in the purification of protein drugs is the clinical safety of the final product. In addition, the commercial nature and the scale of the protein pharmaceutical enterprise make cost another objective of great importance (Heinrikson and Tomasselli, 1991). This has led to the adaptation of older techniques to production scales as well as the development of newer methods.

Purity of a protein is a relative criterion and the limits of purity are dictated primarily by the efficacy of the purified product, and its safety from being the cause of side-reactions or other diseases. The cost of purification adds to the overall cost of the product, and determines the feasibility of launching a product (Spalding, 1991b). Fortunately, the use of rDNA-based systems has resulted in the production of proteins in higher abundance than encountered in natural situations. In addition, rDNA manipulations can be used to engineer proteins to enable their isolation and purification (Brewer *et al.,* 1991). These may include sites for enzymatic or chemical cleavage to release peptides from fusion proteins (Box 3.1) and/or sequences which confer desirable chromatographic properties on the protein.

The steps involved in purification include harvesting of the bioreactor, followed by inactivation of cells and concentration of the starting material, which is the cells, or the medium when the product is secreted. Concentration is achieved by using centrifugation or membrane filter systems by ultrafiltration. Cells are disrupted using the physical, chemical or enzymatic method that is best suited to the particular situation (Hopkins, 1991; Papoutsakis, 1991).

Further purification of the proteins is achieved through the conventional methods of column chromatography and affinity chromatography, but on a larger scale. Several new developments in the instrumentation and chromatographic matrices have occurred in the wake of the needs generated by the advances in the production of pharmaceutical proteins. Systems capable of processing large volumes associated with production operations have been developed (Heinrikson and Tomasselli, 1991; Poutsakis, 1991). These advances have led to significant cost reduction in the purification of proteins. Downstream processing of proteins is estimated to often cost as much as five times the purification cost of drugs made by the traditional way, and may account for at least half the total production cost of a protein drug (Spalding, 1991b).

Assessment of purity and the characterization of purified proteins

Several biochemical and biophysical techniques are used for the characterization of purified proteins. The goal of characterization is to establish that the purified protein is identical or very similar to a predetermined standard preparation. Further, to meet the requirements of regulatory agencies, different preparations of the recombinant protein have to be shown to be equivalent to the standard material by all the specified criteria. The standard is usually the natural material purified from the conventional source, but there are difficulties associated with the establishment of such standards. Wide variations in activity and a slow loss of activity, often not reflected in the chemical and/or structural properties, can occur in the case of the standard. Furthermore, a high degree of intrinsic variation may be encountered with the natural product, and the recombinant product may be more homogeneous (Geisow, 1991). These factors notwithstanding, the comparative characterization of the purified lots is an essential step in the manufacture of protein drugs in compliance with the regulatory guidelines. In addition to the physicochemical characterization, biological activity measurements to ascribe specific activities are also an integral part of protein drug production.

The common analytical techniques used in the characterization of proteins and the nature of the information they provide are listed in Table 3.4. The biotechnology literature is replete with examples of application, of these techniques to the characterization of rDNA-derived proteins; some examples can be found in Heinrikson (1988), Hancock *et al.* (1988), and Rinas *et al.* (1990).

Table 3.4. Protein characterization techniques

Technique	Nature of information
SDS–gel electrophoresis	Subunit composition Molecular weight(s) Purity
HPLC	Purity and homogeneity (small proteins)
Isoelectric focusing	Isoelectric point Charge changes (e.g. deamidation)
N-terminal sequencing	Correct expression Removal of secretion signal
C-terminal sequencing	Integrity of the C-terminus
Amino acid analysis	Overall composition
Peptide mapping	Structure comparisons
Oligosaccharide analysis	Carbohydrate structure
Mass spectrometry	Molecular weight (post-translational modifications)
Optical spectroscopy (UV, CD)	Composition, structure
2-D NMR	Structure comparisons

Giesow, 1991; Deutscher (Ed.), 1990.

The techniques listed in Table 3.4 are useful for the determination of purity and the presence of contaminating proteins. In addition to the physicochemical characterization and assays for bioactivity, the detection of undesirable biological activities arising from the protein product itself, and from contaminating proteins and other biomolecules is important, and is required by regulatory agencies.

Regulatory issues

Safety and efficacy are the two criteria that are used by regulatory agencies in the approval of all drugs. Previous experience with biologicals such as vaccines and blood products has had considerable influence on the development of the rationale for approval of protein therapeutics produced through biotechnology. FDA in the US regards the use of methods of biotechnology as an extension and refinement of older techniques, and therefore, considers new statutes unnecessary (Miller, 1988). Thus, biotech products are expected to fulfil the same criteria established previously for biologicals produced by older methods. Major criteria for evaluation in these cases were fidelity of bacterial or viral growth, fidelity of replication of animal cell substrates, occurrence of spontaneous mutations, constancy of media composition, pathogenic viral contaminants in sera, purity, stability, and immunogenicity (Esber, 1988). Clearly, all or many of these same criteria are applicable to products of rDNA and hybridoma technologies. Additional considerations for biotechnological products arise from their production in heterologous "unnatural" hosts, which results in gross changes in the nature of contaminants and in the post-translational modifications. The processes used to introduce DNA into host cells may lead to mutations resulting in changes in the primary sequence of the protein. In addition, rDNA techniques can also be used to produce novel proteins that have not been encountered in nature heretofore. Nonetheless, the evaluation criteria used for pre-rDNA biological drugs appear to be sufficient to deal with the special situations encountered with rDNA-based products. Therefore, FDA has espoused a "product-specific" rather than a "technology-specific" approach to the review of all biologicals, and a "case-by-case" approach to the evaluation of every protein drug. Guideline documents titled "Points to Consider" have been issued by the FDA for the production of proteins and Mabs. The current FDA approval process has been recently summarized (Fradd, 1992b). However, newer analytical techniques are being developed as biotechnology advances (Hodgson, 1991c) and this trend is expected to continue, requiring periodic reevaluation and redefinition of regulatory assessment criteria. Regulatory agencies in Europe and Japan follow nearly the same approach to regulation (Bangham, 1988; Sjodin, 1988; Hayakawa, 1988). The properties currently considered in assessing the efficacy and safety of biologicals are listed in Table 3.5.

Physicochemical methods used for the determination of the purity and homogeneity of proteins have been discussed before. The major concerns regarding contaminating proteinaceous and non-proteinaceous materials are addressed by the choice of appropriate purification procedure and validation of these protocols to meet preestablished criteria. Purity in excess of 95% "when examined by all available analytical techniques" is recommended for proteins used in therapy. In addition, the protein should be free of pyrogens, prominent among which is the endotoxin of gram-negative bacterial hosts such as *E. coli* (Poole, 1991). Levels of contaminating DNA, originating from the production host cell, should be below 10 picograms per dose administered to the patient (Petricciani, 1985; Garg *et al.*, 1991). Other contaminants of concern are substances introduced during the expression and purification processes.

These include antibiotics and antimetabolites such as methotrexate used to stabilize expression vectors, and chemicals used in the induction of expression of the genes. Chemicals leaching from purification columns, and antibodies released from affinity purification columns, are also possible contaminants.

Table 3.5. Criteria for regulatory approval of biological drugs

A. Purity and homogeneity
Contaminating proteins and non-proteins
Contaminants specific to production process
Mutant proteins
B. Potency, efficacy, toxicity
Specific activity differences
Pharmacokinetics
Acute toxicity
C. Safety
Oncogenic DNA and proteins
Bacterial and mycoplasma contamination
Exogenous and endogenous viral contamination
D. Immunogenicity
Variations in primary sequence
Variations in post-translational modifications

A protein drug should be efficacious for the intended application. Its therapeutic dose is determined by its potency (activity per milligram, etc.). It should be free of toxicity generated by the main protein component, or protein and non-protein contaminants. While physicochemical methods establish purity and homogeneity, they are not always good indicators of potency and toxicity. Thus, the biological activity and potency has to be determined using biological assays (Storring, 1988). *In vitro* bioassays are useful because of their rapidity, but they fail to take into account the pharmacokinetics which influences the *in vivo* efficacy, potency, and toxicity. Thus, whole animal assays are necessary for proper evaluation, but even these may not reflect the ultimate pharmacological behavior of the protein in humans. The action of some proteins such as interferon is species-specific and, therefore, non-primate animals may not show the appropriate pharmacological response or toxicity related to the dose of the drug. However these animal models may be sufficient to detect toxicity generated by contaminants. Where the primary sequence of test-animal homolog of a protein differs from the primary sequence of its human counterpart under test, the test animal may mount an immune response resulting in the distortion of both the efficacy and toxicity profiles, especially in tests involving long-term administration (Breckenridge, 1988; Marafino *et al.,* 1988; Dayan, 1991).

From the standpoint of regulatory agencies, consistency between batches of a protein drug in its physicochemical characteristics and biological activity is an important criterion to establish that the production system is under control (Hodgson, 1991c).

A safe drug should not introduce a new disease while curing the disease it is intended for. In the case of protein drugs these concerns arise from contaminating adventitious live disease agents such as bacteria, mycoplasma and viruses. They may be derived from the source materials such as the mammalian cell line used in production, or may be introduced in the production process. Mammalian cell lines, notably the myeloma cells used in the creation of hybridomas, harbor and produce endogenous viruses. In addition, many mammalian cells are natural hosts for the replication of exogenous viruses. The richness of media used in the production processes and the chemical composition of proteins themselves make them suitable substrates for the growth of microorganisms. Low-level contamination of proteins with live infectious agents capable of multiplication in the patient are not detectable by physicochemical techniques. This is exemplified by the contamination of cadaver-derived human growth hormone preparations by the Creutzfeldt–Jakob virus (Osborn, 1988). Therefore, a battery of tests for relevant viruses and other microorganisms is a routine procedure in the production of biological drugs.

Segments of DNA derived from mammalian cells possess oncogenic potential, and their removal is crucial from a safety standpoint. Based on many theoretical considerations, a limit of 10 picograms of contaminating DNA per dose of a biological drug has been set as a standard by the FDA (Petricciani, 1985; Ramabhadran, 1987).

Proteins as a class are capable of eliciting antibody responses when they are seen as "foreign" by the patient's immune system. Exogenously administered proteins may be immunogenic or allergenic. Immunogenicity of a protein drug can lead to the need for continually increasing doses of the protein to counteract the effects of neutralization and elimination produced by antibody binding. Reversible binding to antibodies can sequester the protein temporarily thereby distorting the pharmacodynamics of the protein. Immune complexes produced during the therapy may produce toxic side-effects such as allergy, tissue damage, and renal failure (Konrad, 1989). Unfortunately, studies in lower animals are poor predictors of immunogenicity in man. Factors which contribute to the immunogenicity of a protein are listed in Table 3.6.

Amino acid differences arising from the use of protein from non-human sources have been encountered during the use of therapeutic proteins before the advent of rDNA production methods. Porcine insulin, which differs from human insulin in a single amino acid, bovine insulin, which differs from human insulin in three amino acids, and salmon calcitonin, which differs from its human counterpart in nearly half the amino acids, have been used in therapy with varying degrees of immunogenicity in accordance with the degree of difference (Konrad, 1989; Stebbing, 1988). Immune reactions are also seen in the use of mouse monoclonal antibodies in humans as described earlier. One of the benefits of rDNA-based production is the availability of therapeutic proteins with authentic human sequences. However, the methods used for production may also result in differences in amino acids at the termini, causing immunogenicity. This has been the case with the human growth hormone, where the presence of an additional methionine at the amino terminus rendered the molecule immunogenic in patients (Chiu and Sobel, 1988). Furthermore, the power of rDNA has made feasible the production of novel and ''unnatural'' proteins, such as mutants and chimeras, with improved or novel characteristics. Immunological consequences of the use of such entities will have a great bearing on their use in therapy.

Table 3.6. Factors determining the immunogenicity of protein drugs

Amino acid sequence
Species differences
Novel recombinant proteins
Post-translational modifications
Lack of modification
Incorrect modification
Physical structure alterations
Denaturation
Aggregation
Individual patient response
Sex
Genetic background
Administration route
Intravenous
Intramuscular
Oral
Other

The use of a heterologous host cell system in the production of proteins leads to differences in post-translational modifications. The most prevalent, and therefore the best studied of these, is protein glycosylation (Berman and Lasky, 1985), which, as discussed earlier, can vary highly depending on the host cell used for production. Expression in *E. coli* produces unglycosylated proteins. While some of these may be biologically active, exposure of amino acids that are normally concealed by carbohydrates can make proteins appear foreign, and hence cause an immune reaction. Use of yeasts or insect cells as production hosts results in the attachment of carbohydrates that differ grossly from those found in mammalian cells with attendant immunogenicity (see Box 3.3).

Because glycoprotein therapeutics are generally of mammalian origin, their production in mammalian cells results in glycosylation that most resembles the natural situation. However even here, the fine structure of the sugar chains attached by mammalian cells is influenced by several factors such as the source organ of the cell, its transformed nature, and by growth conditions and the composition of the growth medium (Goochee *et al.,* 1991; Van Brunt, 1990). The presence of glycosylation at some sites in a protein can also vary with cell type. Furthermore, glycoproteins produced by the same cell type can have slightly varying sugar structures generating "microheterogeneity". For instance, the carbohydrates of t-PA molecules produced by two different engineered mammalian cell lines were different from each other as well as from those produced by two non-engineered cell lines (Parekh *et al.,* 1989). The microheterogeneity profiles of Mabs are influenced by the conditions used in the growth of the hybridoma (Maiorella *et al.,* 1993). Some degree of microheterogeneity is found to occur naturally in glycoproteins from conventional tissue sources. The consequences of microheterogeneity on immunogenicity and other properties of proteins are not well understood, and the factors which influence the microheterogeneity are not understood well enough to allow its manipulation. Therefore, at present the regulatory criteria are focused on the efficacy of the glycoprotein, and the consistency of the sugar profile between lots (Hodgson, 1991c; Ratner, 1991). Wide variations in the oligosaccharide profile may mandate equivalency studies to satisfy the regulatory agencies.

Box 3.3. Structure of carbohydrates in glycoproteins

Synthesis of N-linked oligosaccharide chains involves the *en bloc* addition of a preformed sugar oligomer to the asparagine residues in proteins. Asparagine residues that are acceptors for carbohydrate chains occur in the sequence context Asn–X–Ser or Asn–X–Thr, where X is any amino acid excluding proline. Addition of the preformed block oligosaccharide is followed by trimming back and rebuilding of the sugar chains by a host of glycosyl transferase enzymes to produce oligosaccharides which have two, three, four or five branches or "antennae". Involvement of multiple glycosyl transferases results in oligosaccharide structures which reflect the composition and the activity levels of glycosyl transferases present in a cell. Accessibility of the asparagine and/or a linked-oligosaccharide chain to glycosyl transferases can also influence the presence and the final composition of the oligosaccharide chain. O-linked sugars, where the oligosaccharides are linked to the hydroxyl groups of serines or threonines in proteins, are produced by addition of individual sugar moieties, again by a host of glycosyl transferases (Rademacher *et al.,* 1988; Kobata and Takasaki, 1992; Varki, 1992). The diagrams in Fig. 3.6 show some examples of sugar structures encountered in eukaryotic cells. The same protein may contain different members of this family at any given glycosylation site, leading to microheterogeneity. In some cases, the terminal sialic acids may be replaced by sulfate groups. Yeast cells synthesize only high-mannose oligosaccharide with the basic structure as shown in Fig. 3.6, but the number of mannose residues added to the branches is higher (>50 residues depending on the strain of yeast: Bergh *et al.,* 1988).

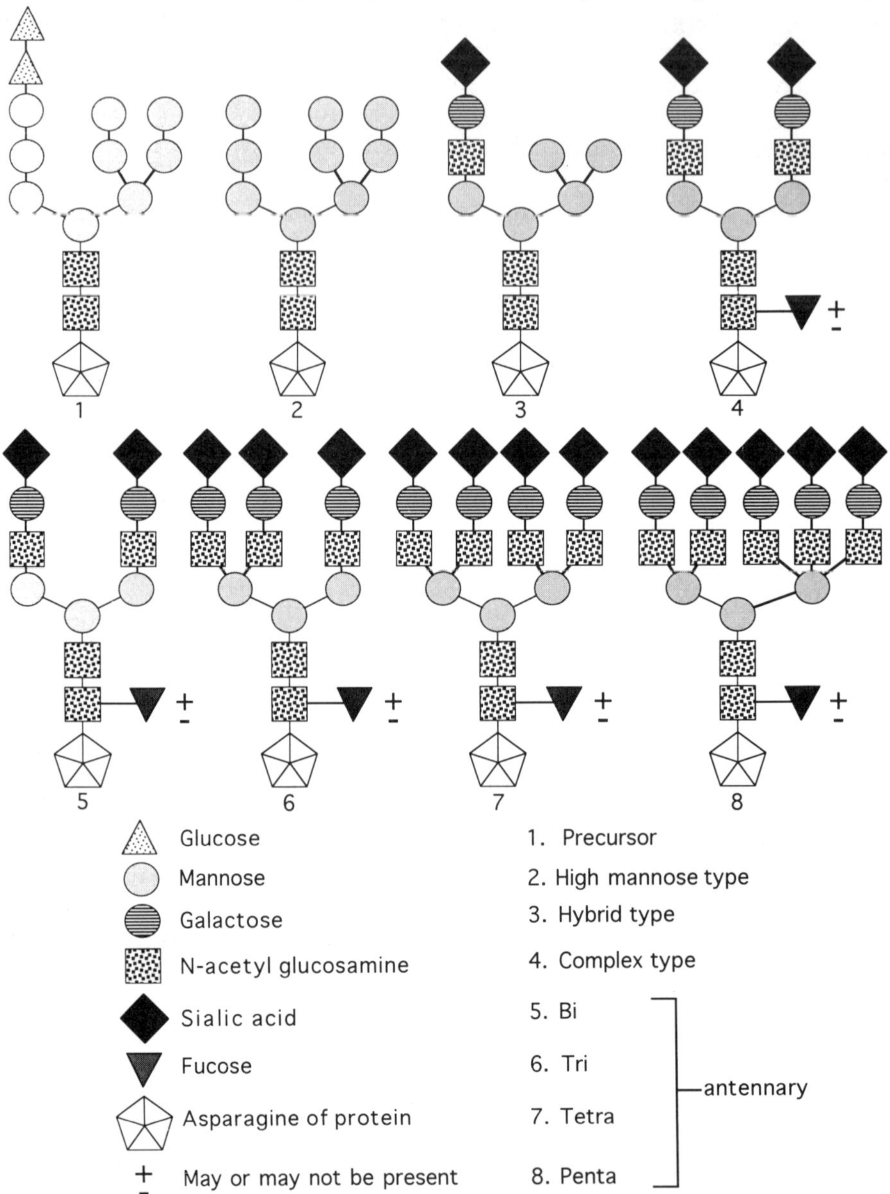

Fig. 3.6. Structure of asparagine-linked carbohydrate chains of mammalian glycoproteins.

The purification process, formulation, and storage may introduce changes in proteins that make them immunogenic or allergenic. These could be proteolysis, chemical modification of amino acids, disulfide bond scrambling, etc. The net effect of these changes is the denaturation and aggregation of proteins, making them immunogenic.

Finally, even with homologous proteins, immunological reactions are seen in some patients as is the case with the production of neutralizing antibodies to conventional or recombinant factor VIII preparations (Schwartz, 1991). The route of administration and the dose may also influence the immunogenic response. Thus, it is likely that all exogenously administered proteins will be immunogenic under some circumstances, but the important consideration in their use is the degree of immunogenicity at the optimal dose and its clinical consequences (Konrad, 1989).

Formulation and delivery

Packaging in a stable form, and introduction into the patients are the final steps in the production and use of therapeutics. A detailed discussion of these aspects of protein drug development falls outside the scope of this book, which is aimed at the molecular biological methods. However, the following brief discussion is included because molecular biological manipulations may be helpful in improving the stability of protein formulations and modifying their properties in a manner suitable for a particular delivery method. Advances in drug delivery technologies, and suitable formulations for these delivery methods, are under intense research because of the biotechnology-induced surge in the number of protein drugs.

As with other aspects of protein drugs discussed earlier, the precedents for formulation have already been set by the protein drugs of the pre-rDNA era. Protein drugs are supplied as ready-to-use liquid formulations, or in a lyophilized form, which requires their reconstitution in the clinic. Proteins are susceptible to a number of chemical and physical changes during storage. These include cleavage of amide bonds, deamidation of glutamine and asparagine moieties, oxidation of methionines, and inter- and intramolecular rearrangement of disulfide bonds. These changes lead to denaturation and loss of biological activity. The shelf-life of a biological drug is determined by the inherent properties of the protein itself and by the physical form of the formulation. Stability is also influenced by pH, ionic strength of the solution, presence of metals and detergents, and the temperature of storage. Components of the solutions such as bacteriostatic agents used in the hydration of lyophilized products can also influence stability. Many formulations contain stabilizing agents such as dextrose, human albumin, mannitol, glycine, glycerol, and polysorbates (Geigert, 1990; Mathias *et al.*, 1991; Ganderton, 1991). The most appropriate formulation for a given protein is determined by trial and error by using accelerated stability tests and through experience gained in the clinic at the trial stages.

From a molecular biological viewpoint, it is possible to facilitate the formulation process by increasing the stability of a protein by changing specific amino acids in the protein. For instance, amino acids which are prone to detrimental chemical changes but are not involved in the biological activity can be replaced to improve stability, if the change does not lead to undesirable immunological consequences. Interleukin-2 (IL-2) and human fibroblast interferon are two proteins in which this strategy has been found beneficial (Wang *et al.*, 1984). Both contain three cysteine residues, two of which are involved in a disulfide bridge, which is required for biological activity, and the third cysteine is dispensable. When these proteins are produced in *E. coli*, the third cysteine, which is normally free, forms intra- and intermolecular molecular disulfide bridges with the other cysteines, lowering the recovery of active product. Replacement of the non-essential cysteine with the homologous amino acid serine (the sulfur atom in cysteine is replaced by an oxygen atom in serine) eliminates the formation of incorrect disulfide bridges improving the yield, and also improves the stability of the proteins against denaturation by disulfide scrambling. It is possible that other directed changes of single or multiple amino acids can be used to improve the formulation properties as the causes of instability are better defined (Shami *et al.*, 1989).

Most currently used protein drugs are delivered through the parenteral route, because the oral route results in the loss of activity due to the acidity in the stomach and due to the presence of proteases in the gut. Parenteral administration requires medical or paramedical facilities and skills, or a high degree of self-administration skills in the user population, restricting its wide use. Therefore, the development of alternative delivery routes is deemed to be important for the wider acceptance of the large number of protein drugs made possible by the application of biotechnology. The frequency of parenteral administration can be reduced by converting the protein or peptide into an insoluble form, often embedded in a variety of inert and/or biodegradable matrices or as lipid encapsulations known as liposomes. Implantable infusion pumps and osmotic pumps also offer means of efficient parenteral delivery (Van Brunt, 1989; Langer, 1990; Ganderton, 1991; Dunn and Ottenbrite, 1991; Sherwood *et al.*, 1992). These methods also offer a more acceptable alternative of sustained and targeted release, compared to the introduction of the drug at high levels into circulation through bolus injections. In addition to these improved parenteral methods, several novel alternative routes of delivery of proteins and peptides into the blood and to the brain are also under investigation (Carrell, 1993; Friden *et al.*, 1993). Prominent among these is the use of the membranes of the nasal epithelium, which appears suitable for the delivery of small peptides. Other routes under investigation include pulmonary, buccal, rectal, and colonic in conjunction with a variety of novel approaches such as receptor-mediated targeting (Ganderton, 1991; Edgington, 1991; Leamon and Low, 1991; Pardridge, 1991). However, the oral route, which has been the key to the success of chemical drugs, remains the dream of major pharmaceutical manufacturers. Approaches towards the goal of oral (and sublingual) delivery using proteinoids are also being pursued actively (Gebhart, 1991). Use of these novel delivery techniques will require suitable developments in formulation methods.

CASE STUDIES

In this section, the development of a few of the currently approved protein drugs is examined with emphasis on the choice of expression system, method of purification, and other factors that have had an influence on their commercialization. At least one drug produced through each of the expression systems is considered to illustrate the rationale for the choice and the influence of this choice on production, purification, and regulatory aspects.

Human insulin

Human insulin produced by rDNA is marketed by Eli Lilly and Company, Indianapolis, under the trade name Humulin. This was the first rDNA therapeutic to gain FDA approval in October, 1982 (PMA Survey Report, 1991).

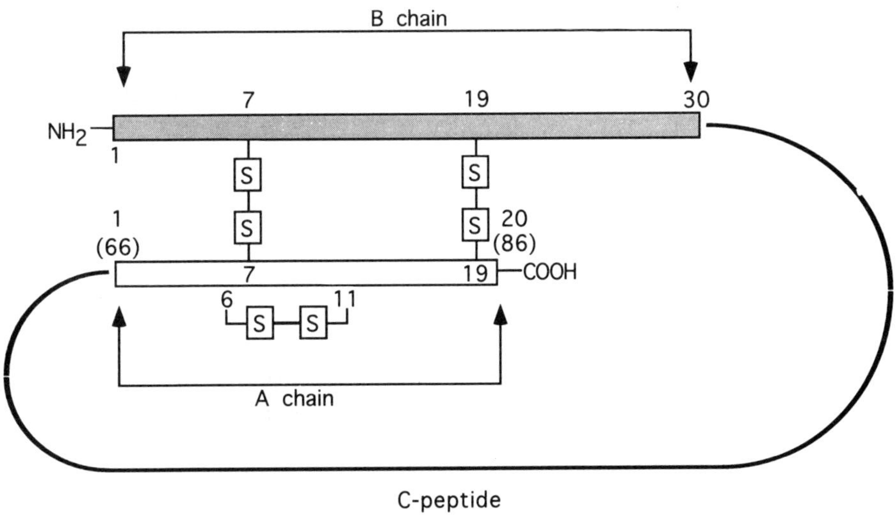

Position	Human	Bovine	Porcine
30 (B30)	Thr	Ala	Ala
73 (A8)	Thr	Ala	Thr
75(A10)	Ile	Val	Ile

Fig. 3.7. Structure and inter-species variation of insulin.

Biological structure and function

Insulin is a protein of 51 amino acids, composed of an A chain of 21 amino acids and a B chain of 30 amino acids, whose complete sequence was well known before the advent of rDNA technology. This made both the chemical synthesis of the gene and the isolation of the proinsulin cDNA one of the earliest milestones in the application of rDNA to the production of therapeutics (Efstratiadis, 1981; Miozzari, 1981). The A and B chains are held together by two disulfide bridges (A7–B7 and A20–B19) as shown in Fig. 3.7. In addition, an intrachain disulfide bridge in the A chain (A6–A11) is also present. A and B chains are derived by the proteolytic cleavage of a single chain prohormone known as proinsulin in which they are linked by a stretch of amino acids known as the C peptide (connecting peptide). The order of the domains in the proinsulin molecule is: amino terminus–B chain–C peptide–A chain–carboxyl terminus (NH_2—B—C—A—COOH). In addition, the cDNA encoding preproinsulin includes the coding sequence of a secretion leader which is removed as the proinsulin enters the endoplasmic reticulum. Bovine and porcine insulins used therapeutically prior to the commercialization of human insulins differ from the human molecule in three (A8, A10, and B30) and one amino acid (B30) respectively, as shown in Fig. 3.7 (Freychet, 1990).

Insulin is secreted by the beta cells of the endocrine pancreas, and is responsible for the regulation of glucose utilization. Insulin deficiency is responsible for some forms of diabetes, where it is used in replacement therapy (Kahn and Shechter, 1990).

Expression and production

The insulin molecule contains no post-translational modifications such as glycosylation. A and B chains expressed independently, or as proinsulin molecule, were obtained in a stable form at high yields by intracellular expression in *E. coli*. However, disulfide bridges are unable to form within the *E. coli* cell, and the chains or proinsulin are found as aggregates in inclusion bodies. This was not a major obstacle because purified chains or the proinsulin molecule could be disulfide-linked *in vitro* successfully. Thus, Humulin is produced in *E. coli*. However, two different production strategies described below have been used in the production of Humulin (Johnson, 1982; Chiu and Sobel, 1988). In both cases, the small size of the A and B chains and of proinsulin required their expression as fusions with other proteins in order to stabilize them against degradation within *E. coli*.

In the first approach, shown in Fig. 3.8A, used before 1986, the A and B chains were expressed independently in *E. coli* as fusion proteins to a 191 amino acid segment of an *E. coli* protein, trpE, with a methionine residue separating the insulin chains from the trpE segment. Chains were released from the fusion proteins by chemical cleavage with cyanogen bromide (CNBr), which cleaves at the carboxyl terminal of methionine residues in proteins. This cleavage strategy was possible only because neither of the insulin chains contained internal methionines. The cysteines in the released A and B chains were modified by

S-sulfonation (oxidative sulfitolysis: Jaenicke and Rudolph, 1989), and the chains were combined under conditions favorable for oxidation of the cysteines. Given

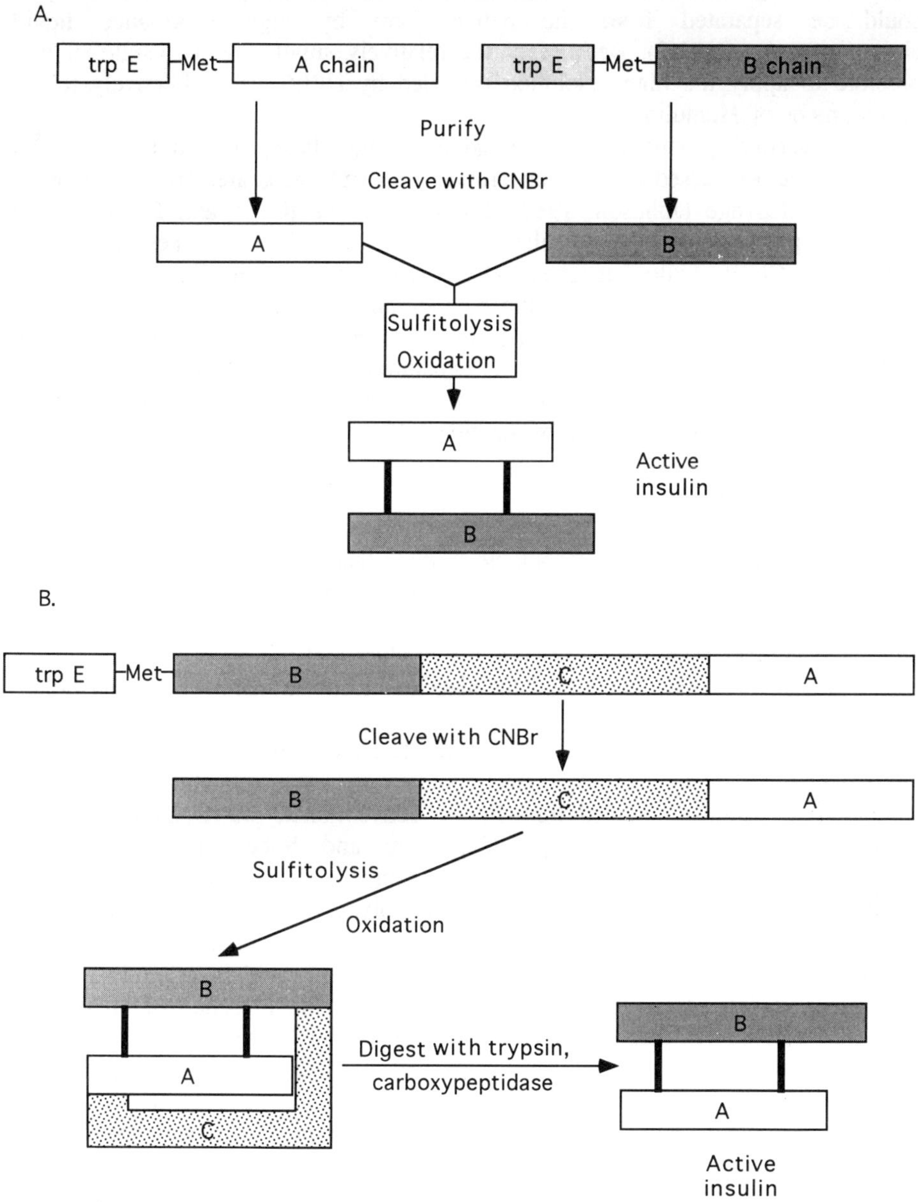

Fig. 3.8. Recombinant production of human insulin in *E. coli*. A. Independent synthesis of chains followed by assembly. B. Synthesis as proinsulin followed by protease digestion.

the total of six cysteines in the two chains, there are, theoretically, 10,395 possible disulfide pairings that can form (Jaenicke and Rudolph, 1989). However, in the laboratory, the desired native insulin structure is obtained at yields of 50–60%, along with only two other disulfide isomers. These undesirable forms could be separated from the native form by high-performance liquid chromatography (HPLC). Because of the relatively small size of insulin, it was possible to apply the high resolution provided by HPLC very effectively to the development of Humulin.

In the second production scheme adopted after 1986, the entire proinsulin molecule was expressed as a fusion protein with trpE, separated by a methionine for CNBr cleavage (Johnson, 1982). Fortunately, like the A and B chains, the C-peptide present in the proinsulin is also devoid of methionines, making it resistant to CNBr. Following chemical cleavage, crude proinsulin was subjected to oxidative sulfitolysis, oxidized under conditions favorable for the formation of disulfide bridges. Presence of the C-peptide has been known to facilitate correct folding and disulfide formation in denatured proinsulin (Freychet, 1990). Following high-yield refolding, the C-peptide was removed enzymatically by using proteases, trypsin and carboxypeptidase B, as shown in Fig. 3.8B.

Regulatory aspects

Humulin was approved rapidly in a 2–3-year period between 1980 and 1982. This rapid approval is partly attributable to three factors: the vast prior experience with insulin as a drug, its being a normal endogenous protein, and its use in a deficiency state. Thus the FDA deemed extensive animal toxicity studies and prolonged clinical trials unnecessary if the product met the criteria of the correct chemical structure, high purity, and the absence of contaminants (Chiu and Sobel, 1988).

Purified insulins from the two schemes described above were subjected to physicochemical tests and biological potency assays, in which they were compared to insulins obtained through the conventional, pre-rDNA route or to semisynthetic insulins (Johnson, 1982; Chiu and Sobel, 1988). Chemical equivalence was established by HPLC elution profile, HPLC fingerprint analysis of proteolytic fragments, circular dichroism, polyacrylamide–gel electrophoresis, and isoelectric focusing. Biological equivalence was established in the rabbit hypoglycemia model. Acute toxicity studies were performed in mice, rats, dogs, and monkeys for 14 to 30 days. Pyrogenicity and the presence of endotoxins were assessed by temperature elevation in rabbits, by limulus amebocyte lysate (LAL). Immunological assays were developed to detect contaminating *E. coli* proteins in product lots. The sera of patients in clinical trials were also tested for antibody response to *E. coli* proteins. Nucleic acid from *E. coli* was not a major concern for the FDA because of its lack of oncogenic potential and its elimination in the purification process: thus process validation demonstrating the removal of DNA was considered adequate (Chiu and Sobel, 1988). Mutagenicity tests were performed, and, based on the lack of mutagenicity, carcinogenic tests were waived. Patients transferred from animal insulins to human insulin were not found to produce antibodies against human insulin although a mild antibody response was elicited in naive patients. Recombinant human insulin was found to have faster absorption characteristics. The development of Humulin also benefited from the prior formulation and delivery experience with animal insulins.

Recently, however, an unexpected complication has been associated with the use of human insulin. The transfer of patients from porcine insulin to human insulin has been suggested by some investigators to cause the death of diabetics due to a phenomenon named "hypoglycemia unawareness", where there is a loss of sensation in the patient due to a drop in the blood glucose to dangerously low levels. This phenomenon is not associated with porcine insulin, probably due to its better penetration of the blood–brain barrier because of the difference in one amino acid. The experimental evidence is controversial at this time, but will lead to a reevaluation of the safety of human insulin (Wolff, 1992).

Human growth hormone (hGH)

Approved for clinical use in the US as Protropin (1985, Genentech) and Humatrope (1987, Eli Lilly), this is a notable example of a protein where one of the production processes resulted in hGH (Protropin) with an additional amino acid. This hormone is also under development by other companies under trade names Biotropin (Bio-Technology General), Norditropin (Novo Nordisk), Siazen (Sereno Laboratories), and Genotropin (KABI Pharmacia).

Structure and function

The human growth hormone (hGH) is composed of 191 amino acids and contains four cysteine residues involved in two disulfide bonds (53–165 and 182–189). No post-translational modifications have been found in the protein backbone. hGH is produced by the somatotroph cells in the pituitary which release it in a pulsatile fashion under the control of hypothalamic peptides, growth hormone release factor and somatostatin. In addition to the 191 amino acid form, pituitaries produce variant molecules which account for 10 to 20% of the hGH in the pituitaries. However the 191 amino acid form is the predominant circulating form. Growth hormone stimulates the growth of skeletal and soft tissues by inducing the production of insulin-like growth factors (IGFs) in the liver. All forms of growth hormone found in the pituitary are derived from a single gene by alternate splicing. The mRNA for growth hormone encodes a secretion signal which precedes the hGH coding sequences (Kelly, 1990).

Unlike animal insulins, which are active in humans, animal growth hormones are inactive in humans and, therefore, the growth hormone used therapeutically had to be obtained from human cadavers. Fortunately, however, the fact that hGH is active in lower mammals has been useful in testing the activities of the human hormone preparations. Common assays used in the development of hGH include radioimmunoassay, receptor assay using liver membranes from lactating rabbits, and the stimulation of weight gain and tibial growth in rats (Olson *et al.,* 1981; Weilburski, 1991).

Expression and production

The methods used for the expression of hGH in bacterial and mammalian cells are shown in Fig. 3.9. Expression of hGH coding sequences in *E. coli* led to the accumulation of high levels of the hormone, which could be purified in an active form from the intracellular compartment of *E. coli* (Olson *et al.*, 1981; Goeddel *et al.*, 1979; Martial *et al.*, 1979). The gene used in expression was constructed by replacing the sequence coding for the secretion signal in the hGH cDNA with an oligonucleotide containing bacterial translation signals and a methionine codon used for the initiation of protein synthesis in *E. coli* (Miozzari, 1981). This resulted in the expression of hGH in the intracellular compartment of *E. coli* from where it was purified and refolded to produce the active hormone.

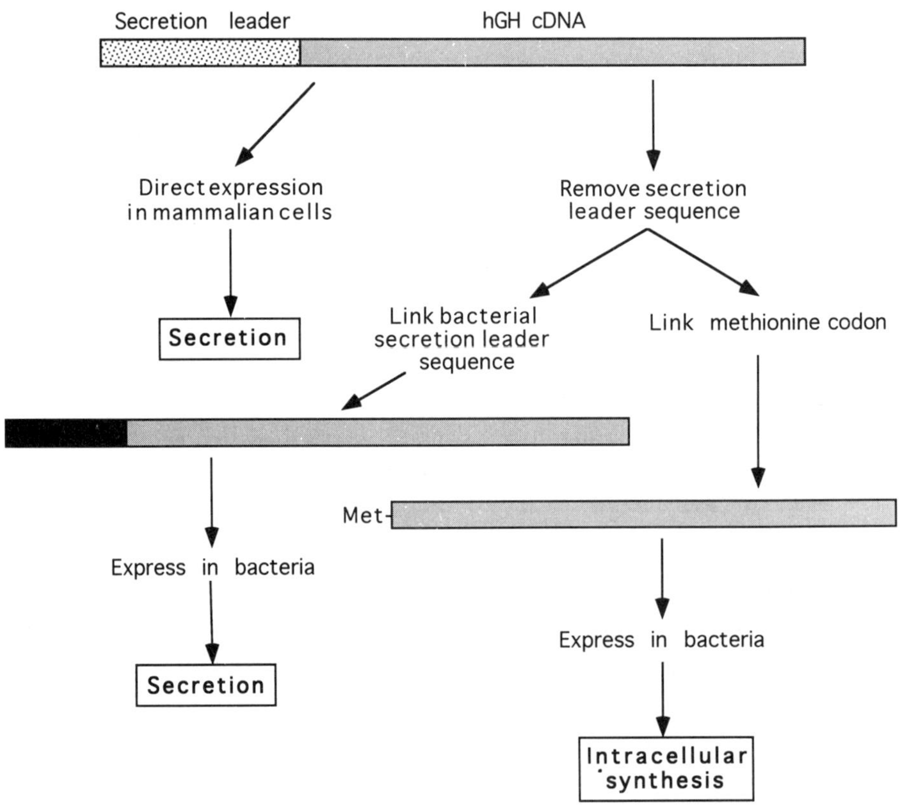

Fig. 3.9. Three alternative routes used for the commercial production of human growth hormone in bacterial and mammalian cells.

Another manufacturer (KABI) has substituted the sequence of a bacterial secretion signal for the eukaryotic secretion signal in the hGH cDNA. In this case, hGH is routed to the bacterial periplasm as described in Chapter 2, and is folded and disulfide-bonded very efficiently (Weilburski, 1991). Mammalian cells engineered with cDNA or gene encoding hGH also secrete high levels of authentic growth hormone efficiently (Pavlakis and Hamer, 1983). This expression system is used commercially by Serono Laboratories for the production of hGH, which is nearing approval under the brand name Saizen (PMA Survey Report, 1991; Hernandez *et al.,* 1991). hGH is produced in mammalian cells in a fashion closest to its natural production, and is easier to purify from the supernatants of cell cultures. However, the economic disadvantages of cell culture production and the regulatory issues associated with the use of mammalian cells are of concern when compared to hGH produced in the prokaryotic expression systems.

Regulatory issues

The use of pituitary-derived hGH was discontinued in the US the in wake of the occurrence of Creutzfeldt–Jakob disease (CJD), which was traced to the viral contamination of hGH preparations (Chiu and Sobel, 1988; Aldhous, 1992). Therefore, the development of recombinant hGH acquired a high priority, and this led to the rapid approval of recombinant hGH. Protropin was approved even though it differed from the native GH by the presence of an extra methionine at the amino terminus. This methionine results as a consequence of intracellular expression in *E. coli.* As discussed in Chapter 2, initiation of the synthesis of all proteins occurs with a methionine. This methionine is removed from the intracellular protein by methionine amino peptidases (Ben-Bassat, 1991). (In the case of secreted proteins, the initiating methionine is part of the secretion signal and the entire signal peptide is removed.) However, in the case of hGH expressed in *E. coli*, the amino-terminal methionine is not removed. Met-hGH was efficacious but was more antigenic than the pituitary-derived hGH, especially in naive patients. Since the antigenicity led to no overt immune disease, and since only one patient developed antibodies which interfered with growth response, the safety issue was of less concern than the risk of CJD infection. Shortly after the approval of Protropin, Eli Lilly gained approval for Humatrope, where the amino terminal methionine of met-hGH was removed by using a methionine amino peptidase. Humatrope was found to be less immunogenic than Protropin (Chiu and Sobel, 1988). Other versions of hGH produced by secretion in bacteria or mammalian cells also have primary sequences identical to pituitary hGH, and, therefore, should be devoid of undesirable immunological reactions.

Hepatitis B vaccine

Recombivax (Merck), Engerix B (Smith-Kline Beecham) and Bimmugen (Kaketsuken) are the commercial hepatitis B virus (HBV) vaccines. This is the first recombinant human vaccine to receive approval world wide. All of the above brands of the vaccine are produced in the yeast *Saccharomyces cerevisiae.*

Antigen structure

Early hepatitis B vaccines derived from human plasma were composed predominantly of a protein of 226 amino acids named "S antigen" (surface antigen) or HBsAg, which aggregated spontaneously into particles of 22-nanometer diameter. Complete sequencing of the hepatitis virus genome of 3.2 kilobases revealed that the S protein was the carboxyl terminal part of a larger polypeptide composed of three domains, preS1 (108 amino acids), preS2 (55 amino acids) and S (226 amino acids) arranged as preS1–preS2–S. Each domain begins with a methionine codon that can function as a translational initiation site (Raney and McLachlan, 1991; Ellis and Kniskern, 1991). S protein is the major product during viral infection, and is produced in excess of the amounts needed for viral assembly. The free S proteins bud through the endoplasmic reticulum and aggregate into 22-nanometer particles which are secreted by mammalian cells. The S protein is N-glycosylated at the asparagine at position 146; however, glycosylation is variable, and therefore the 22-nanometer particles are a mixture of glycosylated and unglycosylated S proteins. The S protein assembled into these particles is the major component of hepatitis B vaccines derived from the plasma of infected humans who are chronic carriers of HBV.

Expression and purification

Attempts to express the surface antigen in *E. coli* were unsuccessful because of the instability of the expressed protein and its inability to assemble into particles. However, the S antigen was expressed successfully by rDNA methods in the yeast, *Saccharomyces cerevisiae*, and in mammalian cells. In yeast, the S protein is expressed intracellularly, but the formation of disulfide bridges and the assembly into 22-nanometer particles occurs during cell disruption and purification. Mammalian cells, on the other hand, secrete the assembled particles into the culture medium. The S protein derived from intracellular expression in yeast, unlike those derived from carrier serum or from engineered mammalian cells, is not glycosylated because it does not pass through the endoplasmic reticulum where glycosylation occurs (Chapter 2); nonetheless it is equally efficacious (Ellis and Conley, 1991; Yoneyama, 1990). The choice of yeast as the production system on a commercial scale was based on past experience in yeast fermentation and the economy of the process. Although mammalian cells secreted the antigen in an assembled, easily purifiable form, the overall cost of mammalian cell production and concerns associated with the use of continuous mammalian cell lines with oncogenic potential made yeast the system of choice.

Yeast cells engineered to express HBsAg are grown in stirred-tank fermentors, and the protein is purified to >99% purity by conventional protein chemistry techniques. HBsAg folds and assembles into 22-nanometer particles during purification, and is formulated with an alum adjuvant. The use of different strains of *S. cerevisiae* has led to the subsequent isolation of high-producing seed stocks. The strain improvement, combined with changes in the purification procedure, has resulted in the final product with significantly increased immunogenicity (Ellis and Conley, 1991; Ellis and Kniskern, 1991).

Regulatory aspects

The sera of HBV-infected chronic carriers is an abundant source of the HBsAg in the 22-nanometer particle form. These particles could be purified relatively easily and treated to inactivate HBV and HIV viruses, which are major risk factors in plasma products. However, the shortage of suitable plasma donors and the justifiable uneasiness associated with the use of blood products in general were the major factors which made the development of the recombinant vaccine desirable. Although yeast-derived HBsAg is not glycosylated, it is efficacious, and the immunological consequences of the structural difference, if any, would only be expected to increase the efficacy. Tests showed the immune responses elicited by the yeast-derived vaccine to be equivalent to that of the plasma-derived vaccine by several biochemical criteria. The vaccine is administered in 5 to 20 microgram doses, and has been tested in a large population of healthy individuals who were seronegative for HBV (Peetermans, 1991; Ellis and Conley, 1991; Ellis and Kniskern, 1991).

Erythropoietin

Although tissue plasminogen activator (t-PA) was the first product produced from engineered mammalian cells to be approved, erythropoietin produced by similar methods has been a greater commercial success (Bluestone, 1992). Erythropoietin is currently approved under trade names Epogen (Amgen), Procrit (Ortho Biotech), and is in development as Marogen (Genetics Institute) for the treatment of anemia associated with renal failure, and anemia in HIV-infected patients.

Structure and function

Human erythropoietin (hEpo) is a glycoprotein of 36,000 daltons, produced by the kidney in response to hypoxia. It regulates the rate of production of mature erythrocytes by stimulating the proliferation and differentiation of erythroid precursor cells. Renal failure leads to lack of this growth factor which, in turn, leads to anemia (Hillman, 1990; Cotes and Spivak, 1991).

Human Epo is composed of 165 amino acids. Prior to its production by the rDNA method, hEpo was isolated from human urine. Circulating levels of Epo in human plasma are 0.1 to 100 nanograms per milliliter of serum compared to 70 milligrams per milliliter of total protein. hEpo has been isolated from the urine of patients with aplastic anemia, where the levels are elevated. The cDNA of hEpo encodes a protein of 193 amino acids with 27 amino acids at the amino terminus constituting the secretion signal which is cleaved during secretion. hEpo isolated from human urine lacks the carboxyl terminal arginine encoded in the cDNA. The hormone contains four cysteine residues with two disulfide bridges between positions 7 and 161, and 21 and 33. The carbohydrate of the N- and O-linked types constitutes approximately 39% of the total mass of hEpo. Asparagines 24, 38, and 83 serve as substrates for the attachment of N-linked sugar chains, and serine 126 serves as an acceptor for the O-linked sugar chain. Carbohydrate chains attached to natural hEpo show a varied composition and are composed of predominantly tetraantennary chains (65%). The remaining sugar chains are triantennary (24%) and biantennary (9%). All the branches terminate with sialic acids (Egrie and Browne, 1991; Goldwasser, 1991). Attachment of carbohydrate is essential for the synthesis, secretion and biological activity of hEpo. While deglycosylated or desialated hEpo retains its receptor binding ability and *in vitro* biological activity, the presence of sialic acid and the degree of branching are important in determining the *in vivo* biological activity, by preventing rapid clearance of the molecule from the blood (Spivak and Cotes, 1991). Erythropoietin interacts with a cell-surface receptor found on erythroid precursor cells to elicit the proliferative response (Sawyer, 1991).

Expression and purification

Because the carbohydrate chains and their sialic acid termini in hEpo were required for activity, the expression system of choice was mammalian cells (bacteria do not glycosylate, and carbohydrates attached by yeast or insect cells are not sialated). hEpo cDNA has been expressed successfully in a variety of established mammalian cell lines. For commercial production, Chinese hamster ovary (CHO) cells engineered with an amplifiable DHFR-based expression vector were used to secrete the hormone in high levels (Vapnek *et al.,* 1988). An increase in expression is obtained by inducing amplification of the vector in the transfected cells by selecting for their ability to grow in the presence of an increasing concentration of the antimetabolite methotrexate. hEpo was purified from the culture medium of the transfected CHO cells grown in large batches by standard chromatographic procedures.

Regulatory issues

With recombinant hEpo (rhEpo) being a product derived from established mammalian cells, the purification procedures had to be validated to meet the guidelines for product safety on criteria such as absence of adventitious pathogens, mammalian DNA, and contaminating proteins, established by regulatory agencies. CHO cells had been used previously to produce t-PA, which was approved by the FDA prior to the approval of Epo (PMA Survey Report, 1991), and this provided useful regulatory background on the expression system.

Because the activity of Epo was known to be influenced by the composition of the oligosaccharide chains, there were concerns regarding the authenticity of the recombinant material. Therefore extensive physicochemical comparisons were made between the recombinant Epo and urinary Epo (Vapnek *et al.,* 1988). Like the urinary Epo, recombinant hEpo lacked the carboxyl terminal arginine and thus the protein backbones were identical. The carbohydrate compositions of the two Epos were compared by digestion with a series of glycosidase enzymes which cleave between specific residues in the carbohydrate chain. Digestion with single or multiple glycosidases resulted in identical changes in electrophoretic mobilities indicating very similar carbohydrate composition between the two molecules. No differences could be detected in UV absorbance, and in CD and fluorescence spectra. However, differences in the fine structure of carbohydrates in rhEpo have been observed, but the glycosylation pattern in natural Epo isolated from the urine of different individuals also shows some variability (Spivak and Cotes, 1991). rhEpo had nearly twofold higher specific activity in bioassays, and this difference is attributed to the difference in purification procedures used in the two cases. The two molecules behaved similarly in immunological assays, and no antibody response to rhEpo was seen over the one year of its use. Thus, by most criteria, rhEpo was identical to natural urinary Epo (Vapnek *et al.,* 1988). rhEpo has been on the market under the brand name Epogen since mid 1989.

NOVEL PROTEINS

A major technical prowess provided by rDNA technology is the ability to alter primary sequences of proteins to create new molecular entities that may have novel properties. This aspect has already been touched upon in the preceding sections in the discussion of chimeric antibodies and immunoconjugates. Protein backbones have been modified in several ways, as shown in Table 3.7, to improve the activities of known therapeutic proteins and to create new molecular entities. One of the major concerns in the use of the novel proteins in therapy is the immunological consequences resulting from the new antigenic determinants created in the manipulation. Nonetheless, several exciting developments are occurring in this area as discussed below.

Table 3.7. Directed modification of proteins

- Amino acid substitutions
- Deletion of segments or modules
- Chimeras between functional domains
- Chimeras between full-length proteins

Modular structure of proteins

A concept that is central to the creation of chimeric proteins, particularly using segments of individual proteins, is the modular architecture of proteins, where independent functional ''domains'' or ''modules'' are linked to produce multifunctional proteins. The recent increase in the availability of sequence information and the availability of sequence comparison algorithms have revealed the high degree of prevalence of such repeated sequence modules in vertebrate proteins. At the gene level, these modules often correspond to single exons (separated by introns), which facilitates the evolution of new proteins by a combination of exons from genes of existing proteins (Baron *et al.,* 1991; Hoffman, 1991). Families of proteins sharing functional modules have been identified. The immunoglobulin superfamily which includes antibodies also

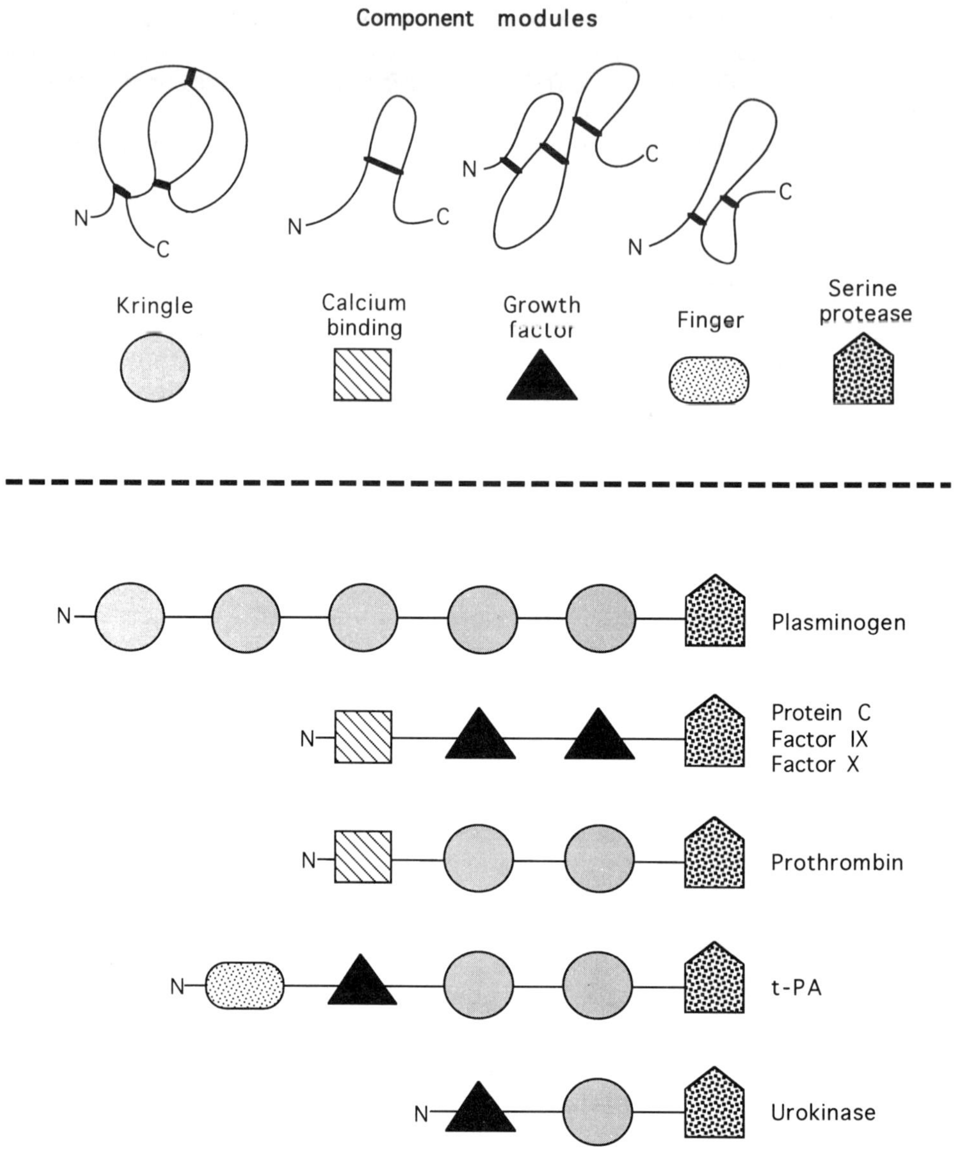

Fig. 3.10. Modular structure of proteins of coagulation and thrombolysis. The shapes of structural motifs, their amino (N) and carboxyl termini (C) and the stabilizing disulfide bridges (bars) are shown on the top. Shown below each module is the schematic symbol used to represent them in the proteins shown.

includes a number of cell-surface proteins. Specific protein modules or domains known as zinc fingers are shared between proteins such as transcription factors that interact with DNA. These proteins also contain other modules and regions conferring other activities on them. A modular theme of protein assembly also occurs within the family of proteins involved in the formation and dissolution of blood clots. It should be pointed out that the conserved modules are not identical in sequence, but in most cases the location of the disulfide bonds is conserved, maintaining the overall conformation of the domain. The functions of many of the domains are not understood. The scheme of assembly of coagulation and the thrombolytic factors, many of which are useful as therapeutics, shown in Fig. 3.10, includes coagulation factors prothrombin, protein C, factor IX, factor X and thrombolytics plasminogen, tissue plasminogen activator (t-PA), and urokinase (Patthy, 1985; Davie *et al.,* 1986; Baron *et al.,* 1991). All of these proteins are proteases which belong to a class known as serine proteases. The domain encoding the protease resides at the carboxyl end of these proteins. Their amino termini contain modules called the C- or gla-domain, which are vitamin K-dependent calcium binding regions, K or kringle domain, G or growth factor module, and F or finger module. These modules regulate the action of the serine protease activity resident at the carboxyl terminal of these proteins. Alterations or deletion of individual modules can be expected to change the regulation of the function. Manipulation of the modular domains of the t-PA gene, in the search for more potent versions of the protein, are discussed below. Alternatively, modules with known functions can be introduced into other protein backbones to obtain chimeric proteins with novel activities.

Point mutations and deletions

The simplest change that can be made in a protein is the replacement of a single amino acid, usually by a single-base mutation in its gene. Such a change may influence the pharmacological characteristics or the production efficiency of a protein drug. Several such proteins, sometimes referred to as ''muteins'', have been constructed successfully.

Proteins that contain multiple cysteines are difficult to refold after high-level production in *E. coli* because of the formation of incorrect disulfide bonds. Replacement of individual cysteines or specific disulfide bonding pairs without compromising the functional activity of the protein can result in increased yield of the correctly folded protein. This technique has been applied successfully to interleukin-2 (IL-2; Wang *et al.,* 1984), human fibroblast interferon (Mark *et al.,* 1984), and basic fibroblast growth factor (b-FGF; Rinas *et al.,* 1992).

IL-2, a protein of 15,000 daltons, contains three cysteines at positions 58, 105, and 125. These amino acids were replaced individually with serine, which causes minimal structural perturbation, because serine resembles cysteine except for the replacement of sulfur in the latter with oxygen in the former. While replacements at positions 58 and 105 led to a loss of biological activity, replacement at position 125 produced no loss in biological activity. This alteration is expected to generate a more stable version of IL-2, which has recently been approved for clinical use (Wang *et al.,* 1984; Table 1.3).

Similarly, human fibroblast interferon β contains three cysteines at positions 17, 31, and 141. Of these, cysteines at positions 31 and 141 appear to be involved in a disulfide bridge, and are required for antiviral activity of the molecule. Replacement of the free cysteine residue at position 17 with serine resulted in a 10-fold increase in the specific activity of interferon β expressed and purified from *E. coli,* which also showed improved stability during storage. These improvements are attributed to elimination of intermolecular aggregation and incorrect disulfide bonds caused by the free cysteine 17 (Mark *et al.,* 1984).

Replacement of appropriate amino acids can alter the interactions of the therapeutic protein with other proteins in ways that may render them therapeutically more effective. Specific amino acids in the B chain of insulin can be replaced to create insulin analogs which show a lesser tendency for aggregation, and are also absorbed 2 to 3 times more rapidly than normal insulin, which aggregates at therapeutic concentrations (Brange *et al.,* 1988). Tissue plasminogen activator (t-PA) molecules resistant to the natural t-PA inhibitor, plasminogen activator inhibitor-1 (PAI-1), have also been created by a single amino acid substitution or small deletions in the t-PA molecule. Existing structural information on the interaction of the t-PA-like serine protease, trypsin with its peptide inhibitor, bovine pancreatic trypsin inhibitor (BPTI), was used to model the interaction between t-PA and PAI-1. Inhibitor-resistant t-PA molecules were designed by using this information (Madison *et al.,* 1989). Deletion of a seven amino acid segment (296 to 302) of t-PA resulted in a t-PA variant with enzymatic activity equivalent to that of wild type t-PA. However, the variant was nearly 100-fold resistant to inhibition by PAI-1. Point mutations altering an arginine at position 304 also produced PAI-1 resistance, although to a lesser degree. These variants may improve the effectiveness of t-PA in thrombolytic therapy.

Replacement of specific amino acids that undergo post-translational modifications can alter the overall composition of a protein and its pharmacological properties. Glycosylation of asparagine residues is one of the common post-translational modifications found in proteins. Replacement of asparagines which are normally glycosylated results in the absence of glycosylation at that site. This approach has been used to create long-acting variants of human uterine t-PA, which is a glycoprotein with three asparagine-linked glycosylation sites. t-PA activates the thrombolytic enzyme plasmin specifically in the vicinity of clots thereby limiting the generalized cleavage of thrombin in the blood. t-PA contains three asparagines at positions 120, 187 and 451, which are potential glycosylation sites (Fig. 3.13). Replacement of the asparagines individually and in combination with a related amino acid, glutamine, which is not glycosylated resulted in seven variants. One of these variants, the glutamine 451 mutant, showed thrombolytic activity equivalent to that of the wild-type molecule, but had a significantly longer *in vivo* half-life. While native t-PA showed a monophasic clearance with a half-life of 3 minutes, the glycosylation variant showed biphasic clearance rates of 0.9 and 20 minutes with each component representing 50% of the total injected t-PA (Lau *et al.,* 1987).

Manipulation of domains

As discussed above, domains in modular proteins represent independent functions. Thus, deletion of specific modules or inclusion of functional modules of other proteins to form chimeras has been used to create novel proteins. This approach has already been touched upon in the preceding discussions of human–mouse chimeric antibodies, antibody variable regions, Fabs, and some antibody toxin conjugates, and is further elaborated here. Additional examples of t-PA domain mutants and chimeras involving the AIDS virus receptor, CD4 and other chimeras, are discussed.

Chimeric and humanized antibodies

One of the highly visible applications of chimera creation by domain shuffling is the construction of chimeric and humanized antibodies. As discussed in Chapter 2, antibodies contain two regions, the variable region which binds antigen, and the constant region which determines the interaction with the effector cell of the immune system. Both the heavy and the light chains of the antibody consist of variable and constant segments. The segments encoding the variable and constant region of each antibody produced by an animal are assembled by gene recombination during lymphocyte maturation. Because the variable and constant regions of antibodies function independently, they can be manipulated by rDNA methods to combine any variable region with any constant region. Thus, the constant regions of a mouse antibody can be replaced with the corresponding or a different constant region from human antibodies, to produce chimeric antibodies (Winter and Milstein, 1991; Seabrook and Atkinson, 1991). This process eliminates all of the mouse-derived antigenic determinants of the constant region which lead to the production of antibodies (HAMA response) in human patients. Chimerization also provides the opportunity to change the isotype of an antibody. The constant region of a mouse antibody can be replaced with the constant region corresponding to any of the different isotypes of the human antibodies. This allows us to choose the constant region which provides the most appropriate effector functions.

Chimeric antibodies are produced by linking the DNA encoding the variable regions of the heavy and light chains of a mouse antibody to the DNA encoding the constant regions of human antibodies as shown in Fig. 3.11. The linkage is made in such a manner that the codons encoding the constant region are in the same translational reading frame as the codons for the variable region. Translation begins at the normally used initiating methionine of the variable region and proceeds through the segment encoding the constant region. In effect, the human constant regions simply replace the mouse constant regions. The chimeric expression vectors can be constructed either using the genes containing introns, or using cDNAs in which the introns have been spliced out. In the former case, the introns are spliced out by mammalian cells when the chimeric genes are expressed in them. Co-transfection of the chimerized gene- or cDNA-vectors for heavy and light chains into mammalian cells results in the secretion of fully active chimeric antibodies.

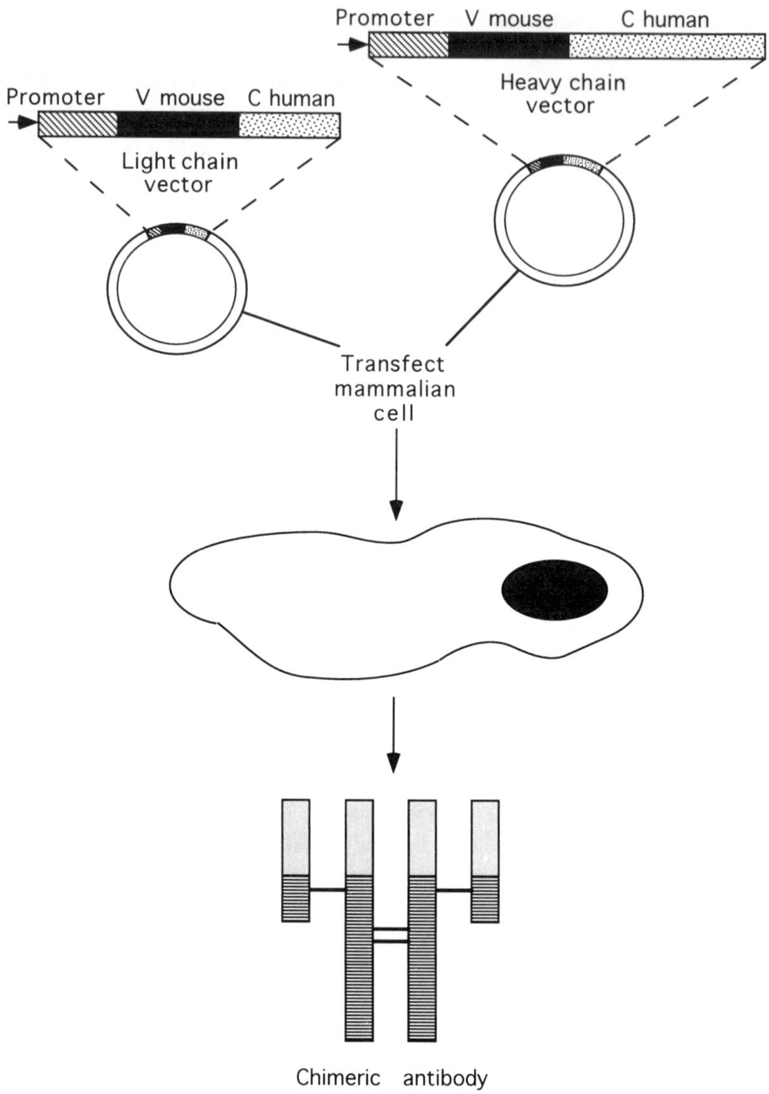

Fig. 3.11. Production of chimeric antibodies. Chimeric genes or cDNA for the heavy and light chains may be assembled into two separate vectors as shown, or may be assembled into a single vector.

The "humanization" of mouse (or other animal) antibodies goes a step further in eliminating the mouse antigenic determinants present also in the variable regions of chimeric antibodies. Examination of the sequences of variable regions of antibodies reveals that, within this antigen binding segment, there are stretches of amino acids which are *relatively* invariant among antibodies of that species, and across species. There are also smaller regions where the amino acid sequence shows a high degree of variability or "hypervariability" (Golub and Green, 1991). The invariant regions are called the "framework" regions. The hypervariable regions determine the interaction of the antibody with the specific antigen and are therefore called "complementarity determining regions" or CDRs. As shown in Fig. 3.12, variable regions of the heavy and light chains of antibodies contain three discrete CDRs that are interspersed within the framework. Using DNA manipulation it is possible to transplant the six CDRs (three each on the light and heavy chains) of a mouse antibody against a desired antigen into the corresponding regions of any human antibody to produce a humanized antibody of desired antigen specificity. This process eliminates all the mouse antigenic determinants which could lead to the HAMA reaction (Winter and Milstein, 1991; Seabrook and Atkinson, 1991).

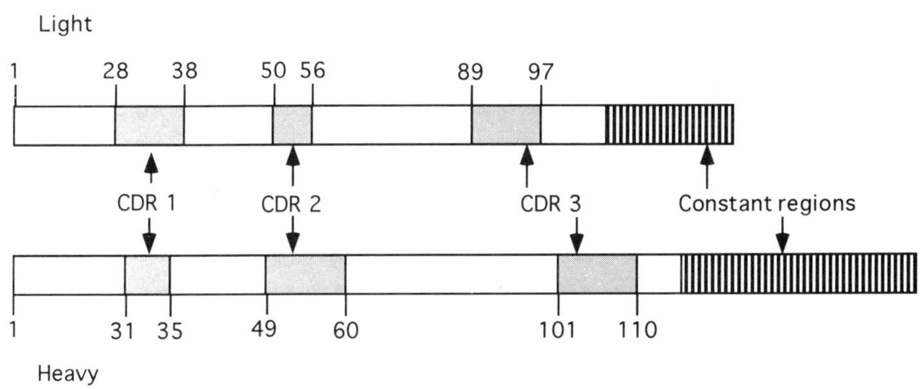

Fig. 3.12. Fine structures of the variable regions of antibody light and heavy chains showing the positions of the CDRs. (Adapted from Hood *et al.* (1984).)

While humanizing is an attractive way to create therapeutic antibodies, the procedure is considerably more laborious and tenuous than the simple chimerization used in the creation of chimeric antibodies. This is because, unlike the variable and constant regions of antibodies which are functionally distinct, there are often interactions between amino acids in the framework region and the CDRs which determine the antigen affinity of the antibody. In such cases, transplantation of the CDRs to a human framework may lower the affinity of the antibody for the antigen. Thus, humanization may require detailed structural information on the atomic interactions between the variable region and the antigen so that the beneficial atomic interactions between the CDRs and framework may be conserved during humanization. This information is obtained through laborious methods of protein structure determination such as X-ray crystallography or computer modeling discussed in Chapter 5. Nonetheless, humanization of a few mouse antibodies has been achieved successfully (Winter and Milstein, 1991; Seabrook and Atkinson, 1991; Co *et al.*, 1991).

Variants of t-PA

Fig. 3.13 shows the modular organization of the t-PA molecule. The potential for use of t-PA in thrombolytic therapy spurred the search for more efficacious proprietary variants for commercialization (Klausner, 1986, 1987). The domains of t-PA were deleted individually and in combination. These studies led to the identification of the domains of t-PA involved in binding to fibrin, the major component of a blood clot, and of the regions responsible for interacting with inhibitors present in blood. Fibrin dependence for activation of plasminogen, restricting the thrombolytic activity to clot vicinity, is the property that makes t-PAs desirable over other earlier thrombolytics like streptokinase. The modular organization of t-PA shown in Fig. 3.13 is: F–G–K_1–K_2–P. The F and K_2 domains were shown to be responsible for fibrin binding (Zonneveld *et al.*, 1986; Pannekoek *et al.*, 1988). A mutant t-PA with a 10-fold increase in circulating half-life was created by eliminating the F and G regions and eliminating the three glycosylation sites (Klausner, 1987).

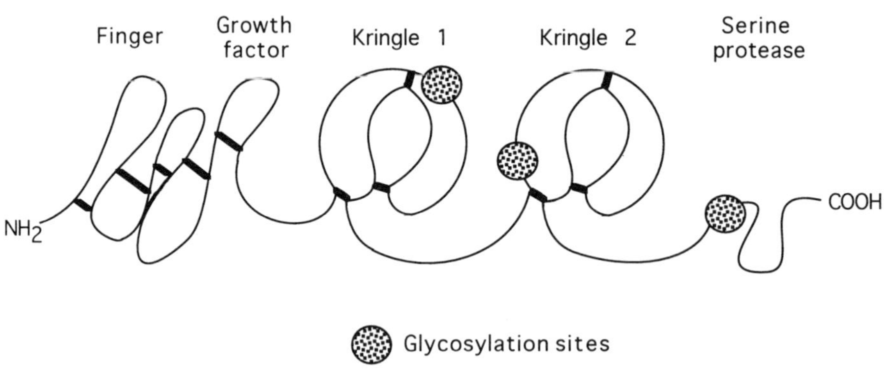

Fig. 3.13. Modular structure of tissue plasminogen activator. Locations of the three asparagine-linked glycosylation sites are shown by closed circles.

Antibody-mediated targeting of t-PA and other members of this thrombolytic family of proteins onto fibrin clots has been used to increase their fibrin specificity in thrombolytic therapy. Targeting is expected to further decrease the side-effects produced by non-specific cleavage of plasma fibrinogen. t-PA chemically coupled to a monoclonal antibody to fibrin was shown to have increased fibrin specificity *in vivo* (Runge *et al.*, 1987). Recombinant molecules where the variable region of the anti-fibrin antibody was fused to a plasminogen activator (single-chain urokinase-type plasminogen activator) led to increases in fibrin specificity and circulating half-life of the chimeric molecule, resulting in a nearly 20-fold increase in the overall thrombolytic activity (Runge *et al.,* 1991). Further progress in the structure–function analysis of t-PA has been slowed because of the reduced interest in second generation t-PAs arising from the controversies relating to the cost–benefit issues with first generation t-PA (Bluestone, 1992; Ratner, 1990).

Immunoadhesins

Chimeric molecules composed of regions of the HIV virus receptor and immunoglobulins, dubbed "immunoadhesins", are under development as therapeutics for AIDS. HIV enters its preferred host cell, the helper T lymphocyte, by interaction between the viral surface glycoprotein, gp120 and a transmembrane protein, CD4, present on the surface of the T cells. The extracellular domain of CD4 was shown to be sufficient to bind to the HIV virus (Berger *et al.,* 1988). Thus, the strategy of containing the spread of HIV infection by saturating the gp120 molecules on the virus surface with soluble CD4 derivatives (amino terminal segment without the transmembrane domain) appeared as an attractive approach to AIDS therapy. However, soluble recombinant CD4 bound the virus only passively, and had no potential for inactivating either the bound virus or the infected cells which express gp120 on their surface. This led to the design of recombinant chimeric proteins containing the gp120-binding region of CD4 and the constant regions of immunoglobulins, wherein the antibody domains would stimulate immune cells. Such "immunoadhesins" are currently in clinical trials (Capon *et al.,* 1989; Palca, 1989).

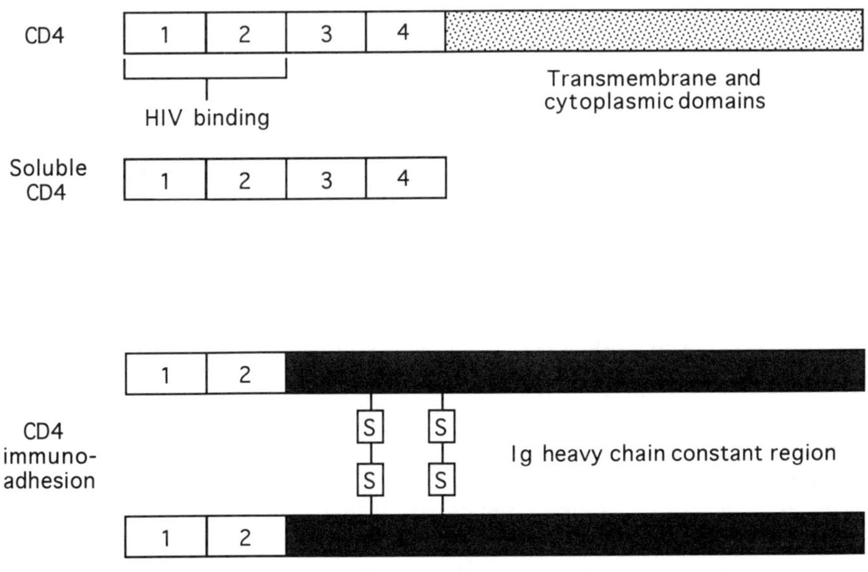

Fig. 3.14. Principle and structure of immunoadhesins. The numbers within the CD4 molecule represent the four domains in the extracellular region.

Immunoadhesin, shown in Fig. 3.14, is composed of the extracellular domain of CD4 fused to the constant region of human IgG_1 antibody. Mammalian cells transfected with the genes for the chimeric protein produced and assembled the molecules into dimers, through disulfide linkages analogous to those found in immunoglobulins (see Chapter 2). The immunoadhesin bound the HIV gp120 and inhibited HIV infection as efficiently as the soluble CD4, but had a circulating half-life of 48 hours compared to the 0.25-hour half-life of soluble CD4. Further, because of its dimeric nature, immunoadhesin was also capable of agglutinating cells which display gp120 on their surface. In addition, like antibodies, the immunoadhesins bound to Fc receptors on cells, thereby stimulating the ingestion of antibody-bound pathogens by phagocytic cells, or their lysis by killer cells (Capon *et al.*, 1989). The CD4–IgG immunoadhesins have recently been shown to protect chimpanzees against HIV infection (Ward *et al.*, 1991). Whether this approach will be pharmacologically and economically feasible in AIDS therapy remains to be determined (Moore and Weiss, 1991).

Other chimeric protein therapeutics

Chimeras between the extracellular domain of CD4 and the cytotoxic segment of *Pseudomonas* toxin or the cytotoxic A chain of ricin have also been designed as therapeutics for AIDS (Palca, 1989). Recently, the extracellular segment of CD4 has been fused to the amino terminus of human serum albumin (HSA) to prolong the circulating half-life of soluble CD4 (Yeh *et al.*, 1992). HSA is an enzymatically inert protein found in high abundance in blood where it acts as a carrier for a number of natural and therapeutic molecules. The HSA–CD4 fusion was expressed and secreted at high levels by transformed yeast, *Kluyveromyces lactis*. The fusion protein exhibited anti-HIV properties similar to soluble CD4. However, the circulating 34-hour half-life of the fusion protein was 140-fold higher than that of soluble CD4. This approach could be generally useful for increasing the residence time of other therapeutic proteins.

Some proteins, like interferons, are members of large families, and offer opportunities for the creation of additional novel members by a combination of existing members. This approach has been used for the design of a mosaic or "consensus" alpha interferon (Johnston, 1991). In humans, 21 subtypes of alpha interferon, with slight differences in primary sequence, are expressed in different tissues. The consensus interferon was designed by using the amino acid most frequently observed at each position among eight members of this family. This molecule has antiviral properties similar to the other members used in its design, but has a higher potency, thereby decreasing the therapeutic dosage and the associated toxicity. This strategy may be applied to other protein families to derive novel therapeutics.

Lastly, the concept of making chimeras by fusing two full-length molecules has also been under exploration. The granulocyte/macrophage colony-stimulating factor (GM-CSF) and interleukin-3 (IL-3), both cytokines which influence the development of hematopoietic cells, were expressed in yeast as fusion proteins linked via a synthetic linker composed of 11 amino acids (Curtis *et al.*, 1991;

Johnston, 1991). Linkage in either order, GM-CSF–IL-3 or IL-3–GM-CSF, produced chimeric molecules which showed receptor affinity, proliferative activity, and hematopoietic colony stimulating activity higher than either IL-3 or GM-CSF alone, or their equivalent combination. This chimera, called PIXY-321, is undergoing clinical testing (Johnston, 1991; Geller, 1993).

While such novel proteins are exciting entities in the research laboratories, their clinical use will depend on the regulatory considerations of immunogenicity and toxic side-effects of the combinations. Nonetheless, the approaches described above bode interesting times in the development of protein therapeutics.

REFERENCES

Abrams, P. (1993). Have monoclonals fulfilled their promise. *Bio/Technology* **11,** 156–157.

Aldhous, P. (1992). Human growth hormone: French officials panic over rare brain disease outbreak. *Science* **258,** 1571–1572.

Bangham, D.R. (1988). Control of new biologicals in the United Kingdom: personal view from a biologist. In *Therapeutic Peptides and Proteins: Assessing the New Technologies.* D.R. Marshak and D.T. Liu, eds. (New York: Cold Spring Harbor Laboratory), pp. 279–292.

Baron, M., Norman, D.G., and Campbell, I.D. (1991). Protein modules. *TIBS* **16,** 13–17.

Behbehani, A.M. (1991). The smallpox story: historical perspective. *ASM News* **57,** 571–576.

Ben-Bassat, A. (1991). Methods for removing N-terminal methionine from recombinant proteins. In *Purification and Analysis of Recombinant Proteins.* R. Seetharam and S.K. Sharma, eds. (New York: Marcel Dekker), pp. 147–159.

Berger, E.A., Fuerst, T.R., and Moss, B. (1988). A soluble recombinant polypeptide comprising the amino-terminal half of the extracellular region of the CD4 molecule contains an active binding site for human immunodeficiency virus. *Proc. Natl. Acad. Sci. USA* **85,** 2357–2361.

Bergh, M.L.E., Hubbard, S.C., and Robbins, P.W. (1988). Glycosylation of heterologously expressed proteins: problems and solutions. In *Therapeutic Peptides and Proteins: Assessing the New Technologies.* D.R. Marshak and D.T. Liu, eds. (New York: Cold Spring Harbor Laboratories), pp. 59–68.

Berman, P.W. and Lasky, L.A. (1985). Engineering of glycoproteins for use as pharmaceuticals. *TIBTECH* **3,** 51–53.

Beutler, B. and Cerami, A. (1991). Cachectin (tumor necrosis factor) and lymphotoxin as primary mediators of tissue catabolism, inflammation, and shock. In *Lymphokines and the Immune Response.* S. Cohen, ed. (Boca Raton, FL: CRC Press), pp. 199–212.

Bluestone, M. (1992). t-PA falls short again. *Bio/Technology* **10,** 480.

Bogosian, G., Kane, J.F., Obukowicz, M.G., and Olins, P.O. (1991). Optimizing protein production in recombinant strains of *Escherichia coli.* In *Recombinant DNA Technology and Applications.* A. Prokop, R.K. Bajpai, and C. Ho, eds. (New York: McGraw-Hill), pp. 285–315.

Booth, W. (1988). CDC paints a picture of HIV infection in the U.S. *Science* **239,** 253.

Brange, J., Ribel, U., Hansen, J.F., Dodson, G., Hansen, M.T., Havelund, S., Melberg, S.G., Norris, F., Norris, K., Snel, L., Sorensen, A.R., and Voigt, H.O. (1988). Monomeric insulin obtained by protein engineering and their medical implications. *Nature* **333,** 679–682.

Breckenridge, A. (1988). Clinical toxicology of biotechnology products. In *Therapeutic Peptides and Proteins: Assessing the New Technologies.* D.R. Marshak and D.T. Liu, eds. (New York: Cold Spring Harbor Laboratory), pp. 163–174.

Brennan, M.J., Burns, D.L., Meade, B.D., Shahin, R.D., and Manclark, C.R. (1992). Recent advances in the development of pertussis vaccines. In *Vaccines: New Approaches to Immunological Problems.* R.W. Ellis, ed. (Boston: Butterworth-Heinemann), p. 23–52.

Brewer, S.J., Haymore, B.L., Hopp, T.P., and Sassenfield, H.M. (1991). Engineering of proteins to enable their isolation in a biologically active form. In *Purification and Analysis of Recombinant Proteins.* R. Seetharam and S.K. Sharma, eds. (New York: Marcel Dekker), p. 266.

Brown, P., Gajdusek, C., Gibbs, C.J., Jr., and Asher, D.M. (1985). Potential epidemic of Creutzfeldt–Jakob disease from human growth hormone therapy. *New England J. Med.* **313,** 728–731.

Burnette, W.N. (1990). The advent of recombinant pertussis vaccines. *Bio/Technology* **8,** 1003–1005.

Campbell, A.M. (1991). *Monoclonal Antibody and Immunosensor Technology* (New York: Elsevier).

Capon, D.J., Chamow, S.M., Mordenti, J., Marsters, S.A., Gregory, T., Mitsuya, H., Byrn, R.A., Lucas, C., Wurm, F.M., Groopman, J.E., Broder, S., and Smith, D.H. (1989). Designing CD4 immunoadhesins for AIDS therapy. *Nature* **337,** 525–531.

Carrell, S. (1993). Novel systems for delivering biotechnology drugs explored. *Genetic Engineering News* **13,** February 15, 1–25.

Chiu, Y-Y.H. and Sobel, S. (1988). Scientific review of the safety of peptide hormones: insulin, growth hormone, and LHRH and its analogs. In *Therapeutic Peptides and Proteins: Assessing the New Technologies.* D.R. Marshak and D.T. Liu, eds. (New York: Cold Spring Harbor Laboratory), pp. 219–228.

Co, M.S., Deschamps, M., Whitley, R.J., and Queen, C. (1991). Humanized antibodies for antiviral therapy. *Proc. Natl. Acad. Sci. USA* **88,** 2869–2873.

Cotes, P.M. and Spivak, J.L. (1991). Erythropoietin in health and disease. In *Erythropoietin: Molecular, Cellular, and Clinical Biology.* A.J. Erslev, J.W. Adamson, J.W. Eschbach, and C.G. Winearls, eds. (Baltimore: Johns Hopkins University Press), pp. 184–211.

Curtis, B.M., Williams, D.E., Broxmeyer, H.E., Dunn, J., Farrah, T., Jeffery, E., Clevenger, W., de Roos, P., Martin, U., Friend, D., Craig, V., Gayle, R., Price, V., Cosman, D., March, C., and Park, L. (1991). Enhanced hematopoietic activity of a human granulocyte/macrophage colony-stimulating factor–interleukin 3 fusion protein. *Proc. Natl. Acad. Sci. USA* **88,** 5809–5813.

Danheiser, S.L. (1993). Regulated protein secretion for bioprocessing. *Genetic Engineering News* **13,** February 1, 1–13.

Datar, R.V., Cartwright, T., and Rosen, C.-G. (1993). Process economics of animal cell and bacterial fermentations: a case study analysis of tissue plasminogen activator. *Bio/Technology* **11,** 349–357.

Davie, E.W., Ichinose, A., and Leytus, S.P. (1986). Structural features of the proteins participating in blood coagulation and fibrinolysis. Cold Spring Harbor Symposia on Quantitative Biology **LI,** 509–514.

Davis, G.T., Bedzyk, W.D., Voss, E.W., and Jacobs, T.W. (1991). Single chain antibody (SCA) encoding genes: one-step construction and expression in eukaryotic cells. *Bio/Technology* **9,** 165–169.

Dayan, A.D. (1991). Toxicity and safety: the testing of genetically engineered pharmaceuticals. In *Polypeptide and Protein Drugs: Production, Characterization and Formulation.* R.C. Hider and D. Barlow, eds. (Chichester: Ellis Horwood), pp. 132–145.

Deutscher, M.P.(ed.) (1990). *Guide to Protein Purification: Methods in Enzymology,* Volume 182 (New York: Academic Press).

Diller, W. (1992). FDA questions effectiveness of Centoxin against sepsis. *Genetic Engineering News* **12,** May 1, 1–28.

DMD (1991). Technology and strategy: blood substitutes and oxygen carriers. *Drug & Market Development* **2,** 87–92.

Drake, P.F. (1990). Clinical advances in biotechnology. *Bio/Technology* **8,** 615.

Dreesman, G.R., Sparrow, J.T., Frenchick, P.J., and Kennedy, R.C. (1985). Cyclic synthetic peptides and immune response to hepatitis B virus. In *High-technology Route to Virus Vaccines.* G.R. Dreesman, J.G. Bronson, and R.C. Kennedy, eds. (Washington, DC: American Society of Microbiology), pp. 55–66.

Dunn, R.L. and Ottenbrite, R.M. (eds) (1991). *Polymeric Drugs and Drug Delivery Systems:* ACS Symposium Series 469 (Washington, DC: American Chemical Society).

Dutton, G. (1991a). Monoclonal therapeutics show promise, yet significant barriers remain. *Genetic Engineering News* July/August, 3–30.

Dutton, G. (1991b). Researchers exhibit increasing optimism over human and chimeric Mab development. *Genetic Engineering News* April, 1–26.

Dwyer, J.M. (1987). Intravenous therapy with gamma globulin. *Adv. Intern. Med.* **32,** 111–136.

Dwyer, J.M. (1992). Manipulating the immune system with immune globulin. *New England J. Med.* **326,** 107–116.

Edgington, S.M. (1991). The anatomy of access: peptide drug delivery. *Bio/Technology* **9,** 1326–1333.

Edgington, S.M. (1992a). Biotech vaccine's problematic promise. *Bio/Technology* **10,** 763–766.

Edgington, S.M. (1992b). Is an AIDS vaccine possible? *Bio/Technology* **10,** 768–771.

Efstratiadis, A. (1981). Preproinsulin sequence: A summary. In *Insulins, Growth Hormone, and Recombinant DNA Technology.* J.L. Gueriguian, ed. (New York: Raven Press), pp. 1–11.

Egrie, J.C. and Browne, J.K. (1991). The molecular biology of erythropoietin. In *Erythropoietin: Molecular, Cellular, and Clinical Biology.* A.J. Erslev, J.W. Adamson, J.W. Eschbach, and C.G. Winearls, eds. (Baltimore: Johns Hopkins University Press), pp. 21–40.

Ellis, R.W. and Conley, A.J. (1991). Recombinant-derived vaccines: models for future development. In *Recombinant DNA Technology and Applications*. A. Prokop, R.K. Bajpai, and C. Ho, eds. (New York: McGraw-Hill), pp. 191–231.

Ellis, R.W. and Kniskern, P.J. (1991). Recombinant hepatitis B vaccines. In *Molecular Biology of the Hepatitis B Virus*. A. McLachlan, ed. (Boston: CRC Press), pp. 307–321.

Ellis, R.W. (ed.) (1992). *Vaccines: New Approaches to Immunological Problems* (Boston: Butterworth-Heinemann).

Emini, E.A. and Putney, S.D. (1992). Human immunodeficiency virus. In *Vaccines: New Approaches to Immunological Problems*. R.W. Ellis, ed. (Boston: Butterworth-Heinemann), pp. 309–326.

Esber, E.C. (1988). Regulatory concerns for biologics: United States perspective. In *Therapeutic Peptides and Proteins: Assessing the New Technologies*. D.R. Marshak and D.T. Liu, eds. (New York: Cold Spring Harbor Laboratory), pp. 265–278.

Fradd, R.B. (1992a). Biopharmaceutical firms put emphasis on biology to cure human diseases. *Genetic Engineering News* January, 26–28.

Fradd, R.B. (1992b). Primer on FDA approvals. *Bio/Technology* **10,** 488.

Freychet, P. (1990). Pancreatic hormones. In *Hormones: From Molecules to Disease*. E-E. Baulieu and P.A. Kelly, eds. (New York: Chapman and Hall), pp. 489–532.

Friden, P.M., Walus, L.R., Watson, P., Doctrow, S.R., Kozarich, J.W., Backman, C., Bergman, H., Hoffer, B., Bloom, F., and Granholm, A.-C. (1993). Blood–brain barrier penetration and in-vivo activity of an NGF conjugate. *Science* **259,** 373–377.

Ganderton, D. (1991). The development of peptide and protein pharmaceuticals. In *Polypeptide and Protein Drugs: Production, Characterization and Formulation*. R.C. Hider and D. Barlow, eds. (Chichester: Ellis Horwood), pp. 211–227.

Garg, V.K., Costello, M.A.C., and Czuba, B.A. (1991). Purification and production of therapeutic grade proteins. In *Purification and Analysis of Recombinant Proteins*. R. Seetharam and S.K. Sharma, eds. (New York: Marcel Dekker), pp. 29–54.

Gebhart, F. (1991). CTA uses proteinoid technology to break into oral drug delivery market. *Genetic Engineering News* May, 6–7.

Geigert, J. (1990). Overview of the stability and handling of recombinant protein therapeutics. *Genetic Engineering News* April, 14.

Geller, M. (1993). Cytokines demonstrate promise as agents to stimulate hematopoiesis after chemotherapy. *Genetic Engineering News* **13,** January 1, 1–16.

Geisow, M.J. (1991). Characterizing recombinant proteins. *Bio/Technology* **9,** 921–924.

Geissler, E. (1990). SV40 and human brain tumors. In *Progress in Medical Virology*, Vol. 37. J.L. Melnick, ed. (New York: Karger), pp. 211–222.

Georgiou, G. and Bowden, G.A. (1991). Inclusion body formation and the recovery of aggregated recombinant proteins. In *Recombinant DNA Technology and Applications*. A. Prokop, R.K. Bajpai, and C. Ho, eds. (New York: McGraw-Hill), pp. 333–356.

Goeddel, D.V., Heyneker, H.L., Hozumi, T., Arentzer, R., Itakura, K., Yansura, D.G., Ross, M.J., Miozzari, R., Crea, R., and Seeburg, P.H. (1979). Direct expression in *Escherichia coli* of a DNA for human growth hormone. *Nature* **281,** 544–548.

Goldwasser, E. (1991). The structure–function relationship of erythropoietin. In *Erythropoietin: Molecular, Cellular, and Clinical Biology*. A.J. Erslev, J.W. Adamson, J.W. Eschbach, and C.G. Winearls, eds. (Baltimore: Johns Hopkins University Press), pp. 41–52.

Golub, E.S. and Green, D.R. (1991). *Immunology: A Synthesis* (Sunderland, Massachusetts: Sinauer Associates Inc.).

Goochee, C.F., Gramer, M.J., Andersen, D.C., Bahr, B.J., and Rasmussen, J.R. (1991). The oligosaccharides of glycoproteins: bioprocess factors affecting oligosaccharide structure and their effect on glycoprotein properties. *Bio/Technology* **9,** 1347–1355.

Goto, C., Akai, K., Murakami, A., Hashimoto, C., Tsuda, E., Ueda, M., Kawanishi, G., Takahashi, N., Ishimoto, A., Chiba, H., and Sasaki, R. (1988). Production of recombinant human erythropoietin in mammalian cells: host-cell dependency of biological activity of the cloned glycoprotein. *Bio/Technology* **6,** 67–71.

Graham, F.L. and Prevec, L. (1992). Adenovirus-based expression vectors and recombinant vaccines. In *Vaccines: New Approaches to Immunological Problems*. R.W. Ellis, ed. (Boston: Butterworth-Heinemann), pp. 363–390.

Griffiths, B. (1992). Closing the culture gap. *Bio/Technology* **10,** 30–32.

Griffiths, J.B. (1985). Cell products: an overview. In *Animal Cell Biotechnology*, Vol. 2. R.E. Spier and J.B. Griffiths, eds. (New York: Academic Press), pp. 3–13.

Grinnell, B.W., Berg, D.T., Walls, J., and Yan, S.B. (1987). Trans-activated expression of fully gamma-carboxylated recombinant human protein C, an anti-thrombotic factor. *Bio/Technology* **5,** 1189–1192.

Hancock, W.S., Canova-Davis, E., Chloupek, R.C., Wu, S-L., Baldonado, P., Battersby, J.E., Spellman, M.W., Basa, L.J., and Chakel, J.A. (1988). The characterization of degradation products of human growth hormone. In *Therapeutic Peptides and Proteins: Assessing the New Technologies*. D.R. Marshak and D.T. Liu, eds. (New York: Cold Spring Harbor Laboratory), pp. 95–118.

Hayakawa, T. (1988). Quality control of biotechnological therapeutic agents intended for use in Japan. In *Therapeutic Peptides and Proteins: Assessing the New Technologies*. D.R. Marshak and D.T. Liu, eds. (New York: Cold Spring Harbor Laboratory), pp. 309–330.

Heinrikson, R.L. (1988). Purification and characterization of recombinant proteins: the example of human renin. In *Therapeutic Peptides and Proteins: Assessing the New Technologies*. D.R. Marshak and D.T. Liu, eds. (New York: Cold Spring Harbor Laboratory), pp. 23–38.

Heinrikson, R.L. and Tomasselli, A.G. (1991). Purification and characterization of recombinant proteins: opportunities and challenges. In *Purification and Analysis of Recombinant Proteins*. R. Seetharam and S.K. Sharma, eds. (New York: Marcel Dekker), pp. 3–28.

Hernandez, M., Nieto, J.A., Sobradillo, B., Pombo, M., Ferrandez, D., and Rejas, J. (1991). Multicenter clinical trial to evaluate the therapeutic use of recombinant human growth hormone from mammalian cells in the treatment of growth hormone neurosecretory dysfunction. *Hormone Res.* **35,** 13–18.

Hiller, S. (1991). A better way to make the medicine go down. *Science* **253,** 1095–1096.

Hillman, R.S. (1990). Hematopoietic agents: growth factors, minerals, and vitamins. In *The Pharmacological Basis of Therapeutics.* A. Goodman Gilman, T.W. Rall, A.S. Nies, and P. Taylor, eds. (New York: Pergamon Press), pp. 1277–1310.

Hodgson, J. (1991a). Making monoclonals in microbes. *Bio/Technology* **9,** 421–425.

Hodgson, J. (1991b). Checking sources: the serum supply secret. *Bio/Technology* **9,** 1320–1324.

Hodgson, J. (1991c). Mastering biology. *Bio/Technology* **9,** 926–928.

Hodgson, J. (1991d). Substitutes for human blood. *Bio/Technology* **9,** 696.

Hodgson, J. (1993). Prestidigitation on the clinic: "magic bullets" — are they homing in on disease or just inducing HAMA horror? *Bio/Technology* **11,** 159–162.

Hoffman, M. (1991). New role found for a common protein "motif". *Science* **253,** 253.

Hood, L.E., Weissman, I.L., Wood, W.B., and Wilson, J.H. (1984). *Immunology* (Reading, Massachusetts: Benjamin/Cummings Co.).

Hopkins, T.R. (1991). Physical and chemical cell disruption for the recovery of intracellular proteins. In *Purification and Analysis of Recombinant Proteins.* R. Seetharam and S.K. Sharma, eds. (New York: Marcel Dekker), pp. 57–84.

Hoyer, L.W. and Drohan, W.N. (eds.) (1991). *Recombinant Technology in Hemostasis and Thrombosis* (New York: Plenum Press).

Jaenicke, R. and Rudolph, R. (1989). Folding proteins. In *Protein Structure: A Practical Approach.* T.E. Creighton, ed. (New York: IRL Press), pp. 191–223.

Johnson, I.S. (1982). Authenticity and purity of human insulin (recombinant DNA). *Diabetes Care* **5** (Suppl. 2), 4–12.

Johnston, J. (1991). Therapeutic frankenkines start clinical trials. *J. NIH Res.* **3,** 36–37.

Kadouri, A. and Bohak, Z. (1985). Production of plasminogen activators by cells in culture. *Adv. in Biotechnological Processes* **5,** 275–299.

Kahn, C.R. and Shechter, Y. (1990). Insulin, oral hypoglycemic agents, and the pharmacology of the endocrine pancreas. In *The Pharmacological Basis of Therapeutics.* A. Goodman Gilman, T.W. Rall, A.S. Nies, and P. Taylor, eds. (New York: Pergamon Press), pp. 1463–1495.

Kang, C-Y., Nara, P., Soulamia, C., Caralli, V., Chen, A., Nguyen, M-L., Yoshiyama, H., Morrow, W.J.W., Ho, D.D., and Kohler, H. (1992). Anti-idiotype monoclonal antibody elicits broadly neutralizing anti-gp120 antibodies in monkeys. *Proc. Natl. Acad. Sci. USA* **89,** 2546–2550.

Kearns, M.J. (1990). Integrated design for mammalian cell culture. *Bio/Technology* **8,** 409–413.

Kelly, P.A. (1990). Growth hormone and prolactin. In *Hormones: From Molecules to Disease.* E-E. Baulieu and P.A. Kelly, eds. (New York: Chapman and Hall), pp. 189–217.

Klausner, A. (1986). Researchers probe second-generation t-PA. *Bio/Technology* **4,** 707–711.

Klausner, A. (1987). Second-generation t-PA race heats up. *Bio/Technology* **5,** 869–870.

Kobata, A. and Takasaki, S. (1992). Structure and biosynthesis of cell surface carbohydrates. In *Cell Surface Carbohydrates and Cell Development.* M. Fukuda, ed. (London: CRC Press), pp. 1–24.

Konrad, M. (1989). Immunogenicity of proteins administered to humans for therapeutic purposes. *TIBTECH* **7,** 175–179.

Kresze, G-B. (1991). Proteases during purification. In *Purification and Analysis of Recombinant Proteins.* R. Seetharam and S.K. Sharma, eds. (New York: Marcel Dekker), pp. 85–120.

Kuret, J.A. and Murad, F. (1990). Adenohypophyseal hormones and related substances. In *The Pharmacological Basis of Therapeutics.* A. Goodman Gilman, T.W. Rall, A.S. Nies, and P. Taylor, eds. (New York: Pergamon Press), pp. 1334–1360.

Kurnick, J.T. and McCluskey, R.T. (1990). Perspectives on cell mediated immunity in vivo. In *Lymphokines and the Immune Response.* S. Cohen, ed. (Boca Raton, FL: CRC Press), pp. 1–28.

Lally, E.V. (1991). Therapeutic application of monoclonal antibodies in the rheumatic diseases. In *Monoclonal Antibodies, Cytokines, and Arthritis.* T.F. Kresina, ed. (New York: Marcel Dekker), pp. 37–56.

Langer, R. (1990). New methods of drug delivery. *Science* **249,** 1527–1533.

Langer, L.J. (1993). Validation issues and the development of new product assays stressed at BioEast'93. *Genetic Engineering News* **13,** February 15, 1–28.

Lau, D., Kuzma, G., Wei, C-M., Livingston, D.J., and Hsiung, N. (1987). A modified human tissue plasminogen activator with extended half-life *in vivo. Bio/Technology* **5,** 953–958.

Le, H.V. and Trotta, P.P. (1991). Purification of secreted recombinant proteins from *Escherichia coli.* In *Purification and Analysis of Recombinant Proteins.* R. Seetharam and S.K. Sharma, eds. (New York: Marcel Dekker), pp. 163–181.

Leamon, C.P. and Low, P.S. (1991). Delivery of macromolecules into living cells: a method that exploits folate receptor endocytosis. *Proc. Natl. Acad. Sci. USA* **88,** 5572–5576.

Leff, D.N. (1991). Monoclonal OKT3 saves transplants, may induce cancer. *J. NIH Res.* **3,** 37–38.

Lerner, R.A., Benkovic, S.J., and Schultz, P.G. (1991). At crossroads of chemistry and immunology: catalytic antibodies. *Science* **252,** 659–667.

Lerner, R.A. and Tramontano, A. (1988). Catalytic antibodies. *Sci. Am.* **258,** No. 3, 58–70.

LoBuglio, A.F., Wheeler, R.H., Trang, J., Haynes, A., Rogers, K., Harvey, E.B., Sun, L., Ghrayeb, J., and Khazaeli, M.B. (1989). Mouse/human chimeric monoclonal antibody in man: kinetics and immune response. *Proc. Natl. Acad. Sci. USA* **86,** 4220–4224.

Madison, E.L., Goldsmith, E.J., Gerard, R.D., Gething, M-J.H., and Sambrook, J.F. (1989). Serpin-resistant mutant of human tissue-type plasminogen activator. *Nature* **339,** 721–724.

Maiorella, B.L., Winkelhake, J., Young, J., Moyer, B., Bauer, R., Hora, M., Andya, J., Thomson, J., Patel, T., and Parekh, R. (1993). Effect of culture conditions on IgM antibody structure, pharmacokinetics and activity. *Bio/Technology* **11,** 387–392.

Marafino, Jr., B.J., Young, J.D., Greenfield, I.L., and Kopplin, J.R. (1988). The appropriate toxicological testing of recombinant human proteins. In *Therapeutic Peptides and Proteins: Assessing the New Technologies.* D.R. Marshak and D.T. Liu, eds. (New York: Cold Spring Harbor Laboratory), pp. 175–187.

Margaritis, A. and Bassi, A.S. (1991). Plasmid stability of recombinant DNA microorganisms. In *Recombinant DNA Technology and Applications.* A. Prokop, R.K. Bajpai, and C. Ho, eds. (New York: McGraw-Hill), pp. 316–332.

Mark, D.F., Lu, S.D., Creasy, A.A., Yamamoto, R., and Lin, L.S. (1984). Site-specific mutagenesis of the human fibroblast interferon gene. *Proc. Natl. Acad. Sci. USA* **81,** 5662–5666.

Martial, J.A., Hallewell, R.A., Baxter, J.A., and Goodman, H.M. (1979). Human growth hormone: complementary DNA cloning and expression in bacteria. *Science* **205,** 602–606.

Masuho, Y. (1992). Passive immunoprophylaxis with human monoclonal antibodies. In *Vaccines: New Approaches to Immunological Problems.* R.W. Ellis, ed. (Boston: Butterworth-Heinemann), pp. 405–430.

Mathias, S.F., Franks, F., and Hatley, R.H.M. (1991). The stabilization of proteins by freeze-drying and by alternative methods. In *Polypeptide and Protein Drugs: Production, Characterization and Formulation.* R.C. Hider and D. Barlow, eds. (Chichester: Ellis Horwood), pp. 120–131.

McKillip, E.R., Giles, A.S., Levner, M.H., Hung, P.P., and Hjorth, R.N. (1991). Growth of transformed C-127 cell in bioreactors for large-scale t-PA production. *Bio/Technology* **9,** 805–812.

Melnick, J.L. (1985). Virus vaccines: an overview. In *High-technology Route to Virus Vaccines.* G.R. Dreesman, J.G. Bronson, and R.C. Kennedy, eds. (Washington, DC: American Society for Microbiology), pp. 1–14.

Mernaugh, R.L., Bright, R.K., and Kennedy, R.C. (1992). Active immunization strategies using anti-idiotypic antibodies. In *Vaccines: New Approaches to Immunological Problems.* R.W. Ellis, ed. (Boston: Butterworth-Heinemann), pp. 391–404.

Micklos, D.A. and Freyer, G.A. (1990). *DNA Science: A First Course in Recombinant DNA Technology* (New York: Cold Spring Harbor Laboratory).

Miller, H.I. (1988). FDA and biotechnology. *Bio/Technology* **6,** 1385–1392.

Miozzari, G.F. (1981). Strategies for obtaining expression of peptide hormones in *E. coli.* In *Insulins, Growth Hormones, and Recombinant DNA Technology.* J.L. Gueriguian, ed. (New York: Raven Press), pp. 13–31.

Moore, J.P. and Weiss, R.A. (1991). Passive primate protection. *Nature* **352,** 376–377.

Moss, B. (1991). Vaccinia virus: a tool for research and vaccine development. *Science* **252,** 1662–1667.

Moss, B. (1992). Vaccinia virus vectors. In *Vaccines: New Approaches to Immunological Problems.* R.W. Ellis, ed. (Boston: Butterworth-Heinemann), pp. 345–362.

Nelson, K.L. (1991). Biopharmaceutical plant design. In *Recombinant DNA Technology and Applications.* A. Prokop, R.K. Bajpai, and C. Ho, eds. (New York: McGraw-Hill), pp. 509–565.

Neta, R., Oppenheim, J.J., and Durum, S.K. (1990). The cytokine concept: historical perspectives and current status of the cloned cytokines. In *Lymphokines and the Immune Response.* S. Cohen, ed. (Boca Raton, FL: CRC Press), pp. 29–42.

Netzer, W.J. (1988). Antibodies that mimic drug receptors: a new tool in pharmaceutical R & D. *Bio/Technology* **6,** 38–40.

News Briefs (1993). FDA approves Cytogen's monoclonal imaging agent. *Bio/Technology* **11,** 136.

Ogra, P.L. and Garofalo, R. (1990). Secretory antibody response to viral vaccines. In *Progress in Medical Virology,* Vol. 37. J.L. Melnick, ed. (New York: Karger), pp. 156–189.

Oldshue, J.Y. and Bajpai, R.K. (1991). Mixing equipment for bioreactors and their scale-up. In *Recombinant DNA Technology and Applications.* A. Prokop, R.K. Bajpai, and C. Ho, eds. (New York: McGraw-Hill), pp. 460–476.

Olson, K.C., Fenno, J., Lin, N., Harkins, R.N., Snider, C., Kohr, W.H., Ross, M.J., Fodge, D., Prender, G., and Stebbing, N. (1981). Purified human growth hormone from *E. coli* is a biologically active. *Nature* **293,** 408–411.

Osborn, J.E. (1988). Viruses as contaminants. In *Therapeutic Peptides and Proteins: Assessing New Technologies.* D.R. Marshak and D.T. Liu, eds. (New York: Cold Spring Harbor Laboratory), pp. 137–149.

Palca, J. (1989). New AIDS drugs take careful aim. *Science* **246,** 1559–1560.

Pannekoek, H., de Vries, C., and von Zonneveld, A-J. (1988). Mutants of tissue-type plasminogen activator (t-PA): structural aspects and functional properties. *Fibrinolysis* **2,** 123–132.

Papoutsakis, E.T. (1991). Product recovery and purification: an overview. In *Recombinant DNA Technology and Applications.* A. Prokop, R.K. Bajpai, and C. Ho, eds. (New York: McGraw-Hill), pp. 357–412.

Pardridge, W.M. (1991). *Peptide Drug Delivery to the Brain* (New York: Raven Press).

Parekh, R.B., Dwek, R.A., Rudd, P.M., Thomas, J.R., Rademacher, T.W., Warren, T., Wun, T.-C., Hebert, B., Reitz, B., Palmier, M., Ramabhadran, T., and Tiemeier, D.C. (1989). N-Glycosylation and *in vitro* enzymatic activity of human recombinant tissue plasminogen activator expressed in Chinese hamster ovary cells and a murine cell line. *Biochemistry* **28,** 7670–7679.

Pastan, I. and FitzGerald, D. (1991). Recombinant toxins for cancer treatment. *Science* **254,** 1173–1177.

Pastan, I., Willingham, M.C., and FitzGerald, D.J.P. (1986). *Immunotoxins. Cell* **47,** 641–648.

Patthy, L. (1985). Evolution of the proteases of blood coagulation and fibrinolysis by assembly from modules. *Cell* **41,** 657–663.

Pavlakis, G.N. and Hamer, D.H. (1983). Regulation of metallothionein-growth hormone hybrid gene in bovine papilloma virus. *Proc. Natl. Acad. Sci. USA* **80,** 397–401.

Peetermans, J.H. (1991). Development and quality assessment of vaccines. In *Polypeptide and Protein Drugs: Production, Characterization and Formulation.* R.C. Hider and D. Barlow, eds. (Chichester: Ellis Horwood), pp. 167–180.

Petricciani, J.C. (1985). Regulatory considerations for products derived from the new biotechnology. In *Large-scale Mammalian Cell Culture.* J. Feder and W.R. Tolbert, eds. (New York: Academic Press), pp. 79–86.

Pluckthun, A. (1991). Antibody engineering: advances from use of *Escherichia coli* expression systems. *Bio/Technology* **9,** 545–551.

PMA Survey Report (1991). *Biotechnology Medicines in Development* (Washington, DC: Pharmaceutical Manufacturers Association).

Poole, S. (1991). Pyrogen testing of polypeptide and protein drugs. In *Polypeptide and Protein Drugs: Production, Characterization and Formulation.* R.C. Hider and D. Barlow, eds. (Chichester: Ellis Horwood), pp. 146–153.

Potera, C. (1992). Somatogen's hemoglobin proves promising. *Genetic Engineering News* April 15, 1–12.

Pramik, M.J. (1991). Conference addresses issues on stabilizing cell cultures. *Genetic Engineering News* June, 1–27.

Prokop, A. and Bajpai, R.K. (1991). Bioreactor design and operation. In *Recombinant DNA Technology and Applications.* A. Prokop, R.K. Bajpai, and C. Ho, eds. (New York: McGraw-Hill), pp. 415–459.

Rademacher, T.W., Parekh, R.B., and Dwek, R.A. (1988). Glycobiology. *Ann. Rev. Biochem.* **57,** 785–838.

Ramabhadran, T.V. (1987). Products from genetically engineered mammalian cells: benefits and risk factors. *TIBTECH* **5,** 175–179.

Raney, A.K. and McLachlan, A. (1991). The biology of hepatitis B virus. In *Molecular Biology of the Hepatitis B Virus.* A. McLachlan, ed. (Boston: CRC Press), pp. 1–37.

Ratner, M. (1990). T-PA trials, tribulations, and litigation. *Bio/Technology* **8,** 385–387.

Ratner, M. (1991). When microheterogeneity matters. *Bio/Technology* **9,** 25.

Rinas, U., Risse, B., Jaenicke, R., Broker, M., Karges, H.E., Kupper, H.A., and Zettlmeissl, G. (1990). Characterization of recombinant factor XIIIa produced in *Saccharomyces cerevisiae. Bio/Technology* **8,** 543–546.

Rinas, U., Tsai, L.B., Lyons, D., Fox, G.M., Stearns, G., Fieschko, J., Fenton, D., and Bailey, J.E. (1992). Cysteine to serine substitutions in basic fibroblast growth factor: effect on inclusion body formation and proteolytic susceptibility during *in vitro* refolding. *Bio/Technology* **10,** 435–440.

Ross, M.J. (1981). Production of medically important polypeptides using recombinant DNA technology. In *Insulins, Growth Hormone, and Recombinant DNA Technology.* J.L. Gueriguian, ed. (New York: Raven Press), pp. 33–48.

Runge, M.S., Bode, C., Matsueda, G.R., and Haber, E. (1987). Antibody-enhanced thrombolysis: targeting of tissue plasminogen activator *in vivo. Proc. Natl. Acad. Sci. USA* **84,** 7659–7662.

Runge, M.S., Quertermous, T., Zavodny, P.J., Love, T.W., Bode, C., Frietag, M., Shaw, S-Y., Huang, P.L., Chou, C-C., Mullins, D., Schnee, J.M., Savard, C.E., Rothenberg, M.E., Newell, J.B., Matsueda, G.R., and Haber, E. (1991). A recombinant chimeric plasminogen activator with high affinity for fibrin has increased thrombolytic potency *in vitro* and *in vivo. Proc. Natl. Acad. Sci. USA* **88,** 10337–10341.

Rybak, S.M., Hoogenboom, H.R., Meade, H.M., Raus, J.C.M., Schwarz, D., and Youle, R.J. (1992). Humanization of immunotoxins. *Proc. Natl. Acad. Sci. USA* **89,** 3165–3169.

Sawyer, S.T. (1991). The physiology and biochemistry of erythropoietin receptors. In *Erythropoietin: Molecular, Cellular, and Clinical Biology.* A.J. Erslev, J.W. Adamson, J.W. Eschbach, and C.G. Winearls, eds. (Baltimore: Johns Hopkins University Press), pp. 115–132.

Schwartz, R.S. (1991). Clinical trials of factor VIII produced by recombinant technology. In *Recombinant DNA Technology in Hemostasis and Thrombosis.* L.W. Hoyer and W.N. Drohan, eds. (New York: Plenum Press), pp. 229–234.

Scott, M.G. and Fleischman, J.B. (1991). Monoclonal antibodies in diagnostic medicine. *In Recombinant DNA Technology and Applications.* A. Prokop, R.K. Bajpai, and C. Ho, eds. (New York: McGraw-Hill), pp. 255–282.

Seabrook, R. and Atkinson, T. (1991). Modified antibodies. In *Principles and Practice of Immunoassay.* C.P. Price and D.J. Newman, eds. (New York: Stockton Press), pp. 53–77.

Shami, E.Y., Rothstein, A., and Ramjeesingh, M. (1989). Stabilization of biologically active proteins. *TIBTECH* **7,** 186–190.

Sherwood, J.K., Dause, R.B., and Saltzman, W.M. (1992). Controlled antibody delivery systems. *Bio/Technology* **10,** 1446–1449.

Sjodin, L. (1988). Regulatory aspects of drugs produced by recombinant DNA technology. In *Therapeutic Peptides and Proteins: Assessing the New Technologies.* D.R. Marshak and D.T. Liu, eds. (New York: Cold Spring Harbor Laboratory), pp. 293–298.

Snape, T.J. (1991). Assuring the quality of plasma products. In *Polypeptide and Protein Drugs: Production, Characterization and Formulation.* R.C. Hider and C. Barlow, eds. (Chichester: Ellis Horwood), pp. 181–188.

Spalding, B.J. (1991a). Cancer immunoconjugates: will clinical success lead to commercial success? *Bio/Technology* **9,** 700–704.

Spalding, B.J. (1991b). Downstream processing: key to slashing production costs 100 fold. *Bio/Technology* **9,** 229–235.

Spalding, B.J. (1991c). A growth market for bioreactors? *Bio/Technology* **9,** 338–341.

Spalding, B.J. (1992). In hot pursuit of an HIV vaccine. *Bio/Technology* **10,** 24–29.

Spivak, J.L. and Cotes, P.M. (1991). The pharmacokinetics and metabolism of erythropoietin. In *Erythropoietin: Molecular, Cellular, and Clinical Biology.* A.J. Erslev, J.W. Adamson, J.W. Eschbach, and C.G. Winearls, eds. (Baltimore: Johns Hopkins University Press), pp. 162–183.

Stebbing, N. (1988). Risk assessment of recombinant DNA-derived proteins. In *Therapeutic Peptides and Proteins: Assessing the New Technologies.* D.R. Marshak and D.T. Liu, eds. (New York: Cold Spring Harbor Laboratory), pp. 189–200.

Sterling, J. (1993). Septic shock products jockey for position after Centocor pulls Centoxin from trials. *Genetic Engineering News* **13,** February 1, 1–16.

Storring, P.L. (1988). The role of biological assays in evaluating purified peptide and protein products. In *Therapeutic Proteins and Peptides: Assessing New*

Technologies. D.L. Marshak and D.T. Liu, eds. (New York: Cold Spring Harbor Laboratory), pp. 119–134.

Stover, C.K., de la Cruz, V.F., Fuerst, T.R., Burlein, J.E., Benson, L.A., Bennet, L.T., Bansal, G.P., Young , J.F., Lee, M.H., Hatfull, G.F., Snapper, S.B., Barletta, R.G., Jacobs Jr., W.R., and Bloom, B.R. (1991). New use of BCG recombinant vaccines. *Nature* **351,** 456–460.

Swanson, M.E., Martin, M.J., O'Donnell, J.K., Hoover, K., Lago, W., Huntress, V., Parsons, C.T., Pinkert, C.A., Pilder, S., and Logan, J.S. (1992). Production of functional human hemoglobin in transgenic swine. *Bio/Technology* **10,** 557–559.

Thanavala, Y. (1989). Anti-idiotype vaccines. *TIBTECH* **7,** 62–66.

Van Brunt, J. (1989). Novel drug delivery systems. *Bio/Technology* **7,** 127–130.

Van Brunt, J. (1990). The importance of glycoform heterogeneity. *Bio/Technology* **8,** 995.

van Leen, R.W., Bakhuis, J.G., van Beckhoven, R.F.W.C., Burger, H., Dorssers, L.C.J., Hommes, R.W.J., Lemson, P.J., Noordam, B., Persoon, N.L.M., and Wagemaker, G. (1991). Production of human interleukin-3 using industrial microorganisms. *Bio/Technology* **9,** 47–52.

Vapnek, D., Egrie, J.C., Browne, J.K., Lai, P., Lin, F-K., Arakawa, T., and Strickland, T.W. (1988). Comparative studies of natural and recombinant human erythropoietin. In *Therapeutic Peptides and Proteins: Assessing the New Technologies*. D.L. Marshak and D.T. Liu, eds. (New York: Cold Spring Harbor Laboratory), pp. 241–256.

Varki, A. (1992). Role of oligosaccharides in the intracellular and intercellular trafficking of mammalian glycoproteins. In *Cell Surface Carbohydrates and Cell Development*. M. Fukuda, ed. (London: CRC Press), pp. 25–69.

Waldmann, T.A. (1991). Monoclonal antibodies in diagnosis and therapy. *Science* **252,** 1657–1662.

Wang, A., Lu, S-D., and Mark, D.F. (1984). Site-specific mutagenesis of the human interleukin-2 gene: structure–function analysis of the cysteine residues. *Science* **224,** 1431–1433.

Ward, R.H.R., Capon, D.J., Jett, C.M., Murthy, K.K., Mordenti, J., Lucas, C., Frie, S.W., Prince, A.M., Green, J.D., and Eichberg, J.W. (1991). Prevention of HIV-1 infection in chimpanzees by CD4 immunoadhesin. *Nature* **352,** 434–436.

Weatherall, M. (1990). *In Search of a Cure* (Oxford: Oxford University Press).

Whitley, R.J. and Meignier, B. (1992). Herpes simplex vaccines. In *Vaccines: New Approaches to Immunological Problems*. R.W. Ellis, ed. (Boston: Butterworth-Heinemann), pp. 223–254.

Wielburski, A. (1991). Genotropin–recombinant human growth hormone. In *Polypeptide and Protein Drugs: Production, Characterization and Formulation*. R.C. Hider and D. Barlow, eds. (Chichester: Ellis Horwood), pp. 197–210.

Wilson, T. (1984). More protein from mammalian cells. *Bio/Technology* **2,** 753–755.

Winter, G. and Milstein, C. (1991). Man-made antibodies. *Nature* **349,** 293–299.

Wolff, S.P. (1992). Trying time of human insulin. *Nature* **356,** 375–376.

Yeh, P., Landais, D., Lemaitre, M., Maury, I., Crenne, J.-Y., Becquart, J., Murry-Brelier, A., Boucher, F., Montay, G., Fleer, R., Hirel, P.-H., Mayaux, J.-F., and

Klatzmann, D. (1992). Design of yeast-secreted albumin derivatives for human therapy: biological and antiviral properties of serum albumin–CD4 genetic conjugate. *Proc. Natl. Acad. Sci. USA* **89,** 1904–1908.

Yoneyama, T. (1990). Hepatitis B surface antigen expressed in murine cells. In *Progress in Medical Virology,* Vol. 37. J.L. Melnick, ed. (New York: Karger), pp. 223–245.

Zonneveld, A-J. von, Veerman, H., and Pannekoek, H. (1986). Autonomous functions of structural domains of human tissue-type plasminogen activator. *Proc. Natl. Acad. Sci. USA* **83,** 4670–4674.

4

Molecular pharmacology

Today's pharmaceutical industry was founded on the productive interactions between the disciplines of synthetic organic chemistry and pharmacology, which occurred at the beginning of the twentieth century. This alliance has led to the production of many small organic molecules with effective therapeutic properties (Weatherall, 1990; Maxwell and Eckhardt, 1990; Silverman, 1992). In contrast, the first phase of pharmaceutical biotechnology was focused primarily on large proteins as drugs. This early phase of biotechnology is undergoing a rapid change as the second phase is spurred forward by the exciting developments in molecular biology and cell biology during the last decade (Gibbons, 1992). These developments are forging a fusion of biotechnology with the traditional methods of drug discovery.

In the early period of drug development, although the concept of molecular or macromolecular "receptors" was widely accepted, receptors were difficult to obtain as isolated, purified preparations. Therefore, pharmacologists could only rely on whole animals and tissue fragments to identify drugs and characterize their action on the putative receptors (Weatherall, 1990; Hodgson, 1992). Advances in biochemistry, enzymology, protein purification methods, and methods of analytical chemistry, although not supplanting the need for whole animal studies, have paved the way for the use of more defined and reproducible receptor preparations for the characterization of drug candidates. However, the development of these defined systems was an arduous process. The advent of rDNA and monoclonal antibody technologies has greatly facilitated this process. This, in turn, has led to the acceleration of the discovery and developments in pharmacology at the molecular level. The approach to drug development using defined molecular receptor components of biological systems in lieu of complex receptor preparations of the past era is termed "molecular pharmacology".

Recent developments in molecular pharmacology hold great promise for the development of novel and specific drugs. The cloning of genes for pharmacologically relevant proteins, revealing their primary sequences and their interrelatedness, has produced structural information on an unprecedented scale. The ability to create cell biological model systems expressing the selected proteins, removed from other closely related proteins of similar function often co-expressed in the natural tissue, has made possible the detailed structural and functional study of receptor macromolecules. By using cloned receptor genes, novel, chimeric assay systems providing easily quantifiable end points and high throughputs are being developed to facilitate the rapid and rational screening of drug candidates (Lester, 1988; Lleonart *et al.,* 1990; Harvey, 1991; Hodgson, 1992; Edgington, 1992a). Highly specific monoclonal antibodies raised against n drug target proteins, and gene probes specific for their mRNAs of these protein targets, have been valuable in delineating the sites of expression. Antibodies are also valuable tools for structure–function studies of proteins (Bahouth *et al.,* 1991; Goldberg, 1991). These biotechnological advances are impacting almost every facet of pharmacological research (Harvey, 1991), and major pharmaceutical firms and smaller start-up companies are applying these tools and approaches to drug development (Netzer, 1990; Brown, 1992; Gibbons, 1992). It is not within the scope and the extent of the discussion here to address all of these aspects in any detail. Therefore, salient examples covering functional groups of proteins are discussed as a means of illustrating the general trends in molecular pharmacology. A few major disease areas wherein the understanding of protein function at the molecular level is paving the way for drug development opportunities are also discussed. Since the drugs sought through the approaches described here are likely to be small organic molecules, the regulatory considerations involved are not different from those already well established for traditional drugs now on the market, and, therefore, merit no special discussion here. Fundamental concepts in molecular and cell biology relating to the topics discussed here can be found in a number of excellent texts such as Alberts *et al.* (1989). Transgenic animals which provide models for deciphering disease mechanisms and for testing of drug candidates also represent a contribution of biotechnology to molecular pharmacology (Kolberg, 1992); this aspect is dealt with in greater detail in Chapter 7.

TECHNOLOGIES AND TECHNIQUES

Cloning of pharmacologically relevant genes and cDNAs

By using the molecular biological techniques described in Chapter 2, it is possible to clone genes or cDNAs for any protein, provided a short stretch of amino acid sequence is known. Oligonucleotide probes based on the amino acid sequence can be used to probe or screen "libraries" to isolate the complete gene or cDNA. More recently, the polymerase chain reaction (PCR) has become a powerful adjunct in gene isolation (Erlich *et al.,* 1991). Sequencing of the isolated gene or cDNA allows the deduction of the complete primary sequence of the protein.

Another strategy used successfully in gene isolation is called "expression cloning" (Sambrook *et al.,* 1989). This method is used when amino acid sequence information required for the design of oligonucleotide probes is unavailable, but an activity assay, an antibody, or a specific ligand to the protein

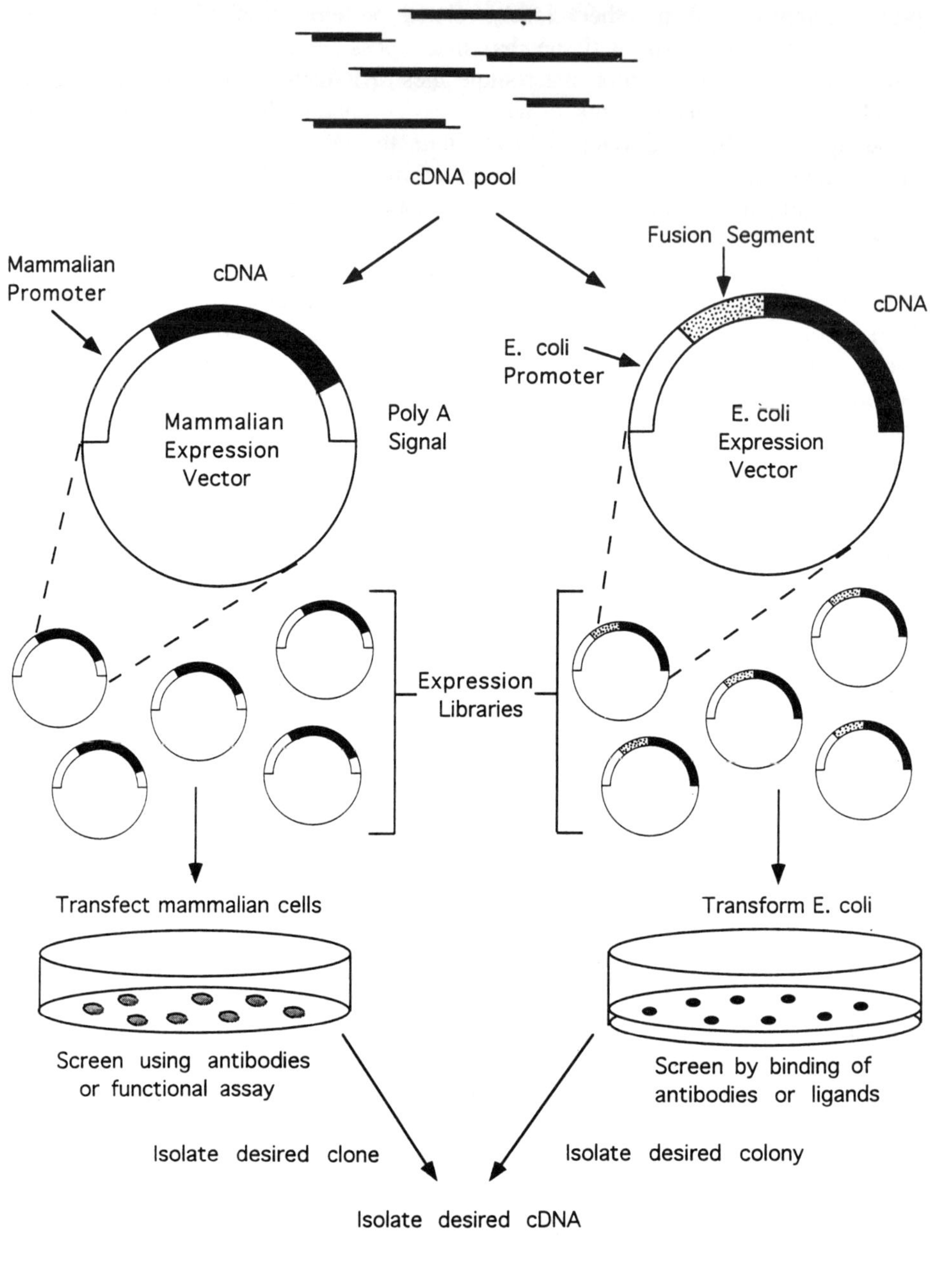

Fig. 4.1. Expression cloning of cDNAs and genes using mammalian and bacterial expression hosts.

of interest exists. Expression cloning depends on the detection of the expression of the protein of interest in cells transfected with a pool of cDNAs obtained from the tissue or cells known to produce the protein, as shown in Fig. 4.1. The method is applicable to genomic DNA fragments as well.

In expression cloning, a cDNA pool is obtained by reverse transcription of the total mRNA derived from a cell line or tissue. The cDNAs are cloned into a vector in such a way that they are transcribed into mRNA when the vector is introduced in the host cell. Alternatively, fragments of genomic DNA (containing introns) may be introduced directly into mammalian cells. The mRNA produced by the cDNA or the genomic DNA fragment is translated by the host to produce the protein of interest in an active form. Expression of the protein is detected by using antibodies or other specific ligands, or by using a functional assay. Some expression cloning systems, such as those using bacterial hosts, produce the protein as a fusion protein (Box 3.1, Chapter 3) which may or may not be biologically active. However, in most cases the fusion proteins retain their immunoreactivity, permitting their detection by using antibodies. The vector containing the cDNA of interest is isolated from the cells and enriched via multiple rounds of expression and purification until a single homogeneous cDNA species is isolated. Expression cloning can be performed by using bacteriophage or plasmid vectors with *E. coli* as host, or by using high-copy-number plasmid vectors or whole cell DNA in mammalian cells (Sambrook *et al.,* 1989), or in frog oocytes (Box 4.2; Snutch, 1988). Once a partial cDNA of interest is isolated, oligonucleotides designed from its sequence can be used to isolate the full-length form by the more conventional method of nucleic acid probing and by PCR methods.

Box 4.1. Specificity of nucleic acid hybridization reactions

Specific intrastrand and interstrand associations in nucleic acids occur through hydrogen bonding interactions between bases as described in Chapter 2. Such interactions occur between two strands of DNA or RNA, or between a strand of DNA and an RNA strand. It can also occur intramolecularly within the same strand of DNA or RNA. The strength of the interaction is dependent on the degree of base-pair complementarity between the strands and the base composition of the strands. A G:C base-pair interaction involving three hydrogen bonds is stronger than an A:T pair held together by two hydrogen bonds. The strength of interaction between strands is measured by the stability of the non-covalent strand association against disruptive forces which break hydrogen bonds and promote strand separation. Such disruptive forces include heat, low ionic strength, and extreme alkaline pH. The process of separation of the hydrogen-bonded strands is known as denaturation.

Hybridization reactions, in which denatured complementary nucleic acid strands are allowed to interact under controlled conditions of temperature, pH, and ionic strength, result in the reassociation of the strands (renaturation) by base pairing. The strength of the association of the renatured double-stranded nucleic acid molecule is determined by the degree of complementarity between the strands; perfectly matched strands are able to withstand a combination of higher temperatures and lower ionic strengths known as conditions of "high stringency". Conditions of "lower stringency" permit strands with varying degrees of base mismatches to associate and remain associated as shown in Fig. 4.2. At very low stringencies hybridization becomes indiscriminate.

Low stringency screening of libraries, or Northern or Southern blotting (Chapter 2) performed under low stringency conditions, using nucleic acid- or oligonucleotide-probes corresponding to a particular gene, permits the detection of related genes which differ from it by several base pairs. This technique has been used extensively in the isolation of members of several gene families.

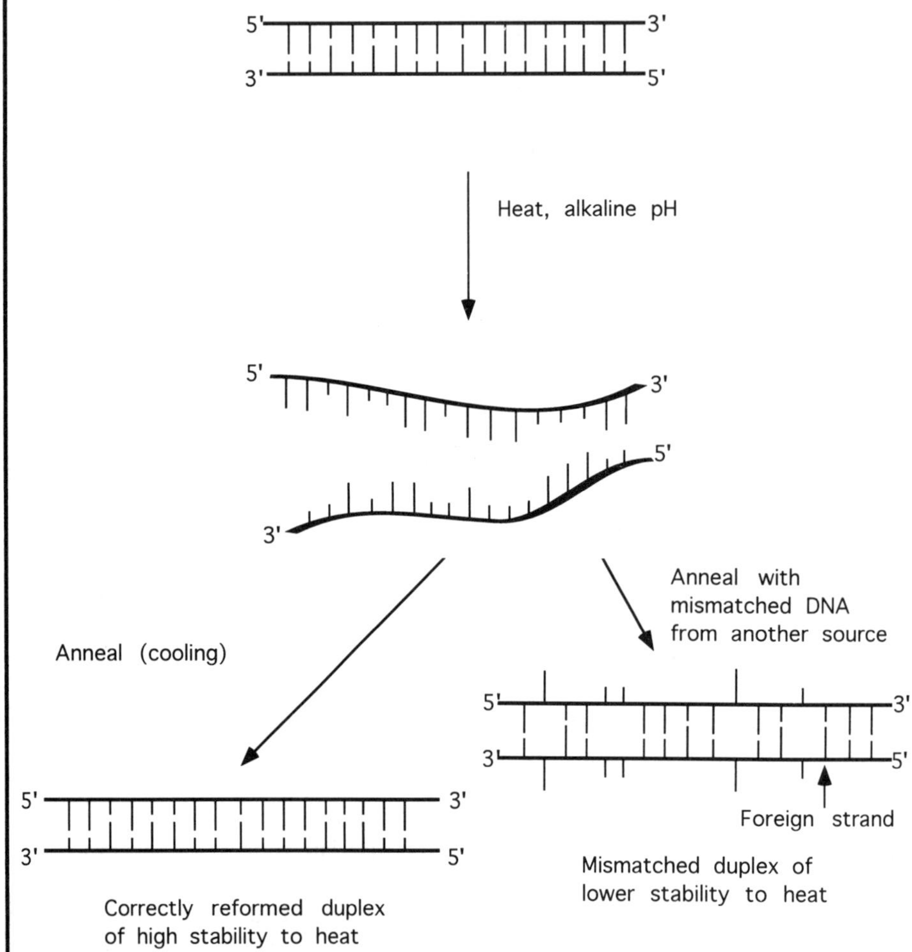

Fig. 4.2. Nucleic acid hybridization: annealing between complementary strands with perfect and partial complementarity.

Isolation of closely related genes belonging to gene families

Many receptors and other pharmacologically interesting proteins are members of families that contain common domains within which the amino acid sequences are identical or highly related. This relatedness is known as homology. Family members may be represented by separate genes in the genome, or may be derived by alternate splicing of the primary transcript of the same gene. Often, the homologies in a protein family extend beyond the family to a larger group of proteins performing a similar function. Such groups are called "superfamilies" (Edgington, 1992a). Thus, for example, the dopamine receptor family, originally thought to consist of two pharmacologically distinct members, has now been shown by cloning to contain five structurally distinct members (Sibley and Monsma, 1992). All the subtypes of the dopamine receptors belong to a larger "superfamily" of G protein-coupled receptors known as "seven pass" receptors because they traverse the cell membrane seven times.

Once a cDNA or the gene for one member of a family is isolated, the sequence similarities at the gene level can be used to isolate other members by probing libraries at lower "stringency" as described in Chapter 2 and detailed in Box 4.1. As noted in Chapter 2, because of the degeneracy of the genetic code, sequence identity at the amino acid level may not translate to sequence identity at the gene level. Therefore, sequence divergence at the gene or cDNA level is always greater than the divergence of amino acid sequence at the protein level.

Structural deductions from sequences

Amino acid sequences of proteins derived from cDNAs can be analyzed for structural features by examining the topological properties of amino acid stretches and by comparison of the sequence for homology to other proteins whose structural features and functions have been established (Green, 1990). Although some structural features may be evident on visual analysis of the sequence, several powerful computer algorithms are used for the detailed analysis of protein sequences. One of the key features detected by such analysis is stretches of hydrophobic amino acids (see Chapter 2) which indicate the presence of transmembrane segments. Multiple membrane-spanning segments, a characteristic of many receptors, ion channels, and pumps discussed below, have been detected by searching for hydrophobic regions in these protein sequences. These regions permit the classification and grouping of newly isolated receptors to families that have similar membrane organization. Comparison of a newly derived sequence with all other protein sequences stored in comprehensive data bases can reveal homologies which often suggest family grouping and possible function. Such comparative analysis also reveals ligand binding sites, potential sites for post-translational modifications, protease cleavage sites, binding sites for cofactors such as calcium ions or nucleotides, and structural motifs such as growth-factor-like domains. Further, some idea of the overall structure of the molecule can also be derived by secondary structure analysis of various regions (see Chapter 5; Green, 1990; Hardie, 1991). While sequence analysis methods are powerful and provide very meaningful insights into the structure of proteins, it is essential to realize that these are only predictive methods and that the predictions require experimental confirmation.

Expression

Cell systems expressing the genes or cDNAs of proteins of pharmacological interest are essential for the characterization of the protein and for the development of assay systems aimed at screening drug candidates. The principles of expression of recombinant genes have been discussed extensively in Chapter 2, but points of specific relevance to molecular pharmacology are further elaborated here. As with the production of protein drugs described in Chapter 3, a variety of expression systems are currently in use in molecular pharmacological studies. However, as the proteins are used in functional assays in this context, there is lesser emphasis on the absolute level of protein production, except in cases where structural studies require large amounts of material.

All expression systems, bacterial, fungal, insect cells, and mammalian cells, are useful tools in molecular pharmacology in different situations (Abbot, 1991; Hodgson, 1992). For many cell-surface molecules and receptors, mammalian cells are the best choice for the functional study of isolated proteins. Further, the use of a mammalian cell line that does not normally express the protein under study is helpful because experiments are not complicated by the endogenous expression of the same or a related protein. Mammalian cells are also appropriate because they are able to perform post-translational modifications and subcellular localizations which may be required for the functioning of some proteins. However, even in the case of mammalian expression, difficulties can be encountered with proteins such as membrane channels which are composed of multiple subunits. In such cases, each subunit has to be expressed at levels appropriate for the correct stoichiometric association and function. In addition, while cells expressing a protein such as a cell-surface receptor are ideal for receptor binding assays, they may be unsuitable for functional assays because they may lack accessory proteins and specific effector systems for eliciting the biological effect which follows the ligand–receptor interaction. Thus, cell lines used for expression require careful consideration based on the anticipated application. Mammalian cells can also be engineered to produce indicator cell systems that are useful in bioassays (Lleonart *et al.,* 1990; Hodgson, 1992).

Oocytes of the frog *Xenopus laevis* (Snutch, 1988; Gurdon and Wickens, 1983) represent an expression system which has been valuable to the isolation and characterization of many receptors and ion channels (Box 4.2). Frog oocytes are particularly useful for studying the function of multisubunit cell-surface proteins because rapid expression can be achieved by injecting a mixture of mRNAs corresponding to the subunits. Oocytes are amenable to electrophysiological studies which allow the functional characterization of expressed channels. Where multiple cDNAs encode slightly different forms of one subunit of a multisubunit receptor or channel, the oocyte system permits expression of the different members of that sub-family and delineation of the pharmacological properties conferred on the channel complex by the particular member subunit. In addition, receptors and channels modified by site-directed mutagenesis can also be characterized rapidly by expression in oocytes.

Oocytes contain many, but not all, of the activities required for the coupling of receptors to their second messenger pathways. However, as with any expression system, there are several important caveats in using oocytes in gene isolation and protein characterization (Snutch, 1988).

Box 4.2. Expression of gene products in *Xenopus* oocytes

Oocytes derived from the African frog *Xenopus laevis* provide an excellent system for the expression of injected messenger RNAs, resulting, in most cases, in the expression of active proteins (Snutch, 1988; Gurdon and Wickens, 1983). Oocytes are relatively large cells of around 1250 micrometers in diameter (compared to 10 to 100 micrometers of a typical mammalian cell). Their size makes them convenient for microinjection and for electrophysiological measurements. Oocytes are found in abundance in the ovaries of adult female frogs from where they can be removed surgically periodically over a few weeks. Harvested oocytes are separated from adherent follicle cell layers prior to the injection of mRNAs. Injection is performed using a micromanipulator setup with glass pipettes which are capable of delivering nanoliter (10^{-9} liters) volumes into the oocyte. Expression is monitored typically between 8 and 36 hours post-injection.

The *Xenopus* oocyte expression system can be used for characterization of products of specific mRNAs transcribed *in vitro* from cDNA isolates. Expression cloning of novel cDNAs, whose function can be assayed following expression, can also be performed using oocytes. In the latter case, as shown in Fig. 4.3, total mRNA is fractionated by size, and expression in oocytes is used to identify mRNA fractions capable of producing the protein of interest. The enriched mRNA fractions are used for cDNA preparation. The cDNA of interest is identified by its ability to select (by hybridization) its mRNA from the total mRNA pool. The selected mRNA is assayed again in oocytes, as shown in Fig. 4.3. Repeated rounds of this procedure with further enrichment of the desired cDNA from the pool leads to the isolation of the cDNA. Alternatively, *in vitro* transcription of the cDNA pool can also be used to generate mRNA for injection and assay. Component cDNAs of the pool that produces the desired proteins can be divided into smaller pools until pure cDNAs are isolated through rounds of repeated screening.

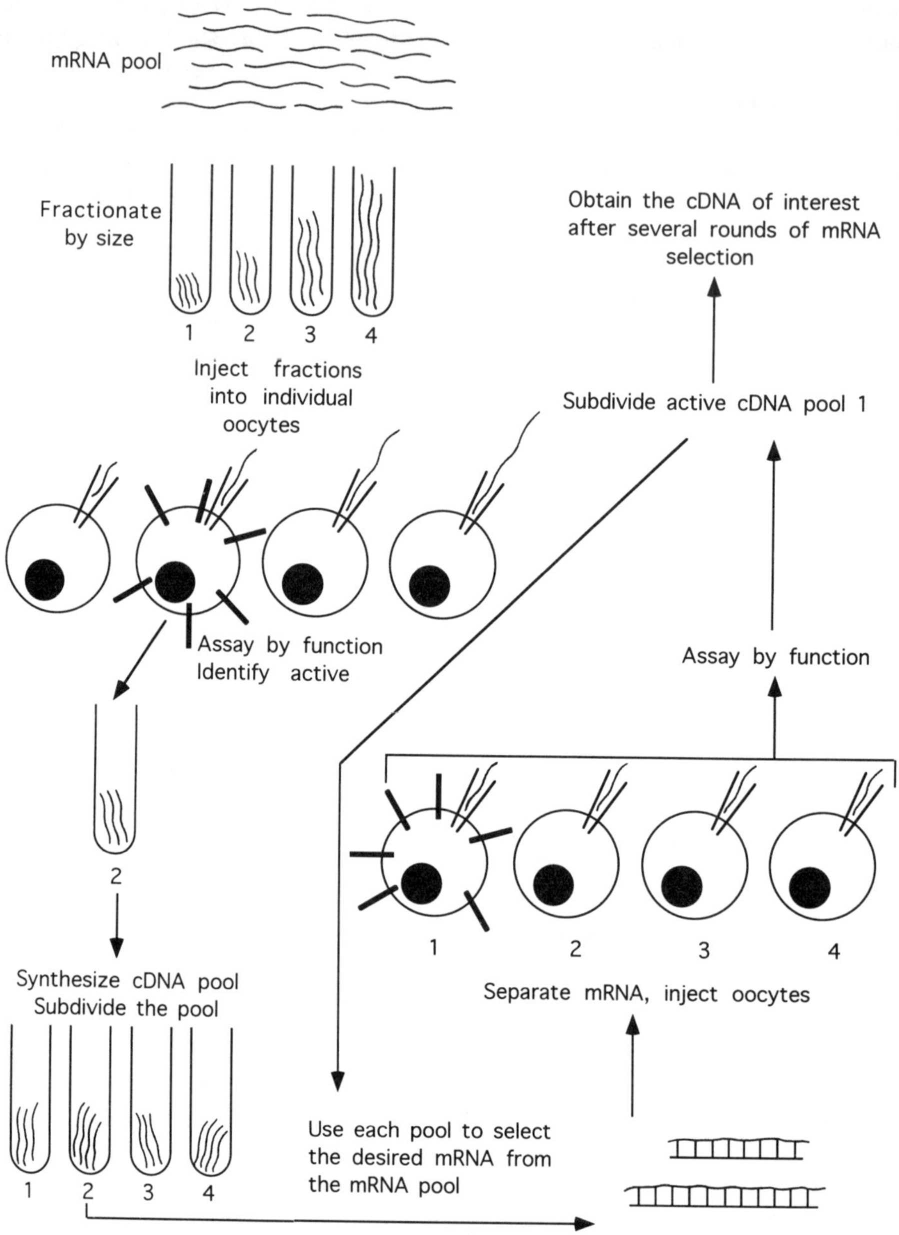

Fig. 4.3. Expression cloning of cDNAs using *Xenopus* oocytes.

Bacterial, fungal, and insect cell systems are useful, and often adequate, for the production and characterization of many intracellular enzymes of pharmacological significance. They are also useful for the production of receptors and other cell-surface molecules for binding studies. Many proteins can be obtained in an active form in these high expression systems in quantities required for structural studies and for the development of screening assays (Abbot, 1991; Hodgson, 1992). For instance, it has been possible to express and purify from *E. coli* the reverse transcriptase and the protease enzymes of the AIDS virus (HIV), which are key therapeutic targets (Graves *et al.,* 1988; Kohlstaedt *et al.,* 1992; Papas, 1990). Cell-surface receptors or their relevant domains can also be produced in high levels in *E. coli,* and can provide an abundant supply for drug screening using binding assays. In addition, genetics of *E. coli* and the yeast *Saccharomyces cerevisiae* are well studied, making these hosts amenable to genetic manipulation that is difficult or impossible in higher eukaryotic cells. Mammalian proteins can be expressed in yeast, and their activity can often be measured by simple enzymatic assays resulting in surrogate assay systems which provide great ease and economy of handling (Harvey, 1991; Abbot, 1991; Hodgson, 1992). For instance, yeast cells have been engineered to express the mammalian β-adrenergic receptor and its cognate mammalian effector protein. The system was so engineered that the agonist binding to the receptor resulted in morphological changes in the yeast colonies and in the induction of the "reporter" enzyme β-galactosidase (King *et al.,* 1990). Design of a typical surrogate assay using the yeast *Saccharomyces cerevisiae* is shown in Fig. 4.4. By using similar principles, other novel assays for studying protein–protein interactions have been developed in yeast cells (Fritz and Green, 1992).

Further, many of the mammalian proteins have counterparts in yeasts, and often mammalian proteins can substitute for the yeast proteins in situations where the resident yeast protein has been inactivated by mutation. In such cases, function of the mammalian protein is obligatory for the growth of the recombinant yeast. Recombinant yeast cells of this type can be used to screen for inhibitors of the mammalian protein by simple tests such as their ability to inhibit the formation of yeast colonies on nutrient agar plates. For instance, an assay based on this rationale has been developed for screening of immunosuppressive compounds which inhibit mammalian cyclophilins (Koltin *et al.,* 1991; Duronio *et al.,* 1992). The study of bacterial and phage genetics has also produced methodologies for the design of high-efficiency screening techniques which are useful for the isolation of receptor-specific peptide sequences and for improving their receptor affinities (Dower, 1992). This and other such novel advances are described in Chapter 9.

Insect cells infected with baculoviral vectors are useful for the high-level production of many proteins in a biologically active form and are finding increasing applications in the biotechnology industry (Glaser, 1993). Being evolutionarily and organizationally closer to mammalian cells than yeast cells, insect cells can perform many of the post-translational modifications found in mammalian cells. It is also possible to express heteromultimeric proteins such as ion channels in an active form. For example, GABA (the gamma amino butyric acid)-activated chloride channel composed of three distinct subunits has been expressed in a functionally and pharmacologically active form in insect cells (Carter *et al.,* 1992). Large amounts of proteins produced in this system can be used for binding and other activity assays, and for structural studies. Baculovirus-infected cells expressing ion channels are also useful in electrophysiological studies.

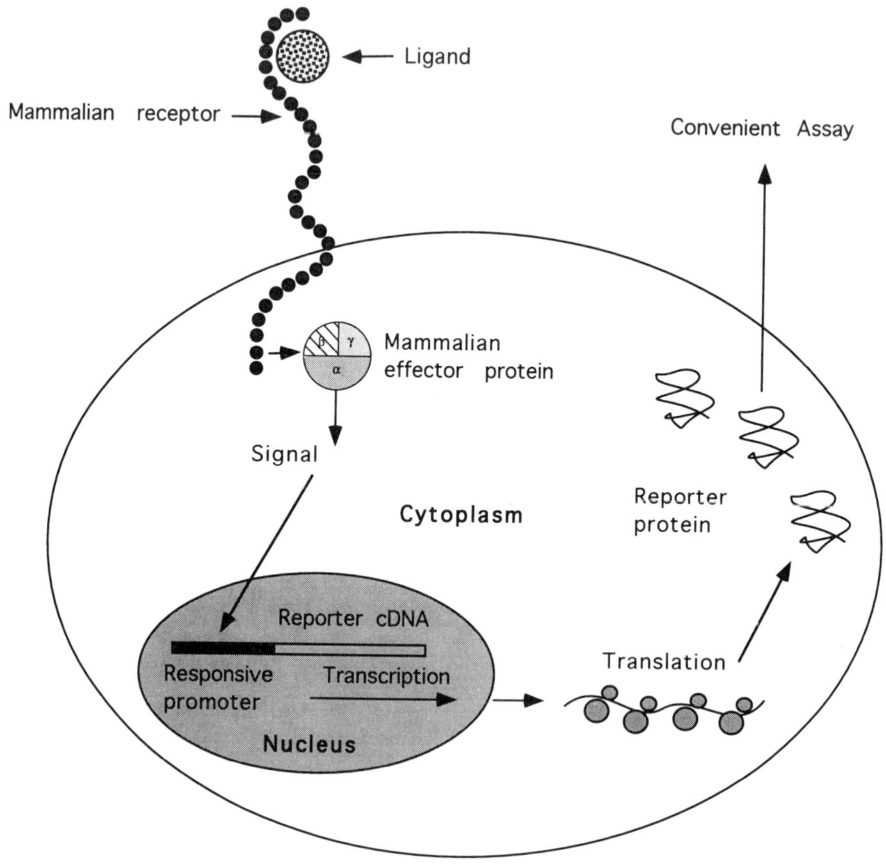

Fig. 4.4. A typical surrogate assay for a mammalian receptor in yeast cells.

In addition, rDNA technology has made possible the cloning of pathways for the production of therapeutic metabolites such as antibiotics and steroids in bacteria, yeasts and plants. These systems provide great economy of production of such therapeutic products (Bialy, 1990; Dixon, 1991; Elander and Chiang, 1991; Moffat, 1992). Because the focus of the chapter is on cellular macromolecules which act as drug receptors, these applications are not discussed here.

Antibodies

While cDNAs and oligonucleotides are useful for studies of the tissue-specific expression of receptor subtypes, the characterization of the receptors at the protein level is essential for defining the sites of expression and localization of proteins (Bahouth *et al.,* 1991). Antibodies bridge the gap between detection of RNA expression and the actual presence of the protein. Usually, such antibodies are raised against short synthetic peptides representing the region unique to a receptor, often inferred from the cDNA sequence. Subtype-specific antibodies raised against peptide regions that are unique to a particular receptor subtype provide sensitive reagents for the study of tissue distribution and quantitation, and for the isolation and characterization of the receptor. Antibodies to different segments of a protein are useful in confirming the topology and orientation of membrane proteins predicted by theoretical sequence analysis (Goldberg, 1991). They are also useful for defining functional interactions between the segments of the proteins under study by their ability to block access of other proteins to their binding region. Antibodies are also valuable for the analysis of normal and abnormal pathways of biosynthesis, modification and trafficking of proteins. Defects in these processes originating from mutations in the protein itself or from defects in other interacting activities are the cause of many metabolic disorders such as Alzheimer's disease and cystic fibrosis (Gandy and Greengard, 1992; Selkoe, 1991; Armstrong, 1992).

MOLECULAR TARGETS FOR DRUG DEVELOPMENT

Any cellular macromolecule of a defined function is in principle a drug target from a molecular pharmacological standpoint. However, the central role and the diversity, and the detailed structural and functional understanding provided by molecular biological approaches have made proteins the prime targets for drug development through molecular pharmacology. Furthermore, even in instances where nucleic acids, carbohydrates, or lipids are targets for drugs, expression of the pharmacological activity involves modulation of the interaction of these macromolecules with proteins (Hodgson, 1991; Van Boeckel *et al.,* 1991). The new field of nucleic acid therapeutics, involving concepts and techniques new to pharmacology and pharmaceutical sciences, is moving ever closer to clinical reality, and also rightfully belongs under the heading of molecular pharmacology (Gibbons, 1992). However, as this represents an entirely different facet of biotechnology, it is dealt with separately in Chapter 6.

Recent progress in protein biochemistry and molecular biology has established that proteins which have similar overall functions contain many common structural features (see also Chapter 3). The theme of the discussion that follows centers around the molecular diversity of key cellular pathways and on the structural details of proteins that have become evident in recent years through techniques of molecular biology and biotechnology. Proteins which carry out key cellular functions interact with other proteins and macromolecules in a cell. A detailed understanding of the structural features of proteins and the mechanisms of their interactions at a molecular level can be used to design novel strategies and specific drugs to pharmacologically manipulate their selected activities. The availability of the genes encoding a protein of interest allows the confirmation of its deduced or inferred functions and mechanisms by site-directed mutagenesis as exemplified by the studies of the β-adrenergic receptor (Medynski, 1992; Ostrowski *et al.*, 1992) and of the cyclic AMP-dependent protein kinases (Taylor *et al.*, 1993). It is also possible to produce receptors or other proteins as chimeras by interchanging gene or cDNA segments among family members that bind different ligands or effectors. Segments of one receptor may be transplanted into corresponding regions of a related receptor, and the resultant chimera is assayed for function. This approach permits the determination of regions of the receptor involved in ligand binding and in interactions with effectors such as G proteins (Ostrowski *et al.*, 1992; Edgington, 1992a).

Historically, many biochemical pathways which could in principle be targeted by therapeutics were found to be ubiquitous; their inhibition at the site of disease while sparing the normal tissues was considered difficult. The recent cloning of components of many such pathways has revealed that they are composed of members of families encoded by multiple genes or alternately spliced messenger RNAs produced from a single gene. These relatives could all function often interchangeably in the pathway, but differences in function are observed depending on the degree of sequence divergence. While pharmacological diversity was well documented before the advent of rDNA, the diversity revealed by molecular cloning has equalled or, in most cases, exceeded the functional diversity previously observed in pharmacological experiments. This diversity is further increased in the case of multisubunit proteins because of the combinatorial possibilities offered by multiple subtypes of individual subunits. Many of these alternate members or their combinations are expressed to varying extents in different tissues, offering hope for modulating their activity in specific tissues through subtype-specific inhibitors. Thus, it may be possible to inhibit disease-related isoforms of protein without affecting other members of a family, thereby avoiding global deleterious effects. The exploitation of these subtypic differences for the design of highly specific drugs is a central goal of molecular pharmacology in the context of pharmaceutical development. The availability of the cloned genes and suitable recombinant expression systems provides the necessary tools towards this goal.

In the following section, the proteins of current pharmacological interest are described in four broad groups, namely cell-surface proteins, intracellular proteins that transduce signals received at the cell surface, transcription factors, and other intracellular enzymatic activities. This is followed by a few specific examples which illustrate the contribution of the knowledge gained in these systems to the advances in the understanding of the diseases and development of therapies.

Cell-surface proteins

The plasma membranes of cells are studded with many proteins and glycoproteins which are unique to each cell type and determine the interaction of a cell with

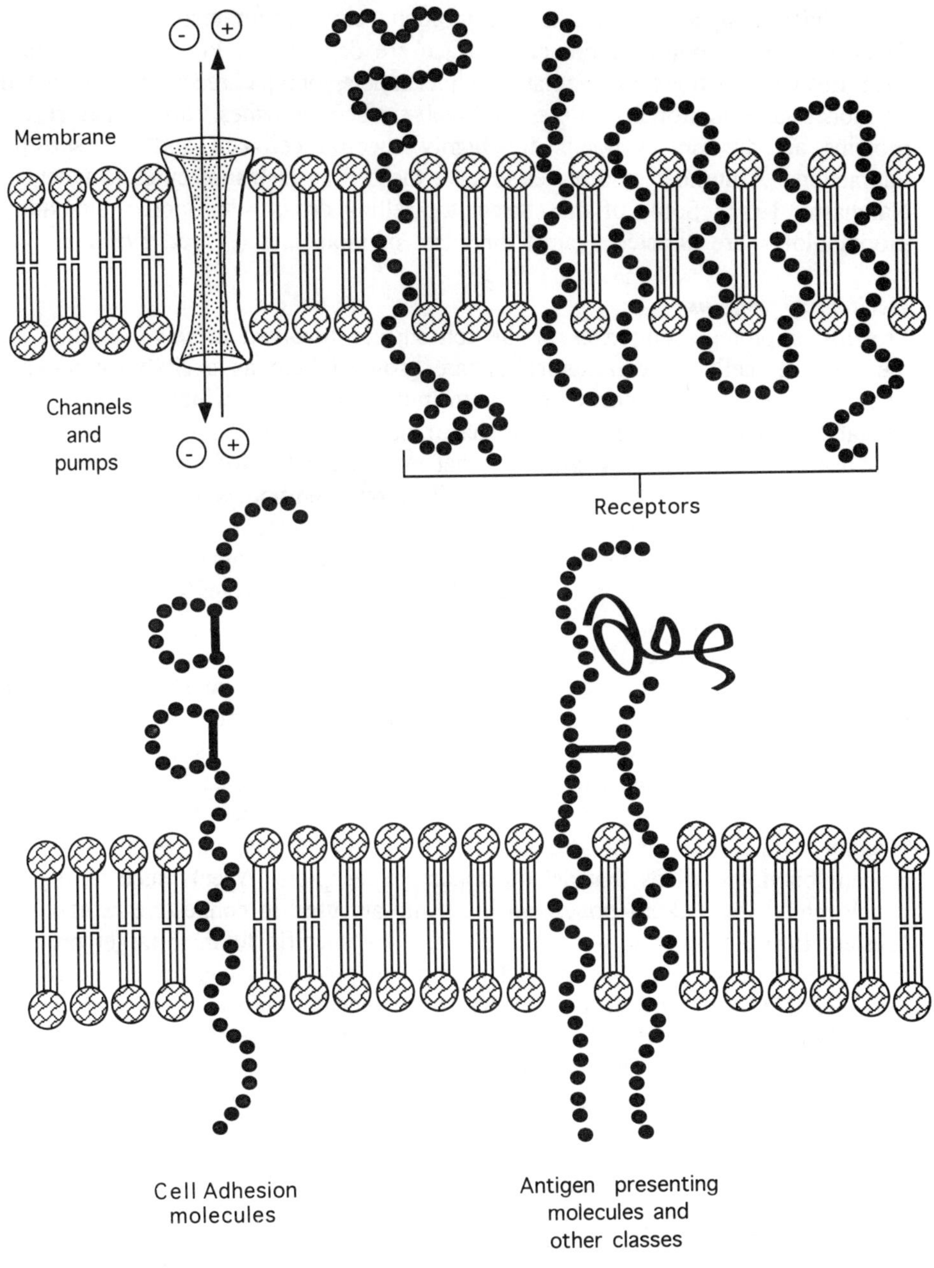

Fig. 4.5. Classes of cell-surface proteins which are possible drug targets.

components of the extracellular fluid, and with other cells of the organism. Many viruses and other pathogens enter cells through interaction with specific cell-surface proteins. Such interactions lead to moderate to drastic changes in the intracellular compartment of the cell through activation of enzymatic pathways. Typical proteins found on the cell surface are depicted in Fig. 4.5. They serve such diverse functions as regulated ion channels, pumps, receptors for peptide hormones and neurotransmitters, and cell-surface enzymes. Some cell-surface proteins act as contact points for highly specific cell–cell and cell–substrate interactions. A number of diseases involve the cell surface molecules (Snyder and Narahashi, 1990). Some of the current top-selling drugs — ranitidine, cimetidine, propranolol — are directed against this class of molecules (Abbot, 1991).

Excitability proteins

Proteins or protein complexes of the cell surface involved in cell excitation and the resultant cell–cell communication are grouped here as excitability proteins. They include ion channels, neurotransmitter receptors which influence the excitability of cells, and ion pumps that transport ions across cell membranes to establish ionic concentration gradients that make excitation of cells possible. Such proteins are found in various combinations on membranes of neurons of the central and peripheral nervous system, and on muscle cells that contract in response to neuronal excitation. They are also found on other cell types which specialize in functions such as secretion. They play vital roles in the specialized functions of these cells.

Members of the excitability class of proteins have been studied extensively, and many of the drugs currently in use are directed against this family of proteins. These include antihypertensive β-adrenergic receptor blockers such as propranalol, and dihydropyridine calcium channel blockers such as nifedipine used in angina pectoris. Also included in this group are benzodiazepines used in the treatment of epilepsy and anxiety acting via the γ-aminobutyric acid (GABA) receptor, and antipsychotic drugs such as phenothiazines, butyrophenones, and diphenylbutylpiperidines that act on dopamine receptors. Agents such as digoxin which inhibit the sodium–potassium ion pump are used in congestive heart failure (Lester, 1988). However, while these drugs are specific to their target proteins, they also interact with other related proteins to produce undesirable side-effects. For example, antihypertensive β-adrenergic receptor blockers, whose desired action is on the cardiovascular system, also interact with neuronal receptors in the central nervous system, causing fatigue and depression (Lester, 1988). A detailed understanding of the structural features of these known receptors and their newly discovered kin, obtained through molecular biological analyses, is expected to lead to the design of drugs that have exquisite specificity for the chosen receptor subtype (Pritchett *et al.*, 1989).

Table 4.1 shows some examples of pharmacologically established excitability proteins and their diversity revealed by isolation of family members through molecular techniques. Different tissues and cell types expressing the same pharmacologically defined receptor may draw the subunits from the repertoire of

Table 4.1. Examples of diversity of excitability protein families[†]

Family	Sub-units	Isoforms	Ref.
Voltage-sensitive channels			
Sodium channel	α, β_1, β_2	4 (α)	(4)
Calcium channel	α_1, α_2, β, γ, δ	5 (α_1)	(9)
Potassium channel	homo-multimeric	>15	(8)
Ligand-regulated channels			
Acetyl choline (nicotinic)			
Muscular	α, β, γ, δ	2–3	(4)
Neuronal	α, β	7 (α), 4 (β)	(1)
$GABA_A$	α, β, γ, δ	6(α), 3(β), 3(γ), 1(δ)	(3)
Glutamate	heteromultimer (3–5 subunits)	9	(5)
G protein-coupled receptors			
Acetyl choline (muscarinic)	1	3	(1)
Adrenergic (α)	1	6 (α_1, α_2)	(2)
Dopamine	1	5	(6)
Glutamate	1	4	(7)
Ion pumps			
Sodium–potassium	α, β multimer	2–4	(4)
Calcium		2	(4)

[†]These are only examples and do not represent the current status.

References: 1. Hall (1992); 2. Harrison *et al.* (1991); 3. Laurie *et al.* (1992); 4. Lester (1988); 5. Mayer (1992); 6. Sibley and Monsma (1992); 7. Tanabe *et al.* (1992); 8. Tsaur *et al.* (1992); 9. Tsien *et al.* (1991).

available subunit subtypes, leading to small, tissue-specific structural and functional differences. Drugs could be aimed at the subtle distributional differences to attain the tissue-specific inactivation or stimulation of the desired excitability function.

Ion channels

The two classes of ion channels found on membranes are: (a) voltage-sensitive channels, whose ion conductance depends on the membrane potential; (b) ligand-regulated channels, whose conductivity is regulated by the binding of specific ligands to the receptor (Cooper *et al.,* 1991; Nargeot, 1991; Hall, 1992). The NMDA class of glutamate receptor channel, which is regulated by both glutamate and membrane potential, forms an exception to this strict grouping (Stevens, 1992a). Both classes of ion channels produce rapid responses when activated by the appropriate stimulus.

The voltage-sensitive ion channel family includes sodium channels, potassium channels, and calcium channels (Hall, 1992; Miller, 1987; Tsien *et al.,* 1991). They are important for the propagation of electrical impulses in neurons and in muscle contraction. These channels are integral membrane proteins that traverse the plasma membrane multiple times. The membrane-spanning α-helical regions form the pores of the channels (Fig. 4.6). Sodium and calcium channel activities reside on large proteins which contains four domains of homology within them. Each domain has a multiple membrane-spanning region that spans the membrane six times. Potassium channels, on the other hand, are produced by a smaller protein that traverses the membrane six times; but the channel is composed of an assemblage of identical subunits forming a homo-oligomeric channel. Injection of the mRNA for the channel proteins into *Xenopus* oocytes is sufficient to produce the particular channel activity. However, the channels isolated from normal tissue may contain additional subunits of unknown functions (Catterall, 1988; Hall, 1992). Toxins and other chemical agents which block these channels have been identified, and these channels are sites of action of drugs currently in use. Local anesthetics act by inactivating the neuronal sodium channels, and the dihydropyridines used in the treatment of hypertension act on the calcium channels of the heart muscle (Murad, 1990; Ritchie and Greene, 1990). The voltage sensitivity of these channels can be regulated by intracellular ligands, or by covalent modifications (such as addition of phosphate groups) activated by other receptor-related intracellular events. Proteins composing the voltage-sensitive ion channels have been shown to belong to larger families, as shown in Table 4.1.

Ligand-regulated or ligand-gated channels regulate the passage of ions across the cell membrane in response to a ligand such as a neurotransmitter which binds to the receptor on the extracellular side. The neurotransmitters may be acetylcholine, GABA (γ-amino butyric acid), dopamine, glutamate, glycine, or others. In addition, intracellular ligands, and/or intracellular post-translational modifications, such as phosphorylation, also regulate the activity of the channels. Ion specificities of ligand-regulated channels vary even among the members of a

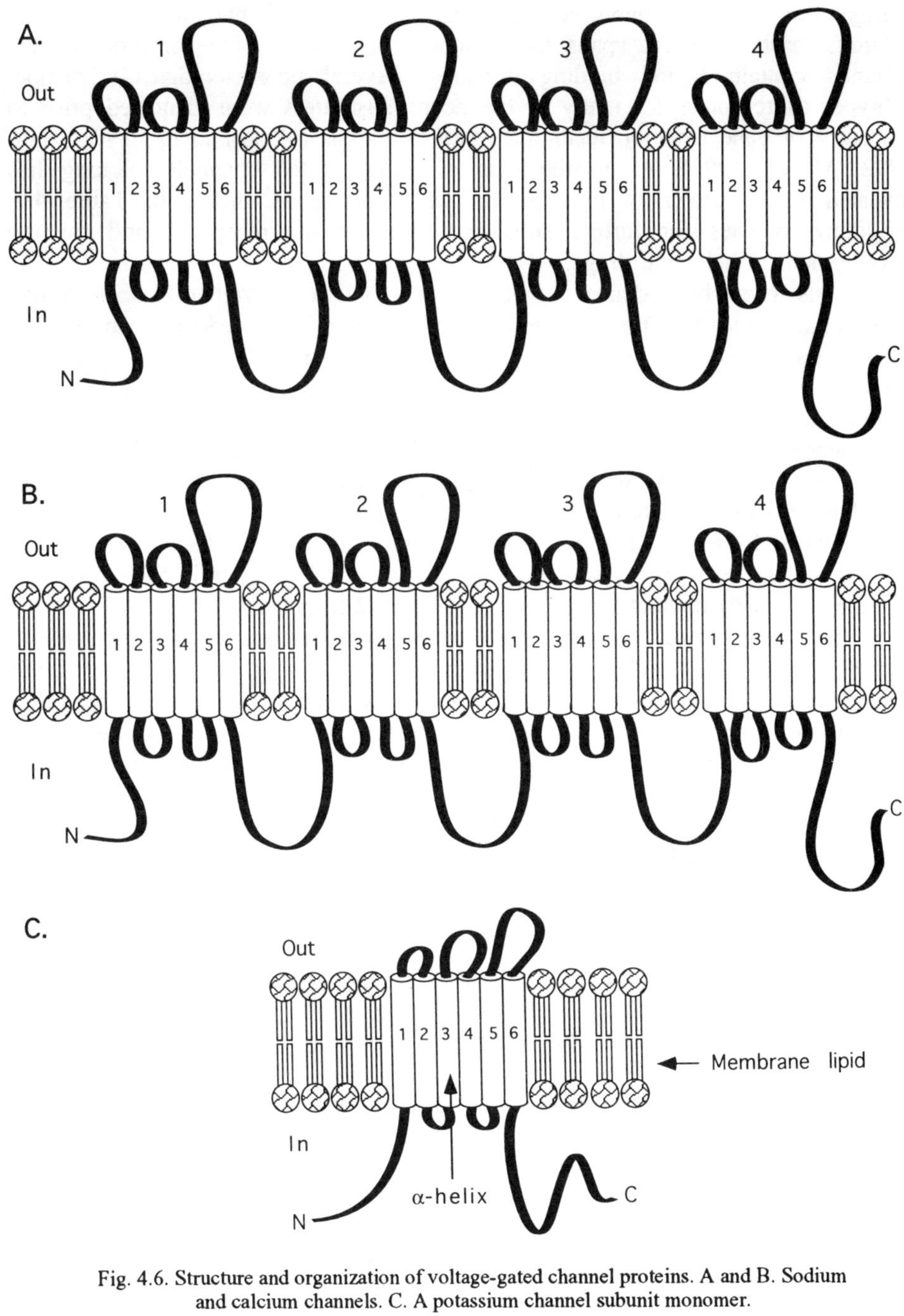

Fig. 4.6. Structure and organization of voltage-gated channel proteins. A and B. Sodium and calcium channels. C. A potassium channel subunit monomer.

family of receptors responding to the same ligand (Hall, 1992; Mayer, 1992). Because these channels respond to their ligands by regulating ion conductance they are also called ionotropic receptors.

Ligand-regulated channels are proteins composed of two to five distinct subunits, each of which spans the membrane four times. One or more of the subunits contain ligand binding domains. Several pharmacologically distinct subtypes of receptors for many of the neurotransmitters were identified prior to the entry of gene isolation techniques into this arena (Cooper *et al.*, 1991; Hall, 1992; Mayer, 1992). As in the case of voltage-gated channels, cloning has revealed further diversity in many of the subunits as shown in Table 4.1, providing avenues for further subclassification of the receptors, and for the development of selective drugs.

For instance, benzodiazepines such as Valium (diazepam) and Xanax (alprazolam), and barbiturates are believed to produce a reduction in anxiety through their action on the GABA-regulated chloride ion channels of the central nervous system (Rall, 1990). While these agents are relatively safe as therapeutics, they produce undesirable side-effects such as sedation and dependence. The GABA receptor is probably a pentamer assembled from four subunits, α, β, γ and δ. So far, six distinct α subunit cDNAs, three each of the β and the γ subunit cDNAs, and a single δ cDNA (totalling 13 members) have been isolated from rats. The combined expression of the cDNAs for the various isoforms of the α, β, and γ subunits in mammalian cells results in the expression of receptors with distinct agonist- and antagonist-response profiles (Pritchett *et al.*, 1989). The number of possible theoretical combinations yielding pentameric receptors from these subunits runs into hundreds. Examination of rat brain sections using oligonucleotide probes specific for each of the thirteen members has revealed region-specific expression of the various subunits (Laurie *et al.*, 1992; Wisden *et al.*, 1992). It may therefore be possible to specifically target the GABA receptors in appropriate brain regions using subtype-specific drugs. This approach is currently being pursued towards the development of more selective GABA channel modulators (Spalding, 1992).

G protein-coupled receptors

The third class of cellular excitability proteins are receptors that are coupled to intracellular second messenger systems through a class of protein complexes known as G proteins, as discussed below. These receptors modulate the excitability of the cells when bound by their respective ligands by initiating intracellular biochemical changes. Some of these changes, in turn, modulate the excitability of the cells by modifying the ion channels and pumps through second messenger action. Others may produce longer lasting changes in gene expression. Because the action of these receptors involves other intermediary steps, the responses generated through the G protein-coupled receptor system are slower compared to those produced by the ligand binding to ion channels, and can often be longer lasting. The G protein-coupled receptors are called "metabotropic" receptors because their effects are metabolic, as opposed to changes in ion permeability induced by ionotropic receptors. This family of receptors includes the muscarinic acetylcholine type, the family of adrenergic receptors which bind to epinephrine and norepinephrine, those for dopamine, GABA, adenosine, serotonin, histamine, and opioid peptides and their analogs such as morphine. A large number (over a hundred) of olfactory receptors, and receptors for many peptide neurotransmitters and some polypeptide hormones such as the fertility hormones belong to the family of G protein-coupled receptors (Cooper *et al.*, 1991; Ross, 1992a; Baulieu, 1990; Iismaa and Shine, 1992). The continuing discovery of other novel G protein-coupled receptors such as the cannabinoid receptor, and the isolation of endogenous ligands such as the lipid ''anandamide'', which binds the cannabinoid receptor, offer exciting avenues for the development of new therapeutics in the future (Barinaga, 1992a).

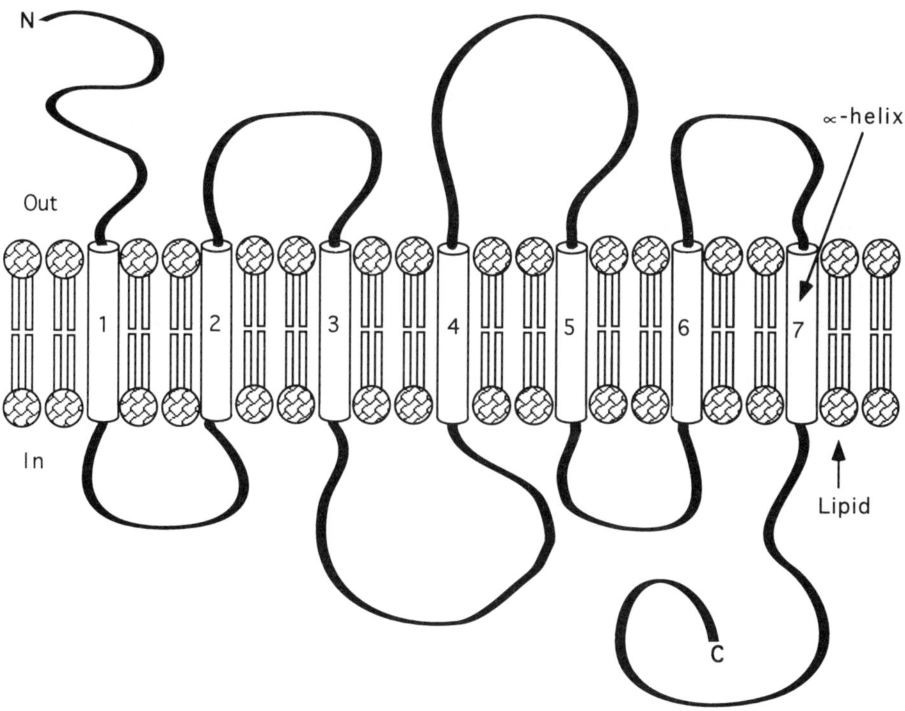

Fig. 4.7. Structure and transmembrane organization of a typical ''seven pass'' G protein-coupled receptor protein.

G protein-coupled receptor proteins are made of a single polypeptide chain that traverses the membrane seven times, with its amino terminus in the extracellular compartment and the carboxyl terminus in the intracellular space as shown in Fig. 4.7. The seven transmembrane domains form the ligand binding pocket for small ligands, which is accessible from the cell exterior. Larger ligands bind to the extended regions of the amino terminus. The segments in the intracellular space interact with protein complexes known as G proteins which are discussed in a following section. There are several species of G proteins, each turning on a distinct set of biochemical events when activated by a receptor. In many cases, G protein activation leads to the production of "second messengers" (the ligand of the receptor being the first messenger) within the cell which, in turn, activate other biochemical pathways. At each step following ligand binding, the response is amplified by an increase in the number of messenger molecules generated. The same ligand binding to different pharmacological and molecular receptor subtypes can produce different biochemical responses determined by the receptor, the particular G proteins expressed by the cell, and the specific G protein-responsive activities present in the cell. This cascade of events leads to activation or inactivation of ion channels and pumps, thereby changing the excitability and other functions of the cell (Nicoll, 1988; Ross, 1992a). Long-lasting changes in gene expression can also occur when G proteins are stimulated (Jackson, 1992). Thus, when triggered by the same first messenger, different cells may produce distinct biochemical responses determined by the unique combination of effector proteins which are assembled from families or subtypes of every protein involved in the cascade.

Ion pumps and other pumps

Ion pumps are cell-surface transmembrane molecules which pump ions across concentration gradients and electrical gradients. They maintain the transmembrane ionic gradients required for the transmission of electrical impulses in neurons and muscles, and for other physiological functions in other cell types (Hardie, 1991). Ions are pumped at the expense of metabolic energy, which is stored in the cell in the "high energy" phosphate bond of adenosine triphosphate (ATP; Alberts *et al.,* 1989). The sodium–potassium ATPase, for example, is a pump that concomitantly moves potassium into the cell and sodium out of the cell using energy released by ATP hydrolysis. Normally, the concentration of sodium is higher in the extracellular space, which is also electrically positive. Thus the sodium ion is moved against its electrical and concentration gradient. This pump is the target for agents such as digitalis drugs and ouabain which are used in cardiac therapy (Hoffman and Bigger, 1990). Ion pumps are also involved in the transport of calcium ions and chloride ions in many cell types of the body. In addition, calcium pumps are present on intracellular membranes, and in organelles such as the endoplasmic reticulum. These pumps, along with the plasma membrane calcium pumps, deplete the cytoplasm of calcium ion which is used as a second messenger in triggering receptor-initiated responses (Hardie, 1991). Thapsigargin, a recently discovered natural sesquiterpene compound, specifically inhibits the intracellular calcium pump of the endoplasmic reticulum while sparing related pumps found in muscle cells (Thastrup *et al.,* 1990); this and other such compounds may have therapeutic applications.

Energy for transport by pumps may be derived from ATP hydrolysis or from the ionic gradients of another ion. This is the case of the sodium/calcium exchanger, which uses the electrical energy stored in the sodium gradient across the plasma membrane to transport calcium out of the cell while harnessing the energy from concerted sodium influx (Komuro *et al.*, 1992).

Ion pump proteins traverse the membrane multiple times and may be composed of multiple subunits (Lester, 1988). These proteins are also members of families within which diversity is created through multiple genes and alternate splicing. In addition, families of transmembrane molecules that pump peptides, sugars and toxic chemicals occur in a wide variety of cells. Molecular pumps known as P-glycoproteins pump out of the cell a diverse group of cytotoxic chemicals used in chemotherapy. During cancer chemotherapy, cells resistant to the chemotherapeutic agent in use arise spontaneously, and, interestingly, these cells show resistance to killing by other chemotherapeutics as well, giving rise to a multi-drug resistance phenotype in cancer cells (Roninson, 1991). The multidrug resistance phenotype is associated with an increase in copy number of the P-glycoprotein genes (Kartner and Ling, 1989; Juranka *et al.*, 1989). This pump has been cloned and consists of a single polypeptide that spans the membrane twelve times. Methods of inhibition of the transport of chemotherapeutics by P-glycoprotein are under development, and these "chemosensitizers" should allow the use of anticancer agents to their full potential. It is becoming increasingly clear that membrane pumps that transport peptides between cellular compartments have vital roles in immune recognition (Sambrook, 1991). Studies of the molecular mechanisms of the action of such pumps hold promise for the development of effective therapeutic strategies for immune disorders.

Hormone-, cytokine-, and growth-factor-receptors

Polypeptide hormones such as insulin and growth hormone, and growth factors such as epidermal growth factor, elicit their effects by binding to specific cell-surface receptors. Many of these receptors are now cloned, and their amino acid sequence and structural features are understood. These receptors are composed of a single protein chain or are homodimers. Each molecule or subunit traverses the membrane only once, with the amino terminal, hormone-binding site in the extracellular space and the carboxyl terminal tail in the cytoplasm (Baulieu, 1990; Hardie, 1991). (Some hormones use the seven-transmembrane receptor system for signaling, as discussed previously.) Table 4.2 is a partial list of this family of receptors and their ligands.

Many members of this class of receptors have an enzymatic activity known as a protein tyrosine kinase within their cytoplasmic segment. This kinase phosphorylates tyrosine residues in the receptors themselves (autophosphorylation), and in other proteins to initiate biochemical cascades. Phosphorylation of tyrosine can be reversed by protein tyrosine phosphatases, which are also present in all cells (Shenolikar and Nairn, 1990). Tyrosine phosphatases form a diverse family of proteins, some of which are cytosolic while others are transmembrane molecules analogous to receptors. Some members of the transmembrane class may be involved in the mechanism of bacterial and viral infections (Tonks, 1991). Thus, kinases and phosphatases together act as "on–off" switches in the activation of receptors and other proteins.

Table 4.2. Single-pass receptors

Receptor	Comment
Containing tyrosine kinase	
Epidermal growth factor-R	Dimerized by ligand EGF
Insulin-R	Present as a homodimer
Insulin-like growth factor-R	Present as a homodimer
Colony stimulating factor 1-R	
Platelet-derived growth factor-R	
Containing no known enzymatic activity	
Growth hormone-R	
Prolactin-R	
Interleukin family-R's	
Erythropoietin-R	
Low density lipoprotein-R	Lipid internalization
Transferrin-R	Iron uptake

R stands for "receptor".
From Aaronson *et al.* (1991); Baulieu (1990).

The tyrosine kinase class of receptors includes receptors for insulin and insulin-like growth factors, and epidermal growth factor. The kinase activity appears to be essential for the activity of these receptors (Cadena and Gill, 1992; Baulieu, 1990). Novel receptor-specific inhibitors of the tyrosine kinase activity are under development. These compounds may have therapeutic utilities where activation or inhibition of tyrosine kinase receptors are involved in disease states (Casnellie, 1991; Levitzki and Gilon, 1991; Powis, 1991). While protein phosphorylation, protein–protein interactions and second messengers (see below) appear to be involved in the signal transduction by these receptors, the exact mechanism(s) by which they elicit their final biochemical responses remains to be clarified (Cadena and Gill, 1992). The cytoplasmic domains of other receptors of this class, such as the growth hormone receptor, have no demonstrable enzymatic activities, and their mechanism of signaling is not well understood. Nonetheless, chimeric receptors constructed by DNA manipulation can be useful for the development of agonists and antagonists to receptors whose mode of action is not known. For instance, a chimeric receptor composed of the extracellular domain of the human growth hormone receptor and the intracellular domain of the granulocyte colony-stimulating factor (G-CSF) has been used to identify agonists and antagonists of the human growth hormone. When expressed in the appropriate cell type, the chimeric receptor binds the growth hormone and its agonists, and stimulates cell proliferation through activation of the intracellular G-CSF portion of the chimera (Fuh *et al.*, 1992).

It has recently been shown that receptors without intrinsic tyrosine kinase activity in their cytoplasmic region may nevertheless activate tyrosine kinases upon ligand binding. Phosphorylation by these kinases may directly influence events such as transcription. Thus, the binding of interferon to its receptor, which lacks an intrinsic tyrosine kinase, results in the phosphorylation of three cytosolic proteins on tyrosines. These factors associate with each other, move to the nucleus, and activate the transcription of genes that are induced by interferon treatment (Marx, 1992a).

Adhesion molecules

The mammalian cell-surface contains a wide variety of transmembrane proteins whose extracellular domains interact with proteins on the surfaces of other cells, and with molecules of the substrates to which the cells attach. These molecules, called cell adhesion molecules, or CAMs, play important roles during embryonic development. They are also involved in normal cell biological processes such as recognition between cells of the immune system, lymphocyte trafficking, wound healing, and hemostasis, as well as in pathological states of tumor metastasis, thrombosis and inflammation. For instance, loss of adhesion molecules reduces the adhesiveness and increases the tumorigenicity of cells. These changes can be reversed by expression of relevant CAM cDNA in the cells by transfection (Hynes and Lander, 1992; Hynes, 1992; Kahn, 1992). Although a large number of adhesion molecules have been identified, many of these molecules can be grouped into four major families whose members perform similar functions. These families, shown in Table 4.3, are (1) cadherins, (2) the immunoglobulin superfamily, (3) selectins, and (4) integrins. Genes and cDNAs for many of the CAMs have been isolated, providing a wealth of structural information. Cadherins are a family of calcium-dependent cell–cell adhesion molecules comprising over a dozen members. They interact with cadherins displayed on the surface of neighboring cells by "homotypic" interaction. Members of the immunoglobulin superfamily (so called because they contain immunoglobulin-related domains) are also involved in cell–cell contact, and interact in homotypic and heterotypic modes. Selectins, expressed by blood cells and/or endothelial cells, interact with specific carbohydrate groups, and their interaction is heterotypic. Lastly, integrins are heterodimers composed of an α and a β subunit. They are derived from pairing between one of the eight β subunits with one of the thirteen α subunits. However, while such combinations predict over a hundred pairs, only about twenty integrins are known. While some of the integrins found on leukocytes and lymphocytes participate in cell–cell interactions, the majority of the integrins interact with molecules of the extracellular matrix (ECM). A number of ECM proteins are known, and they as a group share common modules or motifs (Engel, 1991). The intracellular domains of CAMs interact with molecules of the cellular cytoskeleton, thereby transmitting signals to the interior of the cell (Mosher, 1991; Hynes, 1992). Modulation of the activity of CAMs by using antibodies, peptides, and oligosaccharides promises to offer therapeutic avenues for the treatment of cancer and inflammation. Many large pharmaceutical firms and smaller biotech companies are focusing on this area for the development of novel therapeutics (Edgington, 1992b).

Table 4.3. Cell adhesion molecule families

Family	Function
Cadherins	
E-Cadherin	Early embryonic development Cancer metastasis
N-Cadherin	Embryonic neural development
P-Cadherin	Maternal attachment of embryo
Ig superfamily	
Neural cell adhesion molecule (NCAM)	Axonal growth, cell–cell adhesion
Immune cell adhesion molecule (ICAM-1)	T cell activation, cold virus receptor neutrophil adhesion, binds LFA-1
Selectins	
L-Selectin	Lymphocyte homing
E-Selectin	Neutrophil activation
P-Selectin	Neutrophil adhesion
Integrins (α–β heterodimers)	
LFA-1 ($\alpha_L\beta_2$)	Neutrophil adhesion, lymphocyte homing
LPAM-1 ($\alpha_4\beta_p$)	Lymphocyte trafficking
GPIIb-IIIa ($\alpha_{IIb}\beta_3$)	Platelet adhesion

Compiled from: Hynes (1992); Hynes and Lander (1992).

HIV, the causative agent of AIDS, enters cells by binding to the CD4 protein which is present on the surface of a set of T lymphocytes. The therapeutic use of soluble CD4 and CD4-immunoadhesins in AIDS has been described in Chapter 3.

In addition, one of the members of the immunoglobulin superfamily of CAMs, ICAM-1 (immune cell adhesion molecule), serves as the receptor for the entry of human rhinoviruses, the causative agent of common colds. ICAM-1 is also involved in the endothelial-cell adhesion of erythrocytes infected with the malaria parasite, *Plasmodium falciparum* (Craig and Berendt, 1991). The development of therapeutics for the common cold using soluble, virus-binding regions of ICAM-1 is in progress, although the cost effectiveness of such therapy is still in question (Edgington, 1992c). Many other viruses have also been shown to use cell-surface receptors and other cell-surface proteins as routes of entry into cells (Baulieu, 1990; Delmas *et al.,* 1992; Yeager *et al.,* 1992). Therapeutic approaches similar to those described for AIDS and the common cold may be applicable in these situations as well.

Intracellular signal transduction proteins and second messengers

Components of the intracellular signal transduction systems include a family of proteins known as the G proteins, and low-molecular second messengers that are produced in response to the interaction of the ligand-bound receptors with G proteins. The second messengers in turn activate or inhibit batteries of cellular enzymes, chief among which are protein kinases and protein phosphatases. Protein kinases and phosphatases phosphorylate or dephosphorylate respectively other cellular proteins, such as gene transcription factors, to elicit the physiological effect of the receptor–ligand interaction. While a wide variety of receptors use the G protein-linked pathways of signal transduction, the single-pass receptors (discussed earlier) also trigger their actions, at least partly, through the protein tyrosine kinases. In recognition of the novel avenues for drug discovery provided by these systems, several new biotech companies are focusing exclusively on them as targets (Glaser, 1992; Gibbons, 1992; Watanabe, 1992)

The ultimate biochemical effect of a particular ligand impinging on the extracellular face of the plasma membrane is determined by variations possible at every step down the signal transduction pathway. Many ligands have multiple receptors, each of which leads into a different physiological pathway. For example, the neurotransmitter GABA has a class of receptors, known as $GABA_A$, which are chloride channels (discussed earlier), and another class, known as $GABA_B$, which function through G proteins. A G protein itself may be capable of responding to distinct receptors that bind different ligands, or a receptor may interact with more than one type of G protein. Thus, the physiological response of a cell to a ligand also depends on the presence in the cell of the particular subset of G proteins, their respective targets and the second messengers, the effectors that respond to second messengers, and the targets of the effectors. The presence or the absence of any of the members of this cascade result in different outcomes of ligand binding. The simultaneous presence of multiple, functionally different members of a class of effector protein results in competition between their respective pathways (Ross, 1992b). The biochemical outcome is determined by the relative concentrations of the competing members and their intracellular distributions. Thus, signal transduction pathways provide for a diversity of responses through the activation of singular pathways, simultaneous activation of multiple pathways, and the interactions between pathways along a cascade to achieve a variety of distinct and graded physiological responses. G proteins, kinases, phosphatases, and other components of these pathways are members of families which are further composed of multiple subtypes. For example, upwards of 200 protein kinases belonging to several distinct functional classes have been identified at the gene and the biochemical level (Hanks *et al.*, 1988; Lindberg *et al.*, 1992). Among these, the protein kinase C family has seven or more members which are closely related but are expressed in different tissues (Kikkawa *et al.*, 1989). In exploiting the diversity of second messenger systems in drug development, it is necessary not only to have type- or subtype-specific drugs, but also to ascertain the involvement of the particular species in the disease state.

G proteins

Heteromeric G proteins are membrane-associated proteins consisting of three subunits, α, β, and γ (Spiegel *et al.*, 1991). The activity of these protein complexes is mediated by their interaction with guanosine triphosphate (GTP), hence the name G protein (Ross, 1992a; Kennedy, 1992; Hardie, 1991). The interaction of G proteins with GTP is catalyzed by the cytoplasmic segments of ligand-bound receptors as shown in Fig. 4.8. The cytoplasmic region of the receptors that interact with the G protein may provide a target for the therapeutic modulation of G protein-coupled receptor action (Luttrell *et al.*, 1993).

In the unstimulated state, the three subunits composing the G protein are membrane-associated, and the α subunit is bound tightly to guanosine diphosphate (GDP), which is the hydrolysis product of GTP. Upon contacting the ligand-bound receptor, the GDP in the α subunit is replaced by GTP, and the subunit is released from the β–γ complex. GTP-bound α subunits activate their effectors, which are largely enzymes that produce second messengers. Some G proteins act directly on target protein such as ion channels. The α subunit of G proteins also contains within it the activity to convert GTP to GDP and thereby to cause it to deactivate itself and to reassociate with the β and γ subunits on the membrane, terminating its activated state. Conversion of GTP to GDP may also be enhanced by proteins with which the GTP-bound α subunit interacts; such proteins are known as GTPase activating proteins or GAPs (Marx, 1992b). Many of the effector proteins activated by the α subunit also possess GAP activity. Thus, the time that the α subunits remains active is determined by intrinsic and extrinsic factors (Bourne and Stryer, 1992). A single receptor can activate many molecules of G protein resulting in signal amplification, and the activation of the G protein is transient.

There are several G proteins, each of which is capable of activating distinct, often interconnected pathways (Ross, 1992a,b). Thus, the α subunit varies among different G proteins while the β and γ subunits are common. It is currently believed that the specificity of a G protein resides predominantly in its α subunit. Each α subunit also has subtypes encoded by multiple genes (Bourne *et al.*,

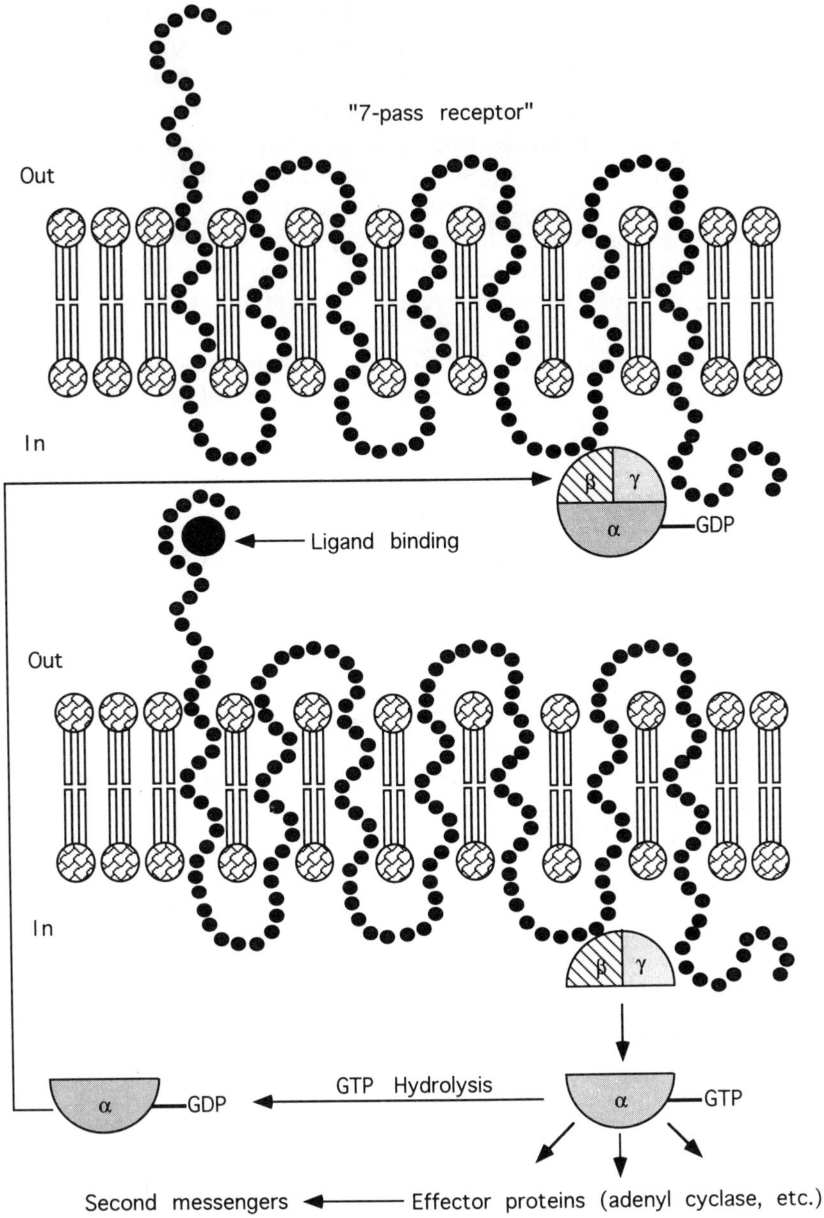

Fig. 4.8. Mechanism of action of G protein-coupled receptors.

1991; Simon *et al.,* 1991). There are at least fifteen different α subunits and four each of the β and γ subunits (Spiegel, 1992). The action of some G proteins is inhibited by pertussis toxin, produced by the bacterium *Bordetella pertussis.* Cholera toxin, produced by the bacterium *Vibrio cholerae,* acts by arresting the α subunit of a G protein in a GTP-bound, activated state (Ross, 1992a; Berridge, 1993). The diversity of the β and γ subunits also adds further diversity to G proteins. Recent experimental observations disagree with the earlier views of the β and γ subunits as inert components of G proteins. It is becoming clearer that the β–γ complex may have roles in signal transduction, and that these roles may be specific to specific combinations of isoforms of β and γ subunits. For instance, certain isoforms of adenylate cyclase, so far believed to respond only to α subunits, are now found to be stimulated by certain β–γ subunit combinations to produce the second messenger cyclic AMP (Lefkowitz, 1992; Kleuss *et al.,* 1993).

Table 4.4 lists some of the G proteins. Their targets, and the second messengers produced by their activation as discussed below, are also shown in Table 4.4.

Second messengers and their production

Many of the effects of a ligand binding to its receptors are mediated through second messengers elicited by the interaction of activated G proteins with intracellular enzymes. The five chief second messengers are: (1) cyclic adenosine monophosphate (cAMP), (2) cyclic guanosine monophosphate (cGMP), (3) inosine triphosphate (IP_3), (4) diacylglycerol (DAG), and (5) calcium ion (Kennedy, 1992). In addition, activation of some G proteins results in the release of arachidonic acid, which is a precursor for the synthesis of prostaglandins and leukotrienes, which act as cellular and extracellular messengers (Piomelli and Greengard, 1990). Recently, nitric oxide (NO) has been shown to be a diffusible intercellular messenger produced by the enzyme nitric oxide synthetase (NOS). Nitric oxide activates the production of cGMP (Snyder, 1992; Stevens, 1992b; Bently and Beavo, 1992). The basis for the well-established efficacy of nitroglycerine patches in the treatment of angina appears to arise from the breakdown of nitroglycerine to the heretofore unappreciated neurotransmitter, nitric oxide.

Cyclic nucleotides (cAMP and cGMP)

Some activated G proteins interact with an enzyme called adenyl cyclase, which converts ATP into adenosine 3′–5′ cyclic monophosphate or cAMP, whose structure is shown in Fig. 4.9A. Adenyl cyclase is a protein that spans the membrane multiple times. The adenyl cyclase family consists of at least four, perhaps six, isozymes, which are expressed in a cell-type specific manner (Bently and Beavo, 1992). cAMP is a cofactor for the activity of a family of kinases known as cAMP-dependent protein kinases (Hanks *et al.,* 1988; Taylor *et al.,* 1993) which phosphorylate target proteins when cAMP concentration in the cell rises. cAMP is hydrolyzed by a group of enzymes known as cAMP phosphodiesterases, terminating the kinase activation event. There are nearly twenty phosphodiesterase isozymes which fall into groups that are regulated by a

Table 4.4. Diversity of the G protein family

α subunits	Receptor (e.g.)	Effector (e.g.)
G_s (four forms)	β-adrenergic	Adenylate cyclase activation
G_{olf}	Odorant	Adenylate cyclase activation
G_{t1},G_{t2} (two genes)	Opsins (vision)	cGMP phosphodiesterase activation
G_{i2}	α2-adrenergic	Adenylate cyclase inhibition
G_{i1},G_{i3}	Dopamine	Adenylate cyclase inhibition
		Potassium and calcium channels
G_0	Acetylcholine (M2)	Potassium and calcium channels
G_z	?	?
G_q,G_{11}	Thromboxane A_2	Phospholipase C-β
G_{14}	?	Phospholipase C
$G_{15/16}$	?	Phospholipase C
G_{12},G_{13}	?	?
β *and* γ *subunits*		
Four variants each	?	?

Adapted from: Spiegel (1992); Ross (1992a).

variety of agents such as calmodulin and cGMP. A similar cycle of production and hydrolysis of cGMP is carried out by guanyl cyclases or cGMP-cyclases, and phosphodiesterase respectively (Fig. 4.9B). There are six isozymes of guanyl cyclase belonging to two major families, namely membrane-bound and soluble (Bently and Beavo, 1992).

Phosphodiesterase inhibitors, which prolong the action of cyclic nucleotides, have been the targets for the development of therapeutically useful compounds. Several selective inhibitors of this class of enzymes have been identified and some are under development for therapeutic purposes (Beavo and Reifsnyder, 1990; Corda *et al.,* 1990).

An attractive approach to the modulation of second messenger levels is to simultaneously manipulate the enzymes that are involved in its production and breakdown. The presence of multiple isoforms of both classes of these enzymes should permit the manipulation of the level of the chosen second messenger by selectively targeting the pair of synthetic and degradative enzymes with sets of subtype-specific modulators. A similar approach should also be applicable to opposing enzyme systems such as protein kinases and protein phosphatases (discussed below), which regulate the net protein phosphorylation in cells.

Inositol triphosphate, diacylglycerol and calcium ions

The interaction of certain members of the G protein family with an enzymatic activity known as phospholipase C results in the hydrolysis of the membrane phospholipid, phosphatidyl inositol, into diacylglycerol (DAG) and inosine triphosphate (IP_3) shown in Fig. 4.9C (Ross, 1992a; Kennedy, 1992; Hardie, 1991). DAG is an activator of the protein kinase C family of enzymes discussed below, and acts by reducing the level of calcium needed for their activation. (Several diacylglycerols, depending on the exact nature of the two fatty acids that are linked to the glycerol, can be produced.) IP_3 interacts with its receptors in the intracellular membranes of calcium-storing organelles, resulting in the release of calcium ions (Irvine, 1992). Several distinct forms of IP_3 receptors are believed to exist in different locations in a cell (Meldolesi, 1992). Under unstimulated conditions, the cytosolic concentration of calcium is maintained at low levels by calcium pumps that transport calcium ions to the outside of the cell and also concentrate it into intracellular membrane compartments such as the endoplasmic reticulum, or the sarcoplasmic reticulum of muscle cells (Lytton and Nigam, 1992). An IP_3-mediated increase in cytosolic calcium results in the activation of kinases, phosphatases, phosphodiesterases and proteases that are calcium-dependent for their activity. These enzymes in turn produce the biochemical event (Berridge, 1993). Drugs such as dihydropyridines, which are clinically used calcium channel blockers, achieve their effects by interfering with the rise of intracellular calcium levels. Sustained high levels of cytosolic calcium ion are toxic to cells. Calcium toxicity has been implicated in phenomena such as neuronal degeneration (Nicotera *et al.,* 1992).

Phospholipase Cs, which produce IP_3 and diacylglycerol, belong to a family consisting of β, γ, and δ types, each with structural distinctions that determine their interactions with proteins that activate them (Rhee, 1991; Berridge, 1993).

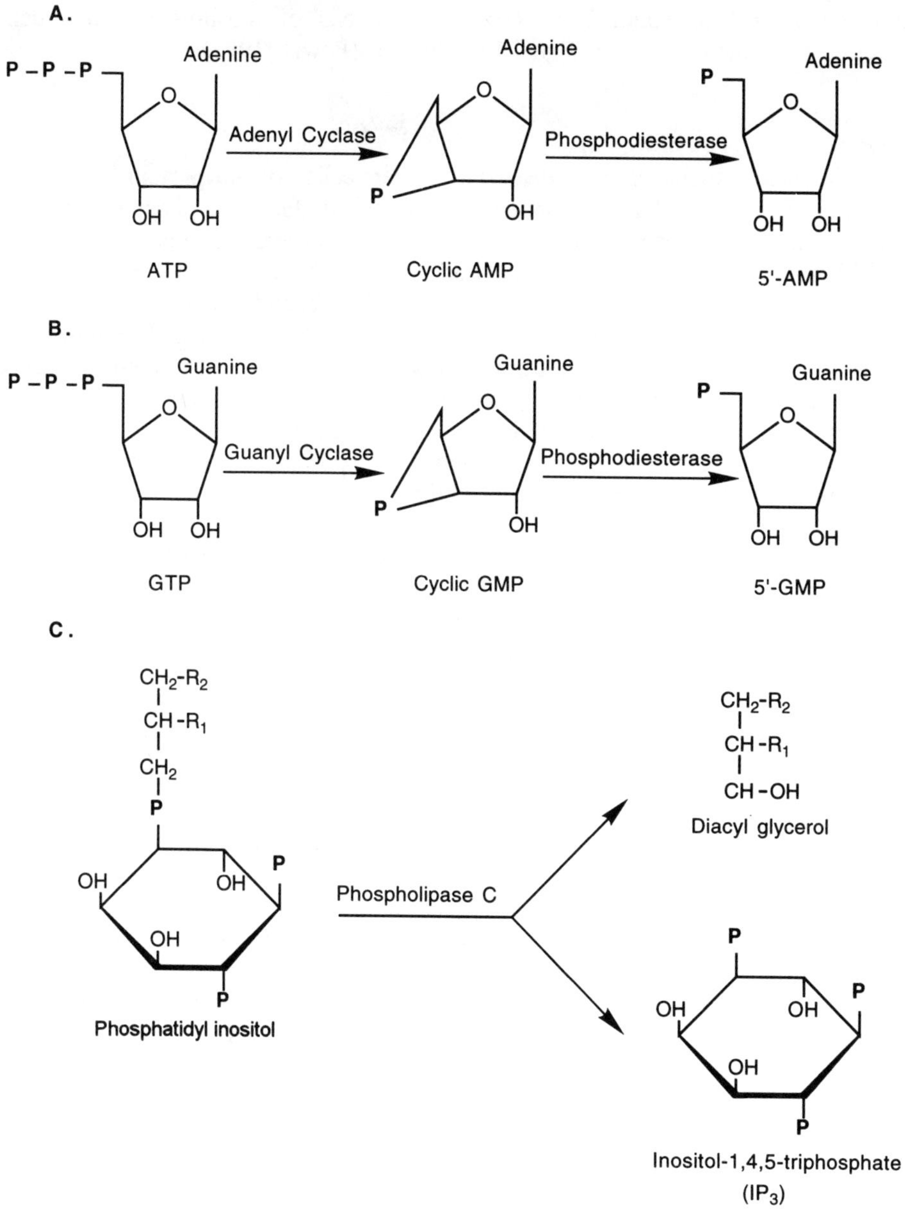

Fig. 4.9. Structures and formation of intracellular second messengers. A. Cyclic AMP (cAMP). B. Cyclic GMP (cGMP). C. Inositol-1-4-5-triphosphate (IP_3) and diacylglycerol.

Each of these groups again contains multiple isoforms which add up to thirteen or more members. Inhibitors and stimulators of phospholipases, and analogs of

IP_3 and DAGs can also be used to modulate the actions of the second messenger pathways. Several anticancer agents currently in development are inhibitors directed against phospholipases. Modified versions of inositols are also being examined for their effect on signal transduction (Powis, 1991).

Protein kinases and phosphatases

In addition to tyrosine kinases discussed earlier, cells contain protein kinases that phosphorylate serines and threonines in proteins. In fact, the phosphorylation of serines and threonines in proteins is a more common event compared to tyrosine phosphorylation. These kinases, as well as phosphatases which remove these phosphate groups, are the major targets for the second messengers (Kennedy, 1992). Kinases and phosphatases are ubiquitous cellular enzymes. The addition of negatively charged phosphate groups to proteins at serines and threonines (and to tyrosines by tyrosine kinases) produces conformational changes in proteins resulting in changes in their activities. Substrates for serine/threonine protein kinases and phosphatases include ion channels, pumps, catabolic enzymes, and transcription factor proteins which are obligate accessories for the transcription of many genes.

Several classes of serine/threonine kinases are known and these enzymes consist of a catalytic domain which transfers phosphate groups from adenosine triphosphate (ATP) to the targets, and a regulatory domain which modulates the activity of the catalytic domain through interaction with second messengers such as cyclic nucleotides, calcium ion, and DAGs. The family of kinases, their activators, and typical synthetic inhibitors are shown in Table 4.5.

Kinases of a given class are also products of multiple genes with high degrees of sequence conservation, and the expression of individual isoforms is often restricted to specific tissues. For instance, the cAMP-dependent protein kinase, PKA, is composed of a regulatory and a catalytic subunit; three isoforms of the catalytic subunit and four isoforms of the regulatory subunit are known. The protein kinase C family consists of seven or more members which show differences in tissue distribution and activation properties (Walsh *et al.,* 1992; Hanks *et al.,* 1988; Kikkawa *et al.,* 1989). A wide variety of structurally unrelated inhibitors of protein serine/threonine kinases have been isolated from natural sources and these have provided starting points for the synthesis of many potent inhibitors (Tamaoki and Nakano, 1990; Casnellie, 1991; Hidaka and Kobayashi, 1992). These inhibitors interact with the catalytic or regulatory domains of kinases to produce their effects. Naturally occurring analogs of physiological activators are also known in the case of members of the protein kinase C family; analogs of diacylglycerols (which are generated by phospholipase C in response to G protein activation), known as phorbol esters, are potent tumor promoters (Gschwendt *et al.,* 1991). The availability of the inhibitors and activators of kinases, coupled with the detailed structural information and the tissue distribution data provided by cloning of the kinase genes, should provide leads for the production of very specific inhibitors and

Table 4.5. Mammalian protein kinases activators, and inhibitors

Kinase	Activator	Synthetic inhibitor (e.g.)
cAMP dependent (α, β)	cAMP	Isoquinoline sulfonamide H-89
cGMP dependent	cGMP	Isoquinoline sulfonamide H-8
Protein kinase C (α, βI, βII, γ, δ, ε)	Calcium, phospholipids diacylglycerols	Calphostin C
CAM kinase I, II, III	Calmodulin, calcium ion	KN-62
Casein kinases	?	CKI-7
Tyrosine kinases	Ligand binding (EGF, PDGF, insulin, etc.)	Tyrphostins

From: Hanks *et al.* (1988); Casnellie (1991); Kikkawa *et al.* (1989).

activators of kinases. Such compounds with possible clinical utility are currently being tested (Powis, 1991; Gibbons, 1992; Glaser, 1992).

Protein phosphatases reverse the action of kinases by removing phosphate groups, and thereby play a role in the regulation of second messenger action. Dephosphorylation of normally phosphorylated proteins may also activate biochemical pathways. Many phosphatases are themselves targets of regulation by protein kinases and second messengers. Multiple classes of protein phosphatases, with further subtypes within a class, have also been documented. Several phosphatase inhibitors have been isolated from natural sources (Shenolikar and Nairn, 1990; Kennedy, 1992). It is interesting that immunosuppressants of the cyclosporin group (described later) seem to achieve their effect by inhibiting a phosphatase, PP2B (protein phosphatase 2B), also known as calcineurin, which appears to be involved in the activation of T lymphocytes (McKeon, 1991; Fruman *et al.*, 1992; Clipstone and Crabtree, 1992). The judicious development and use of activators and inhibitors of kinases and phosphatases appear to hold promise for the treatment of many metabolic diseases including Alzheimer's disease (Gandy and Greengard, 1992).

Transcription factors

With a few notable exceptions, every cell in a multicellular organism contains the genes that encode every protein found in the organism. However, only a small, select set is expressed in a cell type, as determined by its specialized function, its stage in development, and the chemical and physical stimuli that it is subjected to. Expression of a specific subset of proteins from among the large numbers of often related family members described above requires exquisite control of gene expression. While varying degrees of regulation of gene expression occur at every level between a gene and its product protein (mRNA maturation, translation, etc.), initiation of production of the RNA transcript from the gene, or initiation of transcription, is the predominant control point for regulation of gene expression (Stone *et al.*, 1991; Mitchell and Tjian, 1989).

Transcription of a gene begins at a fixed point close to the promoter region of a gene as shown in Fig. 4.10. The enzyme RNA polymerase II, composed of ten subunits, and a set of protein factors which are required for the transcription of *all* genes, is called the ''basal apparatus''. These factors bind to specific sequence motifs in the promoter region close to the starting point of the RNA chain, and position the RNA polymerase to begin elongation of the RNA chain (Lewin, 1990; Stone *et al.*, 1991).

RNA synthesis directed by the basal apparatus is modulated by a host of regulatory protein factors which bind to specific sequence motifs in the region upstream of the initiation point at distances varying between a few bases and thousands of bases. Several such sequence motifs have been identified in various promoter regions. These include sequences that are required for regulation of transcription from the promoter by external stimuli such as metal ions, heat, and steroid hormones. In addition, there are short sequences called ''enhancer sequences'' to which protein factors bind to induce transcription. Similarly, there are "silencer sequences" which, when bound by the appropriate protein factors, reduce or eliminate transcription from the promoter. Proteins which bind to regulatory sequence motifs are called regulatory transcription factors, as they serve to integrate transcriptional activity with various stimuli that a cell is subjected to. Proteins produced by viruses also regulate initiation of transcription from cellular and viral promoters. T-antigen of the SV40 virus and the EIA protein of adenoviruses are examples of viral transcription factors (Mitchell and Tjian, 1989; Hadcock and Malbon, 1991).

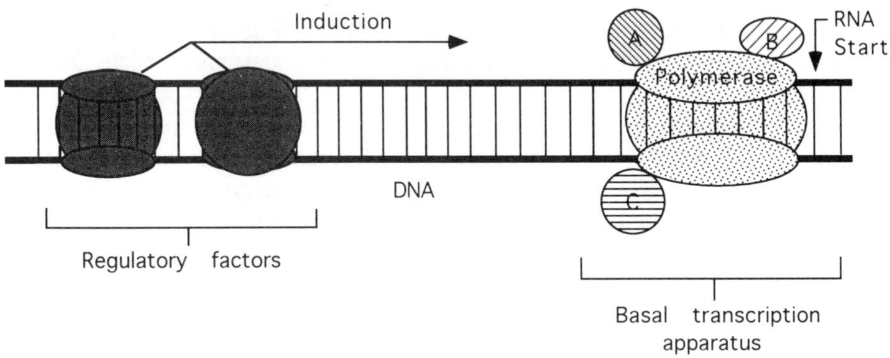

Fig. 4.10. Protein factors and their roles in transcription.

In the last few years, many of the regulatory transcription factors have been purified and their genes have been isolated using standard rDNA techniques. The sequence information from these genes has revealed structural features common to transcription factors. These include regions involved in specific binding to DNA, regions which interact with effectors such as metal ions and hormones, and regions that determine the interactions with other transcription factors and the basal transcription apparatus (Mitchell and Tjian, 1989; Jensen, 1991; McKnight, 1991). DNA binding regions contain several basic amino acids which are positively charged, and interact with DNA (which is negatively charged), but only at specific sequence stretches. The DNA binding domains of transcription factors contain structural motifs known as "zinc fingers", which coordinate zinc ions using a pair each of cysteines and histidines, or two pairs of cysteines. Another set of protein domains have also been demonstrated in the family of transcription factors. This second set of domains determine the transcriptional activation properties of the factors. Here again, several classes of sequence motifs have been found. Often, transcription factors work as homo- or heterodimers. These interactions occur through motifs known as "leucine zippers", which are α helical regions rich in leucines present on both members of the dimer pair (Laudet and Stehelin, 1992; McKnight, 1991). In addition, ligand binding domains are found on factors that activate or suppress transcription in response to a specific ligand. Steroid hormone receptor proteins are a classic example of a class of transcription factors whose ability to activate transcription is regulated by their binding to steroid hormones. These receptors activate transcription of specific genes when bound by glucocorticoids, mineralcorticoids, and reproductive steroids. Under unstimulated conditions, these receptors are predominantly restricted to the cytosol through associations with other specific proteins. Ligand binding releases the receptors, which associate into dimers, enter the nucleus, and stimulate transcription of target genes (Jensen, 1991). This simple picture of ligand-mediated transcriptional activation is rapidly gaining complexity as heterodimeric interactions between these factors are being discovered (Green, 1993). Such complexity provides for fine control and increased specificity to transcriptional regulation, and may provide novel avenues and targets for drug development.

Activity of transcription factors is also regulated through post-translational modifications. Phosphorylation mediated by serine/threonine protein kinases, which are themselves activated by second messenger systems discussed earlier, is a predominant mode of regulation of the transcriptional activity of these factors (Hadcock and Malbon, 1991; Jackson, 1992; Hunter and Karin, 1992). Recently, direct tyrosine phosphorylation of transcription factors (without the involvement of second messengers) has also been shown to activate transcription. Phosphorylation in response to an extracellular signal results in the association of the transcription factors and the migration of the complex to the nucleus, to stimulate transcription of specific genes (Marx, 1992a). Phosphorylation of the RNA polymerase also appears to be involved in the initiation of transcription (Peterson and Tjian, 1992).

In summary, there are many specific DNA–protein and protein–protein interactions involved in the regulation of transcription initiation. Abnormal gene expression is manifested in many disease states. Gene expression, and therefore the infectivity, of many viruses including HIV and the herpes viruses is modulated by viral-specific transcription factors. With a detailed understanding of the physicochemical nature of these interactions, it should be possible to modulate them to turn genes on or off in disease states such as cancer and other proliferative diseases caused by abnormal gene expression, and in viral infections. Therapeutic strategies directed at transcription factors are in the early phases of commercial development (Gibbons, 1992).

Other enzymes and metabolic activities

Recombinant expression of many enzymatic activities at high levels in heterologous hosts has provided systems for large-scale screening operations, with the added benefit of worker safety in cases where these activities were components of high-risk infectious agents. Thus, for example, most of the enzymes required for the replication of the HIV virus have been expressed efficiently in *E. coli*, providing ample supplies of these enzymes for screening of inhibitors and for their structural studies. Other metabolic enzymes such as human renin have also been produced efficiently by this route.

The renin–angiotensin system is involved in the control of blood pressure. Renin, a protease, initiates the production of angiotensin I by cleavage of its inactive precursor angiotensinogen. Angiotensin I is converted by the angiotensin-converting enzyme (ACE) to biologically active angiotensin II, which causes vasoconstriction and an increase in blood pressure. ACE inhibitors such as Captopril and Enalpril are clinically used in the regulation of hypertension (Garrison and Peach, 1990). However, renin, which initiates the production of angiotensin I, has also been considered a target for antihypertensives. Renin, a 340-amino-acid glycoprotein derived from a larger polypeptide, prorenin, is produced and secreted by the juxtaglomerular cells in the kidney. Low blood levels of renin made human renin difficult to obtain in quantities required for drug screens. Early studies of renin inhibition were conducted with renin obtained from mice. Recent cloning and expression of human renin cDNA has provided quantities of human renin for the development of assays for screening renin inhibitors, and for the structural studies for rational design of renin inhibitors (see Chapter 5; Sielecki, 1989).

The RNA genome of the HIV, the causative agent of AIDS, encodes at least nine proteins. Coding sequences of most of these genes, obtained as non-infectious fragments of the viral cDNA, have been expressed in various expression systems to produce the proteins safely for their study as targets for anti-HIV therapy. Notable among the HIV gene products are the reverse transcriptase (see Chapter 2) and an RNA degrading enzyme, RNAase H, which together convert the RNA genome of the invading virus into a DNA copy which integrates into the DNA of the host. HIV also encodes a 99-amino-acid protease which is responsible for cleaving a large precursor protein into the smaller structural proteins required for the assembly of virus particles (Mitsuya *et al.*, 1990). The availability of safe, unlimited supplies of the reverse transcriptase and the protease has led to the development of screening assays for inhibitors of both these enzymes (Mitsuya *et al.*, 1990; Meek *et al.*, 1990; Kohlstaedt *et al.*, 1992). In addition, structural studies of these enzymes combined with mutational analysis has led to the understanding of their mechanisms of action, leading in turn to the rational design of inhibitors as described in Chapter 5 (*ASM News*, 1991; Blundell and Pearl, 1989; Navia *et al.*, 1989).

Fungal products cyclosporin A (CsA), FK506, and rapamycin are potent immunosuppressants that are used in organ transplantation. These agents prevent the activation of the T lymphocytes that are responsible for the rejection of transplants (Chang *et al.*, 1991; Cyert, 1992). They produce their effect by associating with a family of binding proteins known as immunophilins, which are present abundantly in all cell types. The protein that binds CsA, known as cyclophilin, is different from the protein that binds to FK506 and rapamycin, which is known as FK-binding protein or FKBP, and there is no cross binding. However, both cyclophilin and FKBP possess an enzymatic activity known as peptidyl prolyl isomerase or rotamase which catalyzes the *cis–trans* isomerization of proline residues in proteins. This activity may aid the folding of nascent, proline-containing proteins during their synthesis in cells. The prolyl isomerase activity of the immunophilins is inhibited by binding of their respective ligands, and this was initially thought to be the mechansim of immunosuppression. However, immunophilins are a ubiquitous and diverse family of proteins present in high levels in all cells, and CsA and FK506 appear to produce their immunosuppressive action at a concentration well below the levels needed to bind all the immunophilins stoichiometrically. This makes the prolyl isomerase inhibition an unlikely target for the specificity of these compounds in the preferential inhibition of T cell activation. Recent results suggest that the ligand–immunophilin complexes in the cases of CsA and FK506 (but not rapamycin) produce their effect by inhibiting the activity of the protein phosphatase calcineurin (which is also known as protein phosphatase 2B or PP2B). Calcineurin is a heterodimeric enzyme, which is highly conserved among eukaryotes from man to yeast, signifying its key function in cells. Its activity is regulated by the calcium-binding protein, calmodulin, and by the second messenger, calcium ion. There are several subtypes of calcineurins which are expressed in a tissue-specific fashion. Unlike CsA and FK506, however, rapamycin–FKBP complexes are believed to produce their action by interacting with an as yet unidentified enzymatic pathway (Chang *et al.,* 1991; Cyert, 1992).

Isolation of the immunophilin cDNAs has rendered possible the production and the structure–function study of these proteins by site-directed mutagenesis. In addition, yeast strains have been constructed where the endogenous ligands for CsA and FK506 have been replaced with their human counterparts. Such strains provide convenient assay systems for the structure–activity studies of putative immunosuppressants (Koltin *et al.,* 1991). The advances in immunosuppression are yet another salient example of the contributions of molecular biology to drug design and development.

DISEASE TARGETS FOR MOLECULAR PHARMACOLOGY

Recent advances in gene mapping and isolation of defective, disease-causing genes, coupled with the understanding of the molecular mechanisms of the activity of their normal counterparts, have led to the understanding of the genetic and the molecular basis of many diseases. This in turn has provided new angles for the development of therapeutics. In the previous sections, proteins involved in key pathways were discussed as groups. In this section the focus is on the role these proteins, and some others not previously discussed, play in disease states. Gene defects responsible for a number of diseases have been identified, and the genes have been isolated and sequenced. The mechanisms by which these mutations lead to the manifestation of the disease state are also beginning to be understood. The following selected examples illustrate the general trends in understanding disease processes through molecular biological approaches and resultant therapeutic insights.

Cancer

Cancer is a leading cause of death, accounting for half a million deaths annually in the US (Micklos and Freyer, 1990; Henderson *et al.,* 1991). It is a complex disease arising in the cells of many tissues, characterized by uncontrolled growth and multiplication of cells, and their invasion and spread to other organs. It is the added property of invasiveness and spreading, known as metastasis, that distinguishes the malignant cells in cancers from those in benign tumors which also arise because of uncontrolled cell multiplication. The metastatic potential of the cancer cell allows it to enter the blood stream, travel to distant locations in the body, and establish new colonies. Metastasis is the primary cause of death when cancer treatments fail (Liotta *et al.,* 1991; Liotta, 1992).

The uncontrolled growth of cancer cells has been traced at a molecular level to genetic changes which are involved in tumor origin and progression to malignancy. These changes appear to occur in genes encoding key proteins involved in the regulation of normal cell growth and division. The defective genes involved in the process of uncontrolled growth are known as "oncogenes", and anti-oncogenes or "tumor suppressor genes". Activation of an oncogene or inactivation of a tumor suppressor gene leads to loss of growth control resulting in "transformation" (Cooper, 1990; Weinberg, 1991; Aaronson, 1991; Solomon *et al.,* 1991).

In addition, contrary to earlier beliefs, metastasis is now known *not* to be a passive process caused by the mechanical consequences of increasing tumor volume. Tumor metastasis involves active participation of the gene products of the cancer cells which aid the cells to break through the normal barriers that constrain them to their respective tissue locations. At the molecular level, cancer cells use the same invasive mechanisms which are used by normal cells in a controlled fashion during embryonic development, tissue remodeling, wound healing, and homeostasis. Thus, tumor cells produce factors that stimulate the growth of blood vessels in their proximity, and also produce enzymatic activities which break down blood vessel and tissue barriers. Again, there appear to be genes whose activation produces metastatic potential, and suppressor genes whose inactivation also leads to metastatic potential (Liotta *et al.,* 1991; Liotta, 1992). The metastatic potential is also dependent on the ability of tumor cells to evade the immunological surveillance of the organism, using molecular disguises (Kahn, 1992). Many of the chemotherapeutic agents currently in use in cancer therapy are agents which inhibit tumor growth by globally inhibiting the replication and transcription of DNA, the central processes in cell growth (Calabresi and Chabner, 1990). However, since these processes are vital to the normal functioning of the organism, chemotherapeutic agents have narrow therapeutic windows and cause many undesired side-effects. The new information generated by recent molecular biological studies should provide novel approaches to the control of cancer by specific targeting of the defective genes involved in growth and metastasis, and also by stimulating the immune system using cytokines and lymphokines as discussed in Chapter 3. Research into genes controlling programmed cell death or "apoptosis" (by which aberrant cells self-eliminate) is yielding new clues and avenues for cancer therapy (Marx, 1993). These approaches should provide for individualized therapeutic regimens for cancers based on the characteristics and drug response considerations specific for each tumor type.

Oncogenes and tumor suppressor genes

The growth of a cell in a multicellular organism is tightly controlled by the interactions of proteins that stimulate and suppress growth. Both the unregulated activation of a growth-stimulating gene or the loss of a suppressor gene can result in uncontrolled growth. Cells that have lost the growth controls are termed "transformed" (Micklos and Freyer, 1990; Cooper, 1990). While some cancers show a genetic predisposition, a vast majority of them arise through mutations that occur in the population of somatic cells, caused by environmental agents such as chemicals and radiation. These agents damage DNA, causing alterations ranging from point mutations to gross chromosomal abnormalities (Solomon *et al.,* 1991). Transformation is also caused by oncogenic viruses such as papilloma viruses and the hepatitis B virus, which infect a cell and, rather than lysing it, reside in it latently. Transformation is caused by gene products of the virus, or by transcriptional derangement caused by interruption of cellular DNA by incorporation of viral DNA (zur Hausen, 1991). Current evidence suggests that the transformation of a cell is a multi-step event brought about by the activation of more than a single oncogene. Activation of the first oncogene prepares a cell population harboring it to respond to a second activating event. The second event leads to the loss of growth control (Micklos and Freyer, 1990; Cooper, 1990).

Genes whose activation leads to a transformed state in a cell are called oncogenes. Barring the exceptions of viral oncogenes, most cellular oncogenes are modified versions of normal cellular genes known as "proto-oncogenes". Proto-oncogenes are normally involved in key regulatory steps. Their genetic modification into oncogenes, or their overexpression due to accidental gene amplification (increase in gene copy number), leads to unregulated cell growth. Activation of proto-oncogenes occurs also when chromosome breaks occur in the vicinity of these genes and they are joined to transcriptionally active regions on other chromosomes (Solomon *et al.,* 1991).

Oncogenes are derived from every conceivable regulatory pathway in a cell. These include receptors with tyrosine or serine kinase activities, G proteins, and transcription factors (Touchette, 1992; Aaronson, 1991; Cooper, 1990). Gene products of oncogenes confer upon the cell the property of continued multiplication, ignoring the restraining signals from neighboring cells. Large numbers of oncogenes and proto-oncogenes have been identified to date, and the number, not surprisingly, is on the increase. Table 4.6 shows examples of oncogenes, corresponding proto-oncogenes, and their cellular function (Cooper, 1990; Solomon *et al.,* 1991). Activation of oncogenes such as *Ras*, a member of the G protein family, by mutation, and of *Myc* by gene amplification, are encountered in many cancers. Other oncogenes are also amplified in cells from specific tumors (Cooper, 1990). Specific inhibition of the function of the errant

Table 4.6. Oncogenes and their proto-oncogene counterparts

Oncogene	Proto-oncogene	Normal function
Cell-derived		
*erb*B	EGF receptor	EGF signaling
sis	PDGF	Growth factor
trk	NGF receptor	NGF signaling
ras	G protein	Signal transduction
src	Tyrosine kinase	?
raf	Ser/Thr kinase	?
*erb*A	Thyroid hormone receptor	Transcriptional activation
fos	Transcription factor	Transcriptional activation
mas	G protein-coupled receptor	Serotonin receptor
Viral oncogenes		
Adenovirus E1A	—	Transcriptional regulation
SV40 T antigen	—	Transcriptional regulation

From: Baulieu (1990); Cooper (1990); Aaronson (1991).

oncogenes is being explored as a method for the control of the growth of specific tumors. For instance, many oncogenes derived from tyrosine kinases maintain the ability to phosphorylate proteins at tyrosine residues. A number of inhibitors of protein tyrosine kinases are under testing for their antitumor efficacy (Powis, 1991). In another example, the *Ras* function requires association of the protein with the plasma membrane via a lipid molecule that is covalently linked to the protein. Inhibition of lipid addition is a possible way of inhibiting the uncontrolled expression of *Ras* activity. Inhibitors of the cholesterol biosynthetic pathway may be useful in this therapeutic approach (Schafer *et al.,* 1989; Aaronson, 1991).

Many viruses contain oncogenes. In some cases, these are viral genes that interfere with the regulatory function(s) of a normal cellular gene, leading to the loss of regulation. In other cases, the viral oncogenes are cellular proto-oncogenes, modified by mutations and deletions into an oncogenic form, and carried by viruses as a part of their genome (Micklos and Freyer, 1990; Cooper, 1990; zur Hausen, 1991).

In contrast to the activation of oncogenes which causes cell transformation, a group of genes whose *inactivation* leads to transformation has been identified recently. These are known as tumor suppressor genes, as the loss of their activity leads to unregulated growth (Weinberg, 1991). Since all diploid organisms, man included, have two copies of every gene including tumor-suppressor genes, inactivation of both copies of a suppressor gene is usually essential to release a cell from growth restraints. In families with inherited susceptibility to cancers such as retinoblastoma and neurofibromatosis, one member of the pair of suppressor genes is already mutated. Mutation in the remaining normal copy results in a transformation event which leads to retinoblastoma or neurofibromatosis, as the case may be. Independent tumor suppressor genes are found inactivated in different cancers. A suppressor gene known as p53 appears to be a transcription factor which forms complexes with itself and with viral oncogene products. Interference with the functioning of normal p53 through its interaction with viral gene products, or through formation of multimers with mutated copies of p53 protein present in a cell, leads to a transformed state. Function of p53 may be regulated by the levels of the cellular protein MDM2; overexpression of MDM2 can also lead to inactivation of the p53 function. As the detailed mechanisms of action of these proteins are emerging, sharp distinctions between oncogenes and suppressor genes are beginning to blur (Weinberg, 1991; Cooper, 1990; Lane, 1992).

Initial transformation of a cell is believed, in most cases, to involve the co-operation of at least two oncogenes, or the inactivation of both copies of a tumor suppressor gene. Once the property of uncontrolled growth is established in a cell, a tumor develops. The initial transformation events originate in single cells, and, therefore, tumors are clonal. Other mutations that favor invasive and metastatic properties occur subsequently within members of the initial clonal population of tumor cells as they continue to divide. This process of selection gives rise to increasingly virulent populations of cancer cells (Micklos and Freyer, 1990; Liotta *et al.,* 1991).

Genetic mechanisms of cancer metastasis

Metastasis is the progression of cancer that renders treatment difficult, and leads to death. Transformation, while conferring the property of uncontrolled growth, appears insufficient for the ability to metastasize. Metastasizing requires the capacity to perform additional processes required for cell migration. These include the ability to induce angiogenesis (creation of new blood vessels to vascularize the tumor), and the ability to invade and cross tissue boundaries by secreting the proteases required to break down tissue-limiting proteinaceous membranes. The metastasizing cell has to move into the blood stream via the new blood vessels it induced, and move out of the blood vessels to invade the tissue at the site of metastasis. These processes, used by cancer cells in metastasis, are used in normal tissue repair and remodeling, and in blood vessel growth. They require the expression of a variety of gene products by the transformed cell. A gene whose expression is seen to be reducing with increasing metastatic potential (analogous to tumor suppressor genes) has been identified. It appears to be involved in the G protein-mediated pathways of second messenger production (Liotta *et al.,* 1991). A detailed understanding of these phenomena stands to offer therapeutic avenues for the control of metastasis. A new class of compounds called carboxamide aminoimidazoles (CAIs), which alter the flow of calcium ions, appear to inhibit metastasis in animals, possibly by interfering with cell signaling (Liotta, 1992). Analysis of soluble factors which promote angiogenesis is leading to promising insights for the development of therapeutics aimed at the inhibition of angiogenesis induced by cancer cells (Edgington, 1992d).

Cystic fibrosis (CF)

This is an inherited disease whose molecular mechanism has been elucidated in the last few years by locating and isolating the defective gene responsible for the disease (Hooper, 1989). Understanding the function and the mechanism of action of the protein by expression studies and electrophysiology combined with the definition of the nature of the defect in the disease state has provided novel avenues for the therapy of CF (Widdicombe and Wine, 1991; Tsui and Buchwald, 1991; Collins, 1992).

CF is a genetically inherited disorder of the epithelial cells, characterized by excessively salty sweat. It is a recessive, single gene-linked disease which manifests itself when an individual inherits a copy of the defective gene from each parent. The majority of patients die owing to blockage of the airways and pancreatic ducts by accumulation of viscous mucus. The increased viscosity of the mucus is attributed to attenuated transport of chloride ions in sweat ducts and respiratory epithelia of diseased individuals. The frequency of CF varies between ethnic groups, with the highest being 1 in 2500 in certain Caucasian populations.

The average life expectancy of CF patients is currently 29 years, and is on the rise due to the development of effective management techniques.

Molecular biology of CF

The isolation of the CF gene represents a spectacular technological breakthrough in the isolation of disease-causing genes, and has become a paradigm for the isolation of other such genes involved in a variety of diseases (Koshland, 1992). Using genetic linkage analysis of many affected individuals and their normal relatives (discussed in Chapter 8), the gene defect in CF was mapped to human chromosome 7. Further refinement of mapping placed the gene within a 1.5 million base pair region of this chromosome. Techniques of "chromosome walking" and "chromosome jumping", which permit analysis of long stretches of chromosomal DNA sequences, were used to home in on the CF gene (Tsui and Buchwald, 1991). The authenticity of the isolated gene was confirmed by the presence of a specific mutation in 70% of the affected individuals, and by the presence of RNA derived from this gene in the tissues affected by the disease. The CF gene is 250 kilobases long, containing at least 24 exons. The mRNA derived from the gene is 6500 bases long and encodes a protein of 1480 amino acids. Analysis of the primary sequence of the protein revealed the presence of twelve transmembrane segments, suggesting the CF gene product to be a membrane-spanning protein. In 70% of the mutant CF genes, a 3-kilobase deletion bordering on one of the exons causes the loss of a phenylalanine in position 508. The remaining 30% is caused by 170 different mutations characterized to date, which result in in-frame deletions, nonsense and missense codons, frame shifts, and splicing defects (Hooper, 1989; Collins, 1992). These changes may influence not only the functionality of CF protein, but also its synthesis and transport to the appropriate cellular compartments (Armstrong, 1992; Miller, 1993).

Progress in understanding the function of the CF protein came from the expression of the CF cDNA in a variety of cell lines, ranging from *Xenopus* oocytes to mammalian cells, including those derived from the airway epithelia of CF patients. These studies showed that the CF protein influenced the chloride transport in cells, and that the introduction of the normal gene corrected the defect in airway epithelial cells derived from CF patients. Although the protein was believed to be a chloride channel, this thesis was difficult to prove experimentally; the possibility that it was simply an accessory to a chloride channel could not be ruled out. Hence the protein was named Cystic Fibrosis Transmembrane conductance Regulator (CFTR). Recent demonstration of the chloride conductance properties of this protein alone incorporated into artificial membranes has confirmed its function as a chloride channel. However, the structural features of the protein suggest that it may have other functions as well (Widdicombe and Wine, 1991; Collins, 1992; Barinaga, 1992b).

The structure and transmembrane organization of CFTR is shown in Fig. 4.11. It is composed of two homologous domains, each of which contains six transmembrane segments and a nucleotide binding domain known as NBFs (nucleotide binding folds). The two membrane-spanning domains are linked by a domain known as the regulatory or R domain. The phenylalanine deletion found in the majority of CF cases occurs within the first NBF, NBF-1. The functions of the NBFs and the R domains have been examined by expression of mutant CFTR cDNAs created by site-directed mutagenesis. NBFs are binding sites for adenosine triphosphate (ATP), and the R domain contains a number of serines thought to be substrates for phosphorylation by the cyclic AMP-dependent protein kinase, PKA. Deletion of the R domain caused the chloride channel to remain open in the absence of an increase in cyclic AMP (cAMP) levels, indicating the loss of the normal regulation of chloride transport by phosphorylation observed with the wild-type CFTR channel. Thus, the R domain appears analogous to a "plug" that opens and closes the mouth of the transmembrane channel produced by the twelve transmembrane domains. Experimental evidence supports a model for chloride conductance by CFTR in which phosphorylation of the R domain, followed by binding of ATP to NBF domains, results in the opening of the channel. Although the chloride channel function of CFTR is established, its structure is far more complicated than those of typical chloride channels which do not use energy derived from ATP. In this regard, the CFTR structure is analogous to that of pumps such as the multi-drug, resistance-inducing, P-glycoprotein family discussed earlier; like CFTR, P-glycoprotein has twelve transmembrane segments and two NBF domains. Thus, it is believed that CFTR may also have functions other than chloride transport (Hooper, 1989; Collins, 1992).

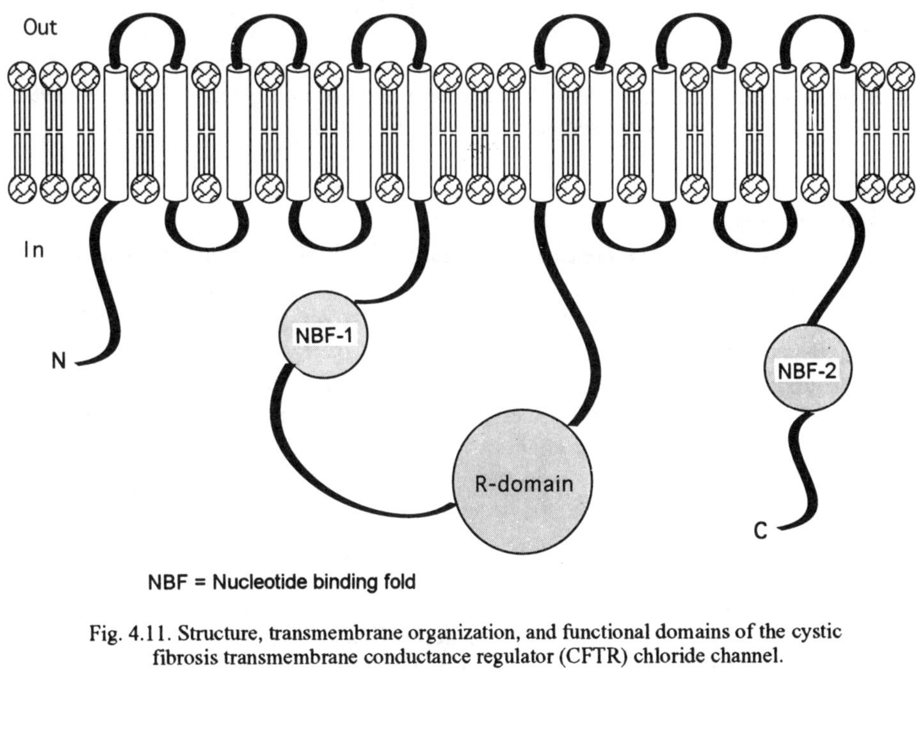

Fig. 4.11. Structure, transmembrane organization, and functional domains of the cystic fibrosis transmembrane conductance regulator (CFTR) chloride channel.

Therapeutic approaches

Therapeutic strategies aimed at several steps in the pathophysiological process are currently used in the management of CF. Since nearly 95% of the morbidity and mortality is a result of pulmonary complications, most approaches to therapy are focused on this aspect of the disease, and not at the CFTR aspect alone. These include relieving the symptoms of the disease by using antibiotics to control bacterial infections as well as decreasing the viscosity of the mucus by using aerosols of the enzyme DNAase, which digests the DNA released from dead white cells congregating at the sites of bacterial infections. Pharmacological agents such as amiloride, which blocks sodium uptake in the respiratory epithelium, are in clinical trials. Application of adenosine triphosphate (ATP) or uridine triphosphate (UTP) to the respiratory epithelial cells has been shown to stimulate the chloride flux, presumably through the activation of a nucleotide receptor. Aerosols of ATP and UTP are currently undergoing clinical trials (Collins, 1992).

Therapeutic approaches directed at the CFTR channel protein are also being considered. Elucidation of the mechanism of action of the CFTR has also led to the initiation of pharmacological strategies to correct the basic defect in CFTR. Elevation of intracellular cAMP has been shown to activate many mutant forms of CFTR. Thus, agents which increase cAMP levels by stimulating adenyl cyclase or inhibiting phosphodiesterases would be useful in therapy. Similarly, phosphatase inhibitors, which increase the net phosphate groups on the CFTR, may also be useful in therapy (Collins, 1992).

Correction of the chloride channel defect in cells explanted from CF patients by the introduction of the normal CFTR cDNA suggests that gene therapy may be beneficial. It may be sufficient to deliver the normal cDNA just to the respiratory epithelial cells. A number of strategies for gene therapy by using viral vectors and other delivery methods are under development and are being tested (Collins, 1992). These approaches are discussed in detail in Chapter 6.

Alzheimer's disease (AD)

This is yet another disease area to which molecular biological analysis has brought unprecedented insights. AD is a major cause of dementia affecting one in ten persons over age 65 and nearly one half of those over age 85. The course of the disease spans a period ranging from two years to over a decade, with an average span of about seven years. Added to the morbidity, the economic impact of AD on the patient and the care-givers, and the impending increase in the over 65 population due to demographic changes, make this disease a clinical and economic challenge of the twenty-first century. Currently there are neither effective therapeutics nor reliable diagnostic tests for AD. Confirmation of the disease is made post-mortem (Aaronson *et al.*, 1991; Selkoe, 1991).

Upon histopathological examination, the brains of AD victims show many changes among which extracellular amyloid plaques surrounding dying neurons and intracellular fibrillar tangles within these neurons are the predominant lesions. The amyloid plaques, unlike tangles which are found in many neurodegenerative diseases, are unique to AD. Both these lesions have been under intense biochemical study for decades, and were shown to contain proteins, but the characterization of their constituents, especially the proteins, was difficult because of the insolubility of plaques and tangles even under harsh extraction conditions. However, progress in the last decade in the isolation and characterization of the protein components of these lesions, and the concurrent developments of rDNA technology, have brought valuable insights into the mechanisms of AD (Selkoe, 1991; Kosik, 1992).

Molecular biology of amyloid plaques

In the mid 1980s, it became clear that the predominant component of the amyloid plaques was a single peptide about 40 amino acids long. When chemically synthesized, this peptide, known as the Amyloid Plaque Core (APC), showed a tendency to form insoluble aggregates similar to those found in amyloid plaques. Based on the sequence of the 40-amino-acid region, DNA probes were synthesized and the cDNA encoding the peptide was isolated. The cDNA sequence revealed APC to be an internal segment of a large protein of nearly 700 amino acids which traversed the membrane once. A schematic diagram of this protein, known as the Amyloid Precursor Protein (APP), is shown in Fig. 4.12. The 12 amino acids at the carboxyl terminus of the 40-amino-acid segment are part of the transmembrane domain of APP (Selkoe, 1991).

Shortly after the isolation of the first APP cDNA, alternative forms of APP cDNAs, all containing APC, and all derived by alternate splicing of a single gene on chromosome 21, were isolated. While no genetic correlates are found in the majority of AD cases, a small fraction (~5%) of the cases were known to be familial. Early attempts to link the APP gene to familial forms of AD were without success. Recently, however, several APP mutations associated with familial cases of AD have been discovered. Though not all cases of AD are accounted for by such mutations in APP, finding that mutations in the APP gene lead to AD was important in establishing the seminal role of amyloids (as opposed to other lesions including tangles) in AD pathology (Tanzi *et al.*, 1991; Joachim and Selkoe, 1992; Kosik, 1992; Gandy *et al.*, 1994).

Cell biological studies expressing the cDNA of APPs in transfected mammalian cells showed that the extracellular, amino terminal segment of APPs was released from the cell by proteolytic cleavage; this was shown to be the case in the brain as well. Intriguingly, the cleavage causing the APP release occurred within APC, precluding its participation in amyloid plaque formation (Fig. 4.12). Thus, the APC found in plaques appears to be derived from the alternative proteolysis of APPs which maintains the integrity of the 40-amino-acid APC segment. Such proteolytic processing has been demonstrated in normal and AD brains. Consequently, events leading to plaque formation in AD brains appear to be regulated by a balance between the alternative pathways of APP proteolysis. Derangement in the processing of APPs can occur through mutational changes in APPs, as has been shown to be the case, or by mutations in proteins that process APP. Alternatively, environmental

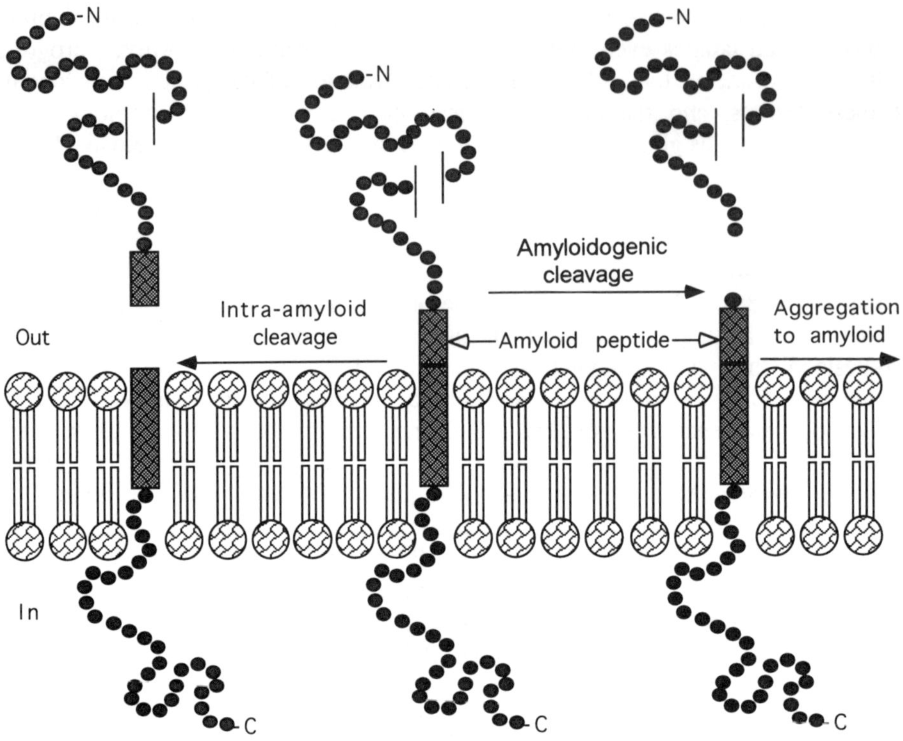

Fig. 4.12. Structure of APP, and its proteolysis through the intra-amyloid and amyloidogenic pathways.

toxins such as aluminum ions, or insults such as head trauma, may influence the metabolism of APP and/or the processing enzymes. The inability to clear the nascent APC aggregates by proteolytic degradation can also lead to the production of amyloid plaques. Overproduction of the APPs, caused by failure of regulation at transcription or other biosynthetic steps in APP production, may also increase the production of amyloidogenic fragments. In this context, it is interesting that brains of patients with Down's syndrome, a disease characterized by the triplication of chromosome 21 on which the APP gene resides, invariably show amyloid plaques similar to those found in AD. Plaque formation in Down's syndrome is attributed to the overexpression of APP due to the extra copy of the gene (Joachim and Selkoe, 1992).

Therapeutic avenues

Current therapies for AD are aimed primarily at combating the deficit of the neurotransmitter acetylcholine, which is reduced in AD brains. This and other such palliative approaches are aimed at treating the symptoms of AD, and have shown marginal success (Erickson, 1991; Joachim and Selkoe, 1992). A further detailed understanding of the molecular mechanisms of APP processing should provide avenues for the inhibition of APC peptide production. Intense activity is focused on identifying and inhibiting proteases that produce amyloidogenic cleavage of APPs (Rennie, 1991). It has been shown that phosphorylation of APP molecules by kinases such as protein kinase C influences the trafficking of APP through the different cellular compartments (Gandy *et al.*, 1991, 1994). Thus, inhibitors and activators of protein kinases and phosphatases directed specifically at kinases and phosphatases modulating APP processing may be useful in diverting the APPs away from the cellular compartments that are responsible for APC-producing proteolytic events (Gandy and Greengard, 1992).

The understanding of the cell biology of APP and the molecular basis of plaque formation is being used in the development of diagnostic tests for AD. Presently, there are no conclusive diagnostic tests available. Because of the risks involved in brain biopsies, the diagnosis of AD is based only on psychometric criteria. This diagnosis of AD is confirmed by a post-mortem analysis of the brain tissue. An accurate, rapid biochemical diagnostic test is vital both for the initial diagnosis and for monitoring the efficacy of therapeutics.

The development of animal models is yet another area impacted by the advances in the understanding of APP molecular biology. Amyloid plaques accumulate in the brains of man, monkeys, and a few other larger mammals in the course of the normal aging process. Similar amyloid plaques have not been observed in the brains of rats, mice, and other rodents which are used routinely in drug testing. Unlike rodents, monkeys and other animals are difficult to use in large-scale drug screens because of factors such as life-span and the availability of animals. The knowledge of APP biology and the mechanisms of plaque formation is being currently used to engineer convenient transgenic animal models for plaque formation (Joachim and Selkoe, 1992).

Other genetic and metabolic diseases

Advances similar to those described in the disease areas discussed above have also been made in the understanding of the genetic and metabolic basis of several other diseases (Caskey, 1992). Muscular dystrophy, Gaucher's disease, myotonic dystrophy, amyotrophic lateral sclerosis (ALS), multiple sclerosis, immunoglobulin deficiency, and diabetes are some examples (Caskey, 1992; Hoffman, 1992; Koshland, 1992; Atkinson and Maclaren, 1990; McNamara and Fridovich, 1993; Vetrie *et al.*, 1993; Potera, 1993). The different genetic mechanisms underlying different types of cancers are being actively investigated and are yielding diagnostic and therapeutic clues (Roberts, 1993). The genetic basis of other less-defined diseases such as schizophrenia and alcoholism is being sought with the aid of the tools that have emerged in the past decade with the advent of rDNA. Rapid advances occurring in the understanding of the molecular basis of diseases hold promise for the identification of new drug targets and for the development of novel drugs using molecular pharmacology.

REFERENCES

Aaronson, M.K., Ooi, W.L., Geva, D.L., Masur, D., Blau, A., and Frishman, W. (1991). Dementia: age-dependent incidence, prevalence, and mortality in the old. *Arch. Intern. Med.* **151,** 989-992.

Aaronson, S.A. (1991). Growth factors and cancer. *Science* **254,** 1146-1153.

Abbot, A. (1991). Receptor screens detect bioactivity. *Bio/Technology* **9,** 694.

Alberts, B., Bray, D., Lewis, J., Raff, M., Roberts, K., and Watson, J.D. (1989). *Molecular Biology of the Cell* (New York: Garland Publishing).

Armstrong, J. (1992). Another protein out in the cold. *Nature* **358,** 709–710.

ASM News (1991). Structural analysis of HIV proteins may lead to drugs. *ASM News* **57,** 446–447.

Atkinson, M.A. and Maclaren, N.K. (1990). What causes diabetes? *Sci. Am.* July, 62–71.

Bahouth, S.W., Wang, H., and Malbon, C.C. (1991). Immunological approaches for probing receptor structure and function. *TiPS* **12,** 338–343.

Barinaga, M. (1992a). Pot, heroin unlock new areas for neuroscience. *Science* **258,** 1882–1884.

Barinaga, M. (1992b). Novel function discovered for the cystic fibrosis gene. *Science* **256,** 444–445.

Baulieu, E-E. (1990). Hormones: a complex communication network. In *Hormones: from Molecules to Disease.* E-E. Baulieu and P.A. Kelly, eds. (New York: Chapman and Hall), pp. 3–170.

Beavo, J.A. and Reifsnyder, D.H. (1990). Primary sequence of cyclic nucleotide phosphodiesterase isozymes and the design of selective inhibitors. *TiPS* **11,** 150–155.

Bently, J.K. and Beavo, J.A. (1992). Regulation and function of cyclic nucleotides. *Curr. Opinion in Cell Biol.* **4,** 233–240.

Berridge, M.J. (1993). Inositol triphosphate and calcium signalling. *Nature* **361,** 315–325.

Bialy, H. (1990). A cloned tyrosinase turns *E. coli* black. *Bio/Technology* **8,** 603.

Blundell, T. and Pearl, L. (1989). A second front against AIDS. *Nature* **337,** 596–597.

Bourne, H.R. and Stryer, L. (1992). The target sets the tempo. *Nature* **358,** 541–543.

Bourne, H.R., Sanders, D.A., and McCormick, F. (1991). The GTPase superfamily: conserved structure and molecular mechanism. *Nature* **349,** 117–127.

Brown, K.D. (1992). Start-up firms take lead in application of advanced technology for drug discovery. *Genetic Engineering News* January, 1–6.

Cadena, D.L. and Gill, G.N. (1992). Receptor tyrosine kinases. *FASEB J.* **6,** 2332–2337.

Calabresi, P. and Chabner, B.A. (1990). Chemotherapy of neoplastic diseases. In *The Pharmacological Basis of Therapeutics.* A. Goodman Gilman, T.W. Rall, A.S. Nies, and P. Taylor, eds. (New York: Pergamon Press), pp. 1202–1276.

Carter, D.B., Thomsen, D.R., Im, W.B., Lennon, D.J., Ngo, D.M., Gale, W., Im, H.K., Seeburg, P.H., and Smith, M.W. (1992). Functional expression of $GABA_A$ chloride channel and benzodiazepine binding sites in baculovirus infected insect cells. *Bio/Technology* **10,** 679–680.

Caskey, C.T. (1992). DNA-based medicine: prevention and therapy. In *The Code of Codes: Scientific and Social Issues in the Human Genome Project.* D.J. Kevles and L. Hood, eds. (Cambridge, Massachusetts: Harvard University Press), pp. 112–135.

Casnellie, J.E. (1991). Protein kinase inhibitors: probes for the functions of protein phosphorylation. *Adv. in Pharmacol.* **22,** 167–205.

Catterall, W.A. (1988). Structure and function of voltage-sensitive ion channels. *Science* **242,** 50.

Chang, J.Y., Sehgal, S.N., and Bansbach, C.C. (1991). FK506 and rapamycin: novel pharmacological probes of the immune response. *TiPS* **12,** 218–223.

Clipstone, N.A. and Crabtree, G.R. (1992). Identification of calcineurin as a key signalling enzyme in T-lymphocyte activation. *Nature* **357,** 695–697.

Collins, F.S. (1992). Cystic fibrosis: molecular biology and therapeutic implications. *Science* **256,** 774–779.

Cooper, G.M. (1990). *Oncogenes* (Boston: Jones and Bartlett).

Cooper, J.R., Bloom, F.E., and Roth, R.H. (1991). *The Biochemical Basis of Neuropharmacology* (Oxford: Oxford University Press).

Corda, D., Luini, A., and Garattini, S. (1990). Selectivity of action can be achieved with compounds acting at second messenger targets. *TiPS* **11,** 471–472.

Craig, A.G. and Berendt, A.R. (1991). The role of ICAM-1 as a receptor for rhinovirus and malaria. In *Integrins and ICAM-1 in Immune Responses. Chemical Immunology,* vol. 50. N. Hogg, ed. (Basel: Karger), pp. 116–134.

Cyert, M.S. (1992). Immunosuppressants hit target. *Curr. Biol.* **2,** 18–19.

Delmas, B., Gelfi, J., L'Haridon, R., Vogel, L.K., Sjostrom, H., Noren, O., and Laude, H. (1992). Aminopeptidase N is a major receptor for enteropathogenic coronavirus TGEV. *Nature* **357,** 417–420.

Dixon, B. (1991). Prostaglandins from yeast could lower cost. *Bio/Technology* **9,** 604.

Dower, W.J. (1992). Phage power. *Curr. Biol.* **2,** 251–253.

Duronio, R.J., Reed, S.I., and Gordon, J.I. (1992). Mutations of human myristoyl-CoA: protein N-myristoyl transferase cause temperature sensitive myristic acid auxotrophy in *Saccharomyces cerevisiae. Proc. Natl. Acad. Sci. USA* **89,** 4129–4133.

Edgington, S.M. (1992a). Superfamily structure and biotech drug development. *Bio/Technology* **10,** 1529–1534.

Edgington, S.M. (1992b). How sweet it is: selectin mediating drugs. *Bio/Technology* **10,** 383–389.

Edgington, S.M. (1992c). Bauhaus biology: biotechnology and the common cold. *Bio/Technology* **10,** 502–507.

Edgington, S.M. (1992d). Angiogenic and angiostatic drugs: reshaping biotech's future. *Bio/Technology* **10,** 981–985.

Elander, R.P. and Chiang, S.J. (1991). Genetics of antibiotic process improvement: from classical genetics to genetic engineering. In *Recombinant DNA Technology and Applications*. A. Prokop, R.K. Bajpai, and C. Ho, eds. (New York: McGraw-Hill), pp. 153–170.

Engel, J. (1991). Common structural motifs in proteins of the extracellular matrix. *Curr. Opinion in Cell Biol.* **3,** 779–785.

Erickson, D. (1991). Love and terror: is a chemical messenger key to treating Alzheimer's? *Sci. Am.* April, 148–150.

Erlich, H.A., Gelfand, D., and Sninsky, J.J. (1991). Recent advances in the polymerase chain reaction. *Science* **252,** 1643–1650.

Fritz, C.C. and Green, M.R. (1992). Fishing for partners. *Curr. Biol.* **2,** 403–405.

Fruman, D.A., Klee, C.B., Bierer, B.E., and Burakoff, S.J. (1992). Calcineurin phosphatase activity in T lymphocytes is inhibited by FK506 and cyclosporin A. *Proc. Natl. Acad. Sci. USA* **89,** 3686–3690.

Fuh, G., Cunningham, B.C., Fukunaga, R., Nagata, S., Goeddel, D.V., and Wells, J.A. (1992). Rational design of potent antagonists to the human growth hormone receptor. *Science* **256,** 1677–1680.

Gandy, S. and Greengard, P. (1992). Amyloidogenesis in Alzheimer's disease: some possible therapeutic opportunities. *TiPS* **13,** 108–109.

Gandy, S.E., Buxbaum, J.D., and Greengard, P. (1991). Signal transduction and the pathobiology of Alzheimer's disease. In *Alzheimer's Disease: Basic Mechanisms, Diagnosis and Therapeutic Strategies*. K. Iqbal, D.R.C. McLachlan, B. Winblad, and H.M. Wisniewski, eds. (New York: Wiley), pp. 155–172.

Gandy, S.E., Caporaso, G., Buxbaum, J., Frangione, B., and Greengard, P. (1994). APP processing, Aβ-amyloidogenesis and the pathogenesis of Alzheimer's disease. *Neurobiol. Aging* **15,** 253–256.

Garrison, J.C. and Peach, M.J. (1990). Renin and angiotensin. In *The Pharmacological Basis of Therapeutics*. A.G. Gilman, T.W. Rall, A.S. Nies, and P. Taylor, eds. (New York: Pergamon Press), pp. 749–763.

Gibbons, A. (1992). Biotech's second generation. *Science* **256,** 766–768.

Glaser, V. (1992). Sphinx Pharmaceuticals takes long look at lipid therapeutics for disease. *Genetic Engineering News* May 15, 9–27.

Glaser, V. (1993). Biotechnology industry's interest grows in baculovirus expression systems. *Genetic Engineering News* **13,** March 15, 10–11.

Goldberg, M.E. (1991). Investigating conformation, dynamics and folding with monoclonal antibodies. *TIBS* **16,** 358–362.

Graves, M.C., Lim, J.J., Heimer, E.P., and Kramer, R.A. (1988). An 11-kDa form of human immunodeficiency virus protease expressed in *Escherichia coli* is sufficient for enzymatic activity. *Proc. Natl. Acad. Sci. USA* **85,** 2449–2453.

Green, N.M. (1990). Structural deductions from receptor sequences. In *Receptor Biochemistry: a Practical Approach*. E.C. Hulme, ed. (New York: IRL Press), pp. 277–301.

Green, S. (1993). Promiscuous liaisons. *Nature* **361,** 590–591.

Gschwendt, M., Kittstein, W., and Marks, F. (1991). Protein kinase C activation by phorbol esters: do cysteine-rich regions and pseudosubstrate motifs play a role? *TIBS* **16,** 167–169.

Gurdon, J.B. and Wickens, M.P. (1983). The use of *Xenopus* oocytes for expression of cloned genes. *Methods in Enzymol.* **101,** 370–380.

Hadcock, J.R. and Malbon, C.C. (1991). Regulation of receptor expression by agonists: transcriptional and post-transcriptional controls. *TINS* **6,** 242–247.

Hall, Z.W. (1992). Ion channels. In *An Introduction to Molecular Neurobiology.* Z.W. Hall, ed. (Sunderland, Massachusetts: Sinauer Associates, Inc.), pp. 81–118.

Hanks, S.K., Quinn, A.M., and Hunter, T. (1988). The protein kinase family: conserved features and deduced phylogeny of catalytic domains. *Science* **241,** 42–52.

Hardie, D.G. (1991). *Biochemical Messengers: Hormones, Neurotransmitters and Growth Factors* (New York: Chapman and Hall).

Harrison, J.K., Pearson, W.R., and Lynch, K.R. (1991). Molecular characterization of α_1- and α_2-adrenoreceptors. *TiPS* **12,** 62–67.

Harvey, A. (1991). New influences of biotechnology in drug discovery: is the rat an endangered species? *TiPS* **12,** 317–319.

Henderson, B.E., Ross, R.K., and Pike, M.C. (1991). Towards the primary prevention of cancer. *Science* **254,** 1131–1138.

Hidaka, H. and Kobayashi, R. (1992). Pharmacology of protein kinase inhibitors. *Ann. Rev. Pharmacol. Toxicol.* **32,** 377–397.

Hodgson, J. (1991). Carbohydrate-based drugs. *Bio/Technology* **9,** 609–613.

Hodgson, J. (1992). Receptor screening and the search for new pharmaceuticals. *Bio/Technology* **10,** 973–980.

Hoffman, B.F. and Bigger, Jr., J.T. (1990). Digitalis and allied cardiac glycosides. In *The Pharmacological Basis of Therapeutics.* A.G. Gilman, T.W. Rall, A.S. Nies, and P. Taylor, eds. (New York: Pergamon Press), pp. 814–839.

Hoffman, E.P. (1992). Stutter, stumble, or fall of a kinase? *Curr. Biol.* **2,** 309–311.

Hooper, C. (1989). Picking the lock on cystic fibrosis. *J. NIH Res.* **1,** 76–81.

Hynes, R.O. (1992). Integrins: versatility, modulation, and signalling in cell adhesion. *Cell* **69,** 11–25.

Hunter, T. and Karin, M. (1992). The regulation of transcription by phosphorylation. *Cell* **70,** 375–387.

Hynes, R.O. and Lander, A.D. (1992). Contact and adhesive specificities in the associations, migrations, and targeting of cells and axons. *Cell* **68,** 303–322.

Iismaa, T.P. and Shine, J. (1992). G protein-coupled receptors. *Curr. Opinion in Cell Biol.* **4,** 195–202.

Irvine, R.F. (1992). Inositol phosphates in cell signalling. *Curr. Opinion in Cell Biol.* **4,** 212–219.

Jackson, S.P. (1992). Regulating transcription factor activity by phosphorylation. *Trends in Cell Biol.* **2,** 104–108.

Jensen, E.V. (1991). Overview of the nuclear receptor family. In *Nuclear Hormone Receptors.* M.G. Parker, ed. (New York: Academic Press), pp. 1–13.

Joachim, C.L. and Selkoe, D.J. (1992). The seminal role of the β-amyloid in the pathogenesis of Alzheimer Disease. *Alzheimer Disease and Associated Disorders* **6,** 7–34.

Juranka, P.F., Zastawny, R.L., and Ling, V. (1989). P-glycoprotein: multidrug-resistance and a superfamily of membrane associated transport proteins. *FASEB J.* **3,** 2583–2592.

Kahn, P. (1992). Adhesion protein studies provide new clue to metastasis. *Science* **257,** 614.

Kartner, N. and Ling, V. (1989). Multidrug resistance in cancer. *Sci. Am.* March, 44–51.

Kennedy, M.B. (1992). Second messengers and neuronal function. In *An Introduction to Molecular Neurobiology*. Z.W. Hall, ed. (Sunderland, Massachusetts: Sinauer Associates), pp. 207–246.

Kikkawa, U., Kishimoto, A., and Nishizuka, Y. (1989). The protein kinase C family: heterogeneity and implications. *Ann. Rev. Biochem.* **58,** 31–44.

King, K., Dohlman, H.G., Thorner, J., Caron, M.G., and Lefkowitz, R.J. (1990). Control of yeast mating signal transduction by a mammalian β-adrenergic receptor and Gs α subunit. *Science* **250,** 121–123.

Kleuss, C., Scherubl, H., Hescheler, J., Schultz, G., and Wittig, B. (1993). Selectivity of signal transduction determined by gamma subunit of heterodimeric G proteins. *Science* **259,** 832–834.

Kohlstaedt, L.A., Wang, J., Friedman, J.M., Rice, P.A., and Steitz, T.A. (1992). Crystal structure at 3.5 Å resolution of HIV-1 reverse transcriptase complexed with an inhibitor. *Science* **256,** 1783–1790.

Kolberg, R. (1992). Animal models point the way to human clinical trials. *Science* **256,** 772–773.

Koltin, Y., Faucette, L., Bergsma, D.J., Levy, M.A., Cafferkey, R., Koser, P.L., Johnson, R.K., and Livi, G.P. (1991). Rapamycin sensitivity in *Saccharomyces cerevisiae* is mediated by a peptidyl prolyl *cis–trans* isomerase related to human FK506-binding protein. *Mol. Cell. Biol.* **11,** 1718–1723.

Komuro, I., Wenninger, K.E., Philipson, K.D., and Izumo, S. (1992). Molecular cloning and characterization of the human cardiac Na^+/Ca^+ exchanger cDNA. *Proc. Natl. Acad. Sci. USA* **89,** 4769–4773.

Koshland, D.E. (1992). Molecular advances in diseases. *Science* **256,** 717.

Kosik, K. (1992). Alzheimer's disease: a cell biological perspective. *Science* **256,** 780–783.

Lane, D.P. (1992). p53, guardian of the genome. *Nature* **358,** 15–16.

Laudet, V. and Stehelin, D. (1992). Flexible friends. *Curr. Biol.* **6,** 293–295.

Laurie, D.J., Seeburg, P.H., and Wisden, W. (1992). The distribution of 13 $GABA_A$ receptor subunit mRNAs in the rat brain. II. Olfactory bulb and cerebellum. *J. Neurosci.* **12,** 1063–1076.

Lefkowitz, R.J. (1992). The subunit story thickens. *Nature* **358,** 372.

Lester, H.A. (1988). Heterologous expression of excitability proteins: route to more specific drugs? *Science* **241,** 1057.

Levitzki, A. and Gilon, C. (1991). Tyrphostins as molecular tools and potential antiproliferative drugs. *TiPS* **12,** 171–174.

Lewin, B. (1990). Commitment and activation at Pol II promoters: a tail of protein–protein interactions. *Cell* **61,** 1161–1164.

Lindberg, R.A., Quinn, A.M., and Hunter, T. (1992). Dual-specificity protein kinases: will any hydroxyl do? *TIBS* **17,** 114–119.

Liotta, L.A. (1992). Cancer cell invasion and metastasis. *Sci. Am.* February, 54–63.

Liotta, L.A., Steeg, P.S., and Stetler-Stevenson, W.G. (1991). Cancer metastasis and angiogenesis: an imbalance of positive and negative regulation. *Cell* **64,** 327–336.

Lleonart, R., Naf, D., Browning, H., and Weissman, C. (1990). A novel, quantitative bioassay for type 1 interferon using a recombinant indicator cell line. *Bio/Technology* **8,** 1263–1267.

Luttrell, L.M., Ostrowski, J., Cotecchia, S., Kendall, H., and Lefkowitz, R.J. (1993). Antagonism of catecholamine receptor signalling by expression of cytoplasmic domains of the receptors. *Science* **259,** 1453–1457.

Lytton, J. and Nigam, S. (1992). Intracellular calcium: molecules and pools. *Curr. Opinion in Cell Biol.* **4,** 220–226.

Marx, J. (1992a). Taking a direct path to the genes. *Science* **257,** 744–745.

Marx, J. (1992b). New genes may shed light on growth control. *Science* **257,** 484–485.

Marx, J. (1993). Cell death studies yield cancer clues. *Science* **259,** 760–761.

Maxwell, R.A. and Eckhardt, S.B. (1990). *Drug Discovery: a Casebook and Analysis* (Clifton, New Jersey: Humana Press).

Mayer, M.L. (1992). Fine focus on glutamate receptors. *Curr. Biol.* **2,** 23–25.

McKeon, F. (1991). When worlds collide: immunosuppressants meet protein phosphatases. *Cell* **66,** 823–826.

McKnight, S.L. (1991). Molecular zippers in gene regulation. *Sci. Am.* **264,** April, 54–64.

McNamara, J.O. and Fridovich, I. (1993). Did radicals strike Lou Gehrig? *Nature* **362,** 20–21.

Meek, T.D., Lambert, D.M., Dreyer, G.B., Carr, T.J., Tomaszek, T.A., Moore, M.L., Strickler, J.E., Debouck, C., Hyland, L.J., Matthews, T.J., Metcalf, B.W., and Petteway, S.R. (1990). Inhibition of HIV-1 protease in infected T-lymphocytes by synthetic peptide analogues. *Nature* **343,** 90–92.

Meldolesi, J. (1992). Multifarious IP_3 receptors. *Curr. Biol.* **2,** 393–394.

Micklos, D.A. and Freyer, G.A. (1990). *DNA Science: a First Course in Recombinant DNA Technology* (New York: Cold Spring Harbor Laboratory).

Miller, C. (1993). Sickly channels in mild disease. *Nature* **362,** 106.

Miller, R.J. (1987). Multiple calcium channels and neuronal function. Science **235,** 46.

Mitchell, P.J. and Tjian, R. (1989). Transcriptional regulation in mammalian cells by sequence-specific DNA binding proteins. *Science* **245,** 371–378.

Mitsuya, H., Yarchoan, R., and Broder, S. (1990). Molecular targets for AIDS therapy. *Science* **249,** 1533–1544.

Moffat, A.S. (1992). High-tech plants promise a bumper crop of new products. *Science* **256,** 770–771.

Mosher, D.F. (1991). How do integrins integrate? *Curr. Biol.* **1,** 394–396.

Murad, F. (1990). Drugs used for treatment of angina: organic nitrate, calcium-channel blockers, and β-adrenergic antagonists. In *The Pharmacological Basis of Therapeutics*. A.G. Gilman, T.W. Rall, A.S. Nies, and P. Taylor, eds. (New York: Pergamon Press), pp. 764–783.

Nargeot, J. (1991). Mixing and matching of calcium channels. *Curr. Biol.* **1,** 350–353.

Navia, M.A., Fitzgerald, P.M.D., McKeever, B.M., Leu, C-T., Heimbach, J.C., Herber, W.K., Sigal, I.S., Drake, P.L., and Springer, J.P. (1989). Three-dimensional structure of aspartyl protease from human immunodeficiency virus HIV-1. *Nature* **337,** 615–620.

Netzer, W.J. (1990). Emerging tools for discovering drugs. *Bio/Technology* **8,** 619–622.

Nicoll, R.A. (1988). Coupling of neurotransmitter receptors to ion channels in the brain. *Science* **241,** 545.

Nicotera, P., Bellomo, G., and Orrenius, S. (1992). Calcium mediated mechanisms in chemically induced cell death. *Ann. Rev. Pharmacol. Toxicol.* **32,** 449–470.

Ostrowski, J., Kjelsberg, M.A., Caron, M.G., and Lefkowitz, R.J. (1992). Mutagenesis of the β_2-adrenergic receptor: how structure elucidates function. *Ann. Rev. Pharmacol. Toxicol.* **32,** 167–183.

Papas, T.S. (Ed.) (1990). *Gene Regulation and AIDS: Transcriptional Activation, Retroviruses, and Transcription* (Advances in Applied Biotechnology Series, Volume 7) (Houston: Gulf Publishing Company).

Peterson, M.G. and Tjian, R. (1992). The tell-tale trigger. *Nature* **358,** 620–621.

Piomelli, D. and Greengard, P. (1990). Lipoxygenase metabolites of arachidonic acid in neural transmembrane signalling. *TiPS* **11,** 367–373.

Potera, C. (1993). Team from Neurocrine Biosciences/Stanford identifies specific T cells linked to MS. *Genetic Engineering News* **13,** March 15, 1–23.

Powis, G. (1991). Signalling targets for anticancer drug developments. *TiPS* **12,** 188–193.

Pritchett, D.B., Luddens, H., and Seeburg, P.H. (1989). Type I and type II $GABA_A$-benzodiazepine receptor produced in transfected cells. *Science* **246,** 1389–1392.

Rall, T.W. (1990). Hypnotics and sedatives; ethanol. In *The Pharmacological Basis of Therapeutics*. A.G. Gilman, T.W. Rall, A.S. Nies, and P. Taylor, eds. (New York: Pergamon Press), pp. 345–382.

Rennie, J. (1991). A plague of plaques. *Sci. Am.* April, 150.

Rhee, S.G. (1991). Inositol phospholipid-specific phospholipase C: interaction of γ_1 isoform with tyrosine kinase. *TIBS* **16,** 297–301.

Ritchie, J.M. and Green, N.M. (1990). Local anesthetics. In *The Pharmacological Basis of Therapeutics*. A.G. Gilman, T.W. Rall, A.S. Nies, and P. Taylor, eds. (New York: Pergamon Press), pp. 311–333.

Roberts, L. (1993). Zeroing in on the breast cancer susceptibility gene. *Science* **259,** 622–625.

Roninson, I.B. (Ed.) (1991). *Molecular and Cellular Biology of Multidrug Resistance in Tumor Cells* (New York: Plenum Press).

Ross, E.M. (1992a). G proteins and receptors in neuronal signalling. In *An Introduction to Molecular Neurobiology*. Z.W. Hall, ed. (Sunderland, Massachusetts: Sinauer Associates), pp. 181–206.

Ross, E.M. (1992b). Twists and turns on G-protein signalling pathways. *Curr. Biol.* **2,** 517–519.

Sambrook, J., Fritsch, E.F., and Maniatis, T. (1989). *Molecular Cloning: a Laboratory Manual* (New York: Cold Spring Harbor Laboratories).

Sambrook, J.F. (1991). Protein traffic: pumping peptides. *Curr. Biol.* **1,** 57–58.

Schafer, W.R., Kim, R., Sterne, R., Thorner, J., Kim, S-H., and Rine, J. (1989). Genetic and pharmacological suppression of oncogenic mutations in *RAS* genes of yeast and humans. *Science* **245,** 379–385.

Selkoe, D.J. (1991). Amyloid protein and Alzheimer's disease. *Sci. Am.* November, 68–78.

Shenolikar, S. and Nairn, A.C. (1990). Protein phosphatases: recent progress. *Adv. Second Messenger and Phosphoprotein Res.* **23,** 1–121.

Sibley, D.R. and Monsma, Jr, F.J. (1992). Molecular biology of dopamine receptors. *TiPS* **13,** 61–69.

Sielecki, A.R., Hayakawa, K., Fujinaga, M., Murphy, M.E.P., Fraser, M., Muir, A.K., Carilli, C.T., Lewicki, J.A., Baxter, J.D., and James, M.N.G. (1989). Structure of recombinant human renin, a target for cardiovascular-active drugs, at 2.5 Å resolution. *Science* **243,** 1346–1351.

Silverman, R.B. (1992). *The Organic Chemistry of Drug Design and Drug Action* (New York: Academic Press).

Simon, M.I., Strathmann, M.P., and Gautam, N. (1991). Diversity of G proteins in signal transduction. *Science* **252,** 802–808.

Snutch, T.P. (1988). The use of *Xenopus* oocytes to probe synaptic communication. *TINS* **11,** 250–255.

Snyder, S.H. (1992). Nitric oxide: first in a class of neurotransmitters? *Science* **257,** 494–496.

Snyder, S.H. and Narahashi, T. (1990). Receptor-channel alterations in disease: many clues, few causes. *FASEB J.* **4,** 2707–2708.

Solomon, E., Borrow, J., and Goddard, A.D. (1991). Chromosome aberrations and cancer. *Science* **254,** 1153–1160.

Spalding, B.J. (1992). Companies target anxiety. *Bio/Technology* **10,** 124.

Spiegel, A.M. (1992). G proteins in cellular control. *Curr. Opinion in Cell Biol.* **4,** 203–211.

Spiegel, A.M., Backlund, Jr, P.S., Butrynski, J.E., Jones, T.L.Z., and Simonds, W.F. (1991). The G protein connection: molecular basis of membrane association. *TIBS* **16,** 338–341.

Stevens, C.F. (1992a). On to molecular mechanisms. *Nature* **358,** 18–19.

Stevens, C.F. (1992b). Just say NO. *Curr. Biol.* **2,** 108–109.

Stone, N., Flores, O., and Reinberg, D. (1991). Transcription initiation: the ultimate target for gene regulation. *Pharmaceutical Technol.* September.

Tamaoki, T. and Nakano, H. (1990). Potent and specific inhibitors of protein kinase C of microbial origin. *Bio/Technology* **8,** 732–735.

Tanabe, Y., Masayuki, M., Ishii, T., Shigemoto, R., and Nakashini, S. (1992). A family of metabotropic glutamate receptors. *Neuron* **8,** 169–179.

Tanzi, R.E., St. George-Hyslop, P., and Gusella, J. (1991). Molecular genetics of Alzheimer disease amyloid. *J. Biol. Chem.* **266,** 20579–20582.

Taylor, S.S., Kinghton, D.R., Zheng, J., Sowadski, J.M., Gibbs, C.S., and Zoller, M.J. (1993). A template for protein kinase family. *TIBS* **18,** 84–89.

Thastrup, O., Cullen, P.J., Dborak, B., Hanley, M.R., and Dawson, A.P. (1990). Thapsigargin, a tumor promoter, discharges intracellular Ca^{2+} stores by specific inhibition of the endoplasmic reticulum Ca^{2+}. *Proc. Natl. Acad. Sci. USA* **87,** 2466–2470.

Tonks, N.K. (1991). Plague, pox and tyrosine dephosphorylation. *Curr. Biol.* **1,** 259–261.

Touchette, N. (1992). Evolutions: cancer genes. *J. NIH Res.* **4,** 92–98.

Tsaur, M-L., Sheng, M., Lowenstein, D.H., Jan, Y.N., and Jan, L.Y. (1992). Differential expression of K^+ channel mRNAs in the rat brain and down regulation in the hippocampus following seizures. *Neuron* **8,** 1055–1067.

Tsien, R.W., Ellinor, P.T., and Horne, W.A. (1991). Molecular diversity of voltage-dependent Ca^{+2} channels. *TiPS* **12,** 349–354.

Tsui, L-C. and Buchwald, M. (1991). Biochemical and molecular genetics of cystic fibrosis. In *Advances in Human Genetics,* Vol. 20. H. Harris and K. Hirschhorn, eds. (New York: Plenum Press), pp. 153–266.

Van Boeckel, C.A.A., Grootenhuis, P.D.J., and Haasnoot, C.A.G. (1991). Specificity in the recognition process between charged carbohydrates and proteins. *TiPS* **12,** 241–243.

Vetrie, D., Vorechovsky, I., Sideras, P., Holland, J., Davies, A., Flinter, F., Hammarstrom, L., Kinnon, C., Levinsky, R., Bobrow, M., Smith, C.I.E., and Bently, D.R. (1993). The gene involved in X-linked agammaglobulinaemia is a member of the *src* family of protein–tyrosine kinases. *Nature* **361,** 226–233.

Walsh, D.A., Glass, D.B., and Mitchell, R.D. (1992). Substrate diversity of cAMP-dependent protein kinase: regulation based on multiple binding interactions. *Curr. Opinion in Cell Biol.* **4,** 241–251.

Watanabe, M. (1992). Ariad Pharmaceuticals, Inc. raises a record $46 million in private placement of its stock. *Genetic Engineering News* April 15, 1–15.

Weatherall, M. (1990). *In Search of a Cure* (Oxford: Oxford University Press).

Weinberg, R.A. (1991). Tumor suppressor genes. *Science* **254,** 1138–1146.

Widdicombe, J.H. and Wine, J.J. (1991). The basic defect in cystic fibrosis. *TIBS* **16,** 474–477.

Wisden, W., Laurie, D.J., Monyer, H., and Seeburg, P.H. (1992). The distribution of 13 $GABA_A$ receptor subunits in the rat brain. I. Telencephalon, diencephalon, mesencephalon. *J. Neurosci.* **12,** 1040–1062.

Yeager, C.L., Ashmun, R.A., Williams, R.K., Cardellichio, C.B., Shapiro, L.H., Look, A.T., and Holmes, K.V. (1992). Human aminopeptidase N is a receptor for human coronavirus 229E. *Nature* **357,** 420–422.

zur Hausen, H. (1991). Viruses in human cancers. *Science* **254,** 1167–1173.

5

Rational design of drugs based on molecular structure

The vast majority of drugs currently in use were identified by a combination of serendipity and mass screening of huge collections of compounds. While this approach has led to the development of unique therapeutic concepts and spectacular drugs, and sometimes to strong patent positions, this process of drug discovery has been a laborious one. For example, it is estimated that only 1 in 40,000 to 100,000 of the compounds initially screened as anticancer agents reach the clinic (Oldham, 1985). Thus, there is great economic benefit to be derived from improving the odds of identifying drug candidates. Rational drug design, where drugs are designed based on the knowledge of three-dimensional structures of the interacting molecules, has always been an attractive alternative and a scientifically satisfying approach; but the technological barriers which faced the structure-based approach were high in the past. This situation has undergone a dramatic change over the last decade, and structure-based drug design is at a stage closer to fruition. This change has been brought about by revolutions in two fields, biotechnology and computer technologies (Hodgson, 1990, 1991).

The term "rational drug design" is used in different contexts with different connotations. For instance, some of the approaches for drug screening described in Chapter 4 utilizing defined receptor systems have been termed rational drug design. While these hypothesis-based approaches are more rational than earlier random-screening approaches, they differ from rational design as used here. Determining the three-dimensional structure of the target macromolecule in atomic detail and using this information to select and optimize compounds that interact with the target receptor protein is how structure-based rational drug design is defined here.

Benefits that derive from the structural understanding at the atomic level are best illustrated by examining the consequences of the elucidation of the three-dimensional structure of double-stranded DNA determined during the 1950s. It would be very difficult or nearly impossible to imagine much of the biotechnology of today without this fundamental discovery. The double-stranded, complementary structure of DNA has provided the basis for understanding the mechanisms of DNA replication, transcription, translation, mutation, recombination, and repair. Our understanding of these mechanisms has been indispensable to the emergence and the continued development of molecular and cell biology, and biotechnology (see Alberts *et al.* 1989).

The structure of DNA and its determination were relatively simple in comparison to those of proteins which are far more complex and diverse in structure. Therefore, the determination of protein structures was relatively more involved and difficult. The determination of the first protein structure, that of the abundantly available muscle protein, myoglobin, reported in 1960, was laborious and complicated, and required large amounts of the pure protein. Unlike DNA and myoglobin, it was difficult to obtain sufficient quantities of many other proteins of interest in a pure form. The problem of availability of proteins has all but vanished with the advent of rDNA methods used in their production. On a different front, determination of the three-dimensional structure involves a large number of complex mathematical computations, and higher resolution structures demand a larger number of computations. Thus, the availability of proteins notwithstanding, the progress in structure determination witnessed today owes as much to the computational power provided by the supercomputers which have been developed over the past two decades (Dambrot, 1992). While protein availability and computational power were the major driving forces, other advances in instrumentation and data-gathering techniques have also contributed to the advances in structure determination.

How a linear sequence of amino acids determines the three-dimensional structure of a protein has been a central problem in molecular biology, and the rules which determine the folding of proteins are sometimes called the ''second genetic code''. Understanding of this code will lead to the ability to predict the complete three-dimensional structure of a protein from its primary sequence data, without resorting to laborious experimental methods. This problem has been addressed on a theoretical level by using *ab initio* quantum mechanical calculations, and thermodynamic calculations, and by using empirical methods. The empirical approaches use the chemical properties of amino acids and the knowledge of their presence, preference or absence in given structural domains of proteins of known sequence and structure. While these methods are far from providing unequivocal structural information, they have led to the development of computational methods which are being applied to drug development. Here again, the computational capabilities of the modern high-power supercomputers are indispensable to the process (Kuntz, 1992).

The following sections provide an overview of the basic techniques and computational methods used in the determination of the three-dimensional structure of proteins and of their complexes with other proteins and with low molecular weight ligands. The goal of this discussion is merely to generate a basic understanding of the techniques and their roles in structure-based drug design. Details of the techniques can be found in the references cited. The discussion on techniques and instrumentation is followed by recent examples of how the structural information is being applied to drug discovery and development.

TECHNIQUES OF STRUCTURE DETERMINATION

Experimental approaches

A host of physicochemical and spectroscopic methods are used for the characterization of proteins (Cantor and Schimmel, 1980). These techniques reveal information about the size, shape, and the chemical and structural composition of proteins. However most of these methods are unable to provide detailed three-dimensional structural information. X-ray diffraction and nuclear magnetic resonance (NMR) are the two major techniques that provide useful structural information on proteins. Application of these techniques has been influenced by rDNA in two ways. First, as mentioned before, many proteins heretofore difficult to obtain from natural sources are available in unlimited quantities through rDNA-based production techniques. Second, the primary sequence information provided by the sequencing of cDNAs is a vital adjunct to arriving at the three-dimensional structure of proteins, as neither X-ray diffraction nor NMR is capable of predicting the complete primary sequence of proteins under study. On the contrary, a knowledge of the primary structures of a protein, obtained by direct sequencing or inferred from the cDNA sequence, is essential for the unambiguous assignment of the three-dimensional structure using diffraction or NMR methods (Branden and Tooze, 1991).

X-RAY DIFFRACTION

Principle of X-ray diffraction

Crystalline arrays of atoms diffract X-ray beams directed at them in a pattern characteristic of the arrangement of atoms in the crystal lattice. Diffracted X-ray beams interfere with each other in a constructive or destructive manner to create a diffraction pattern that contains within it the structural information of the diffracting crystalline array. Experimental, mathematical, and empirical techniques are used to obtain the three-dimensional structure from the diffraction pattern.

The imaging of objects by light microscopy and of macromolecules by X-ray diffraction have similarities permitting the use of imaging by a light microscope as a convenient analogy for understanding some aspects of structure determination using X-rays. Like light, X-rays are electromagnetic radiation which are scattered by electrons in the materials they impinge on and, therefore, the diffraction of light has been used as a useful analogy for understanding the basis of X-ray diffraction (Glusker and Trueblood, 1972). The theoretical resolving power (the minimum separation distance between two microscopic objects for them to be seen as separate entities) of the light microscope is determined by the wavelength of light used. Thus, objects with dimensions near to the wavelength of light used are resolvable. The wavelength of the blue–violet region of the visible spectrum is around 400 nm (1 nm = 10^{-9} m) or 4000

Angstrom units (Å; 1 Å = 10^{-10} m). Therefore the smallest objects amenable to study by light microscopy are of this dimension. The use of a shorter wavelength radiation leads to the ability to image smaller objects. This principle is used in electron microscopes, which utilize high-velocity electron beams which, based on the quantum mechanical principles, have wave-like properties analogous to light and X-rays. The wavelength of an electron beam is much shorter than that of visible light (0.004 nm or 0.04 Å for a 100,000 V electron), and hence the higher resolving power of electron microscopes. Unfortunately, although the wavelength of electrons is theoretically sufficient for resolution at the atomic level, technical problems associated with electron lenses, the poor penetrating power of electrons, and the restrictions on sample preparation set the effective limit of resolution of an electron microscope for biological samples to around 20 Å or about 100 times lower than that of a light microscope (Alberts *et al.*, 1989). Based on the foregoing principle of resolving power, X-rays which have very short wavelengths of the order of 1.0 Å are capable of revealing structure at the atomic dimension. For instance, the carbon–carbon bond in a protein main chain of about 1.5 Å is within the resolving power of X-rays.

However, one major difference between visible light and electron beams, and X-rays, prevents the use of X-rays in the direct imaging of molecules through an X-ray microscope. While lenses are available to focus both light and electron beams, there are no methods available for focusing X-rays. In a light microscope, the light scattered by the object is collected and focused by the objective lens to recreate an image of the object which is recognizable to the human eye. Since no X-ray lenses exist, the X-rays scattered or "diffracted" by individual atoms travel in different directions in space, reinforcing and canceling out those scattered by other atoms in the molecule to produce points of maximal and minimal intensities analogous to bright and dark spots occurring in light diffraction. The process of waves reinforcing and canceling each other is known as "interference", a phenomenon best explained by the wave-like properties of electromagnetic radiation (as opposed to the particle-like properties of photons) such as light and X-rays. The points in space where X-ray beams scattered from a crystal "interfere" to produce maxima or minima are determined by the intensity or strength of the scattered X-rays from different atoms arriving at each point in space, and also by the "phase" of the X-ray waves arriving at that point. The strength of scattering by an atom is directly proportional to the number of electrons in it; the higher the atomic number, the greater the scattering power. The phase, on the other hand, is determined by the position of the atoms. Fig. 5.1 illustrates the concept of interference by using a simple example, where the phase differences between the two beams (of equal amplitude scattered by two atoms) arriving at different points in space determine the final intensity (which is the square of the amplitude of a wave). Whereas waves arriving in-phase add up and reinforce each other fully, those arriving at one-half wavelength out of phase cancel each other completely; intermediate intensities are observed for intermediate phase differences or if the amplitudes of the waves are different. Such reinforcements and annihilations, resulting in alternating bright and dark spots, occur along every plane in space.

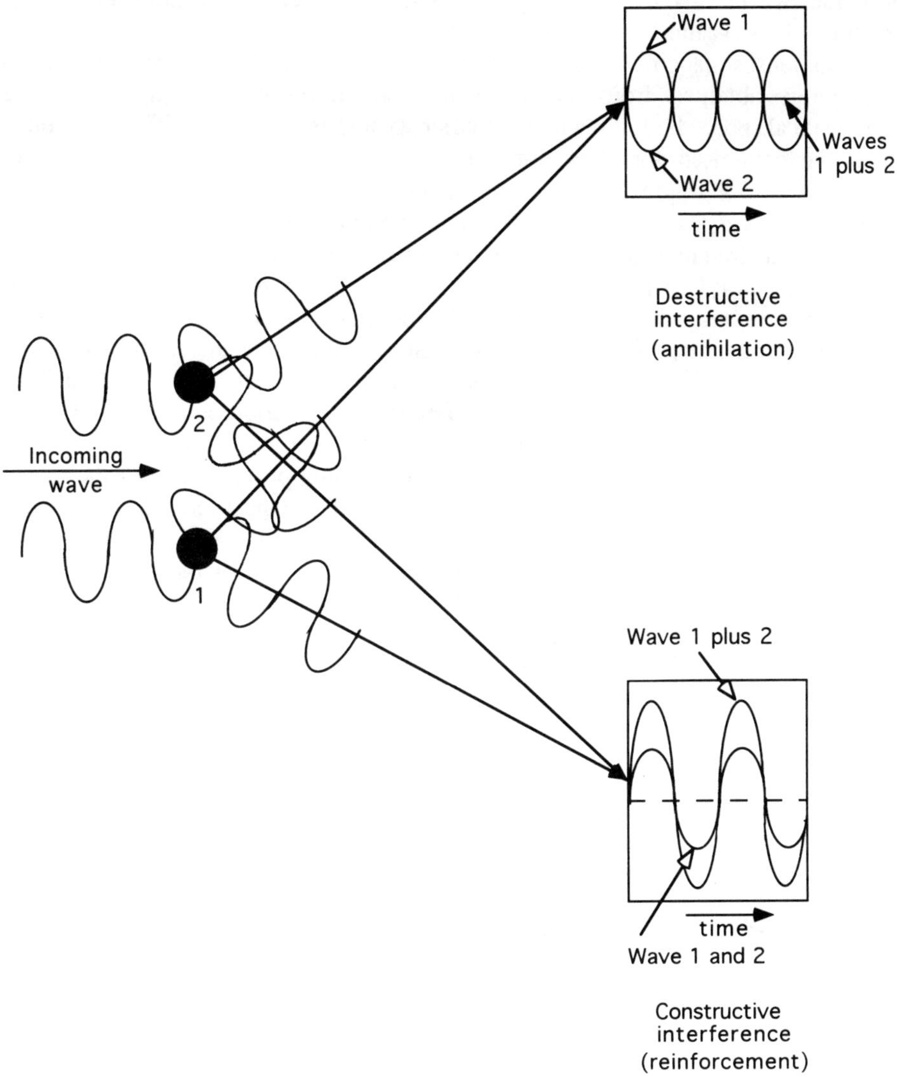

Fig. 5.1. Phenomenon of interference of electromagnetic waves such as light and X-rays illustrated by a simple case of two scattering atoms.

The phase difference between a pair of scattered waves is determined by the relative positions of the scattering atoms with respect to each other. A more complex pattern of intensity maxima and minima is generated by a large assemblage of scattering atoms, as in the case of a macromolecule. The pattern of maxima and minima produced by an object (a macromolecule in this case) is called its diffraction pattern, and can usually be recorded on photographic film which is responsive to X-rays. Knowing the scattering intensities and the relative phases of individual waves arriving at several points in space permits the derivation of the structure of the scattering macromolecule.

As no lenses capable of focusing X-rays are available, the structure of the molecule is obtained from the diffraction pattern by using a highly involved mathematical procedure known as Fourier synthesis. Thus, a diffraction image forms the data used for X-ray structure determination. In principle, the atomic components of a single molecule are capable of yielding a diffracted image. In practice, however, the X-rays diffracted by atoms of a single molecule are too weak to be detected by currently used detection systems. Hence, to increase the intensity of scattered X-rays to measurable levels, it is necessary to use a crystalline array of such molecules wherein the molecule of interest is arranged in a repeating pattern forming lattice structures characteristic of the molecule. A typical crystal may consist of 10^{18} molecules. The basic repeating unit in a crystal is called a "unit cell". The same protein, under different crystallization conditions, can yield crystals of different shapes and hence unit cells of different dimensions. A unit cell may contain one or more protein molecules, depending on the shape of the crystal. The goal of X-ray diffraction is to determine the relative positions of atoms within the unit cell forming a protein crystal. The experimentally recorded X-ray diffraction pattern is a summation of the diffraction pattern of the atoms in a unit cell with the interference properties of the ordered crystalline array of which it is a part. A typical diffraction pattern may consist of 5000 to 1,000,000 spots or "reflections" on a film, depending on the size of the molecule generating the pattern.

Experimental methods

The steps in obtaining the three-dimensional structure of a molecule are shown in Table 5.1. These involve the growth of protein crystals, their exposure to X-rays and collection of the diffraction pattern, and mathematical analysis of the diffraction pattern to obtain the structure.

Table 5.1. Steps in protein structure determination by X-ray diffraction

1. Production, isolation and purification
2. Primary sequence from protein or cDNA
3. Growth of suitable crystals
4. Collection of diffraction intensity data:
(a) with the protein alone
(b) protein with heavy atom replacements
5. Analysis of data for atomic coordinates:
(a) trial structures
(b) homology-based solutions
(c) Fourier synthesis
6. Refinement through iterative comparison

Growth of crystals

The most unpredictable process in X-ray structure determination is the crystallization of the candidate protein into a form suitable for X-ray diffraction. Each protein requires a unique set of conditions to form crystals. Typically 100 mg of highly purified protein is required to determine the conditions that result in usable crystals of 0.1 to 0.3 mm size, although a size of 0.3 to 0.8 mm is preferred. The occurrence of crystals and the rate of crystallization are influenced by many factors such as protein purity, the solvent, concentration of added precipitants, pH, temperature, and the presence of ions and cofactors. The protein solution at a concentration of typically 5 to 20 mg/ml is allowed to slowly reach supersaturation by the removal of or by changing the composition of the solvent by liquid–liquid diffusion or vapor diffusion methods. Microscale methods have been developed to explore several crystallization conditions simultaneously using minimum amounts of the purified protein sample. Recently, use of the ''zero gravity'' atmosphere in space has been explored as a means of facilitating crystallization (Eisenberg and Hill, 1990; Branden and Tooze, 1991; Tomasselli *et al.,* 1991).

Data collection

A satisfactory crystal is exposed to X-rays while held in the vapor phase of the liquid of crystallization or the ''mother liquor'' as shown in Fig. 5.2. The crystal is sealed in a thin-walled glass capillary between two layers of liquid. Orientation of the crystal with respect to the X-ray beam is changed by rotation or oscillation so that the constructive interferences from groups of atoms in different planes of the crystal are recorded by the X-ray detector represented by a sheet of X-ray sensitive photographic film in Fig. 5.2.

X-rays are obtained by the conventional method where accelerated electrons are used to bombard a metal anode. X-rays of higher intensity can be obtained from synchrotrons where they are emitted by accelerating electrons or positrons. The higher X-ray intensity of the synchrotron source is helpful in obtaining larger numbers of diffraction spots or ''reflections'' in shorter exposure times.

Detection of reflections is performed using X-ray-sensitive film where the interference maxima appear as dark spots. Figs 5.3A and B show typical protein crystals of the Krebs' cycle enzyme, porcine heart aconitase, and the diffraction pattern obtained from it. The intensities of the spots on the film are quantified by using a densitometer, and their locations on the film are determined accurately. Alternatively, the interference maxima are also detected and measured by using electronic X-ray detectors. Area detectors, recently introduced, use electronics to simultaneously measure the intensities of reflections over a wide area, and thereby save time both in data collection and in quantitation. Structure determination requires the collection of between 5000 and 100,000 spots (or reflections), depending on the size of the molecule and the degree of precision desired. The analysis of a larger number of reflections over a wider area leads to higher resolution structures. (This is analogous to the higher resolution obtained with a light microscope with objectives of higher numerical aperture; a larger aperture allows the gathering of larger amounts of the light scattered by the object.) For example, structures determined

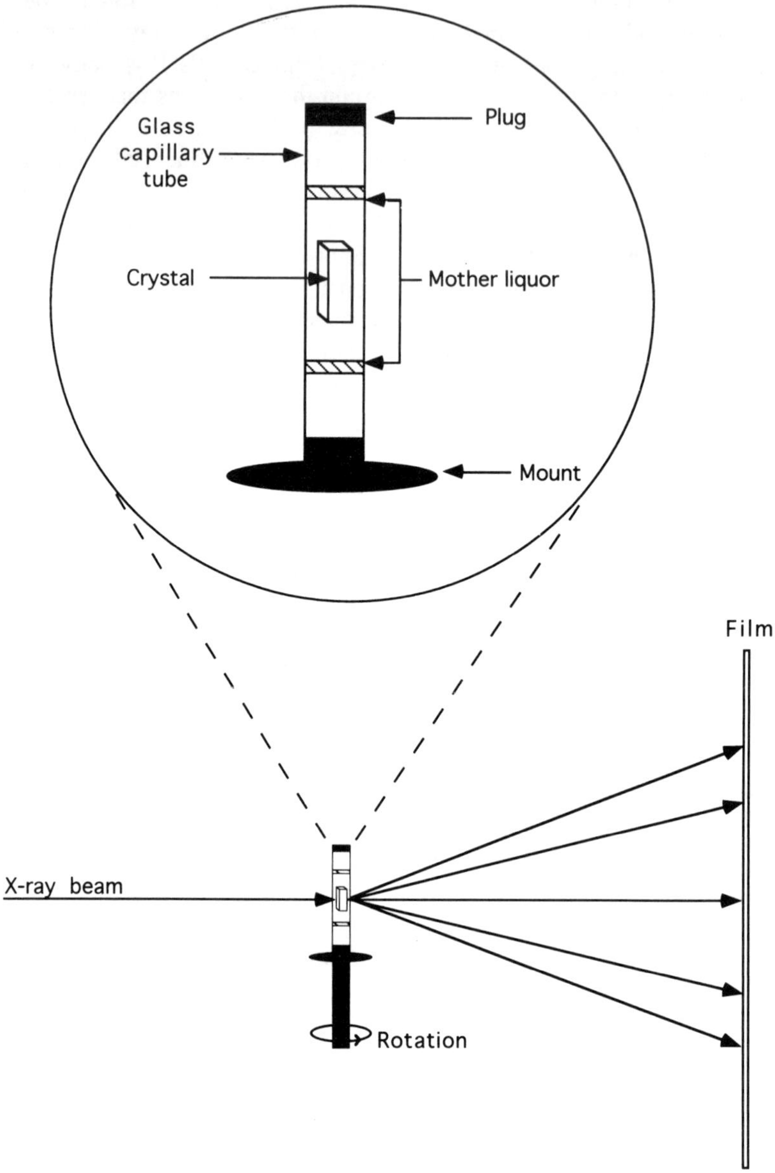

Fig. 5.2. Experimental set-up for obtaining X-ray diffraction patterns of protein crystals.

at 3 Å resolution allow tracing of the main chain and side chain moieties, which allows the determination of the overall structure of the protein. At 2 Å resolution, the side chains and disulfide bonds are clearly visible. However, determination of

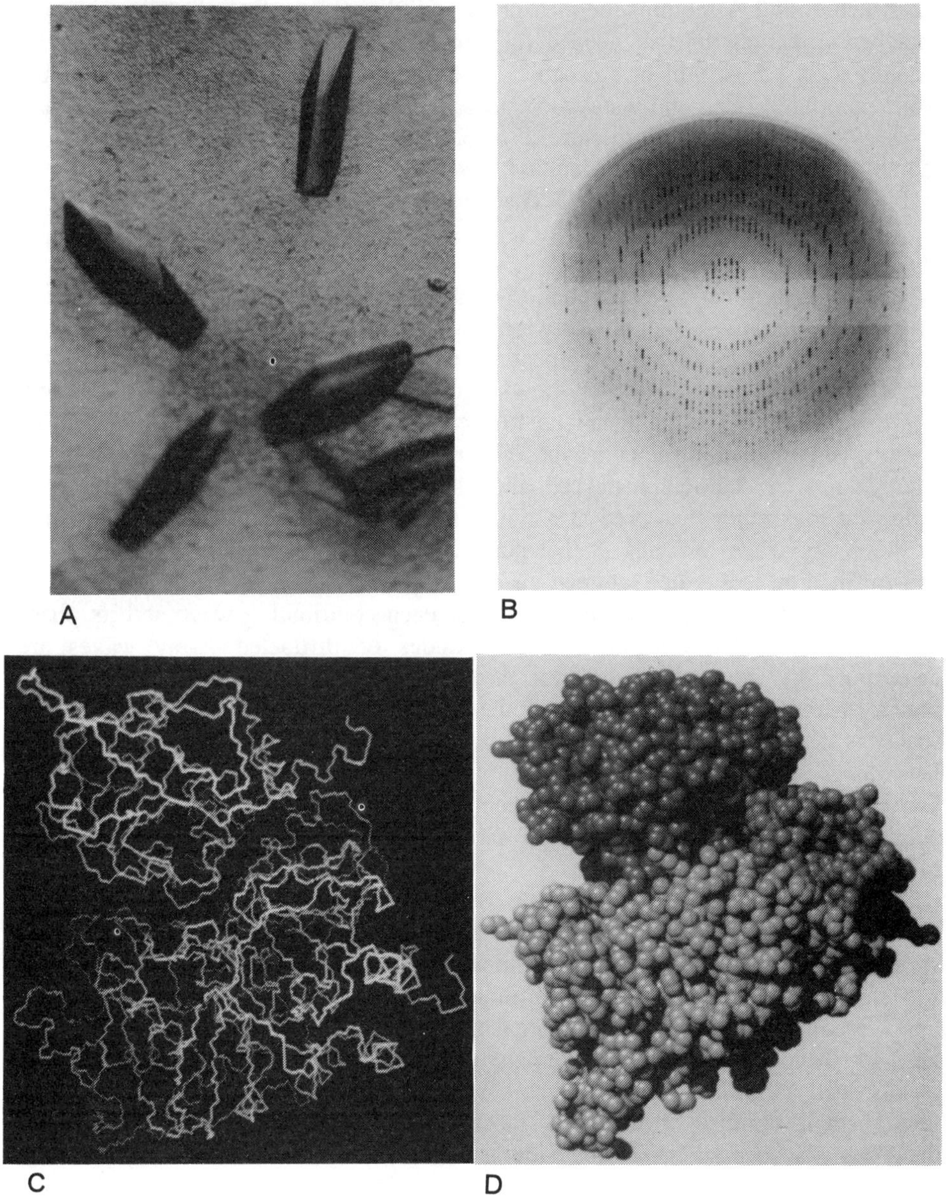

Fig. 5.3. (See colour section.) Protein structure determination by X-ray diffraction. A. Crystals of porcine heart aconitase composed of 754 amino acids. The orthorhombic crystals shown are about 0.5 mm in the longest dimension. B. Film showing the diffraction pattern obtained from the above crystal. These data were used to obtain a 2.7 Å resolution structure shown in two representations in panels C and D. Panel C shows the tracing of the protein backbone, with the small molecule (in red and yellow) in the central region depicting the iron-containing cofactor of the enzyme. Panel D shows the space-filling representation. (Courtesy of Dr Arthur H. Robbins, Miles Pharmaceuticals Inc. For details see: A.H. Robbins and C.D. Stout (1989). *Proteins: Structure, Function, and Genetics* **5,** 289–312.)

the structure at 2 Å requires the measurement and analysis of nearly twice as many spots or reflections as that needed for structure determination at 3 Å. Similarly, resolution of 1.5 Å, which is capable of permitting the visualization of individual atoms, aromatic rings and water molecules, requires the analysis of twice as many spots as a 2 Å resolution structure. Figs 5.3C and D show two representations of the structure of porcine heart aconitase, derived from the diffraction pattern shown in Fig. 5.3C by using the methods described below.

Derivation of structure

While the determination of structures of small molecules from X-ray diffraction patterns is relatively straightforward, it is a laborious task in cases of macromolecules which contain thousands of atoms. Measurement of the spacing between the reflections allows the determination of the unit cell dimensions. However, assigning exact locations to the atoms within the unit cell is a more complicated mathematical endeavor. The crux of this analysis is the solution of what X-ray crystallographers call the "phase problem". The intensity of a reflection maximum measured at a point in space is the result of the summation of the X-ray waves arriving at that point from different atoms in the crystal. As shown in Fig. 5.1, the summed-up intensity is dependent on the amplitude (intensity is the square of the amplitude) of each contributing wave and its phase with respect to the other waves. Amplitudes of diffracted X-ray waves are determined by the scattering power or the atomic number of the atoms which scatter them. The relative phase of the scattered waves arriving at a point in space is a measure of the relative position of the atoms in the unit cell. Knowledge of both phase and intensity is necessary for deriving the structure. Unfortunately, the measurement of spot intensity, which is the square of the amplitude, does not yield phase information. Thus it is necessary to obtain phase information by using analytical and experimental methods. Phases are determined either by purely analytical methods, or by using trial structures to generate theoretical diffraction patterns to match the observed pattern. However, while sufficient for applications to small molecules, these approaches alone are not sufficient when dealing with macromolecules such as a protein composed of many atoms. An experimental approach termed "isomorphous replacement" is used for the determination of the relative phases. In this method, atoms of heavy metals such as uranium, mercury, gold, or lead are introduced into the crystal so that a small number of them are incorporated into the crystal lattice without distorting the overall structure. This is achieved by soaking the crystal in a solution of the heavy metal salt. Owing to their higher atomic numbers, heavy atoms scatter X-rays more intensely than the atoms such as N, C, O, and H found in biological molecules. Because of their intense scattering, it is easier to determine the positions of the heavy atoms in the unit cell, and they serve as landmarks for the determination of the phases of waves generated by the atoms of the protein molecule. A comparative analysis of the diffraction patterns obtained with and without the heavy atoms provides the phase information required to obtain electron density maps which are required to solve the protein structure. In practice, diffraction patterns with at least two independent heavy atom substitutions are required for the unambiguous determination of phases and the structure. Thus, the ability to produce crystals with multiple heavy atom replacements is often necessary for structure determination by X-ray crystallography. However, other methods of phase determination, such as molecular replacement and anomalous scattering, are also applied where possible, and these circumvent the need for heavy atom derivatives. The molecular replacement method uses the known, experimentally determined structure of a related or homologous protein to derive an initial model or "trial structure", and the phases that would result in diffraction by the trial structure (Eisenberg and Hill, 1990). This trial structure is further refined as discussed below.

A mathematical procedure called Fourier synthesis applied to the phase and amplitude (intensity) information yields the electron density maps of the molecule in several planes in the crystal. Electron density maps are analogous to geographical contour maps. Stacking of such contour maps representing each plane results in a three-dimensional electron density map, with atomic nuclei at the centers of electron-dense areas. However, the scattering powers of atoms or chemical groups such as side chains of amino acids are not sufficiently different to allow distinguishing between them at the level of resolution routinely attained in diffraction studies of most proteins. Therefore, a knowledge of the amino acid sequence of the protein becomes essential for the unambiguous assignment of specific atoms or chemical groups to observed electron densities. Protein sequence information is easily inferred from the sequence of the gene.

Refinement of structure

Once a tentative structure or model of the unit cell contents is available, it is possible to calculate the diffraction pattern that would arise from such a structure. A comparison of the calculated pattern with the observed pattern is used to determine the deviation of the predicted structure from the actual structure. This information is used to further refine the deduced structure. This iterative refinement procedure is repeated until the deviation between the calculated and observed diffraction patterns is reduced to a desired level of definition. The deviation of the diffraction pattern of the deduced structure from the observed pattern is measured by a quantity called the "R factor". The R factor measures the correctness of a trial structure and is called the discrepancy index between the observed and the calculated diffraction patterns (for a mathematical definition, see Glusker and Trueblood (1972)). R factors vary from 0.0 for perfect agreement to around 0.59 for total disagreement, with a value of between 0.15 and 0.20 for well-determined structures. The attainment of R factors smaller than 0.15–0.2 is made difficult by limitations of data collection contributed by factors such as slight variations in the conformation of individual protein molecules in the crystal, impurities in the protein preparation, non-homogeneity of crystals, and physical factors such as the thermal motion of atoms. Because of these variations, the determined structure is an average structure incorporating the variations caused by the above physical and chemical factors. While structures with a medium resolution of 3 Å allow the determination of the overall structure of the protein, serious errors are possible at this degree of resolution. Structures at resolutions 2 Å or lower and *R* factors lower than 0.15–0.2 are called "high-resolution structures", and are without major errors. They yield atomic coordinates within an estimated error of between 0.1 and 0.2 Å (Branden and Tooze, 1991). Such highly refined high-resolution structures are essential for structure-based drug design (Appelt *et al.*, 1991).

In addition to the crystal structures of the native, free protein molecule, structures of its complexes with natural inhibitors and other ligands are useful for the rational design of small molecules which influence the activity of the candidate protein. The process of structure-based drug design consists of iterative cycles of using the structural information obtained from the analysis of a protein–ligand complex to design a more effective, tighter-binding ligand. This process is outlined in Fig. 5.4 (Appelt *et al.*, 1991). Although not essential, predicted interactions between chemical groups in the protein and the ligands can be verified by altering the amino acids in the protein via site-directed mutagenesis, thus validating the conclusions derived from the structural model.

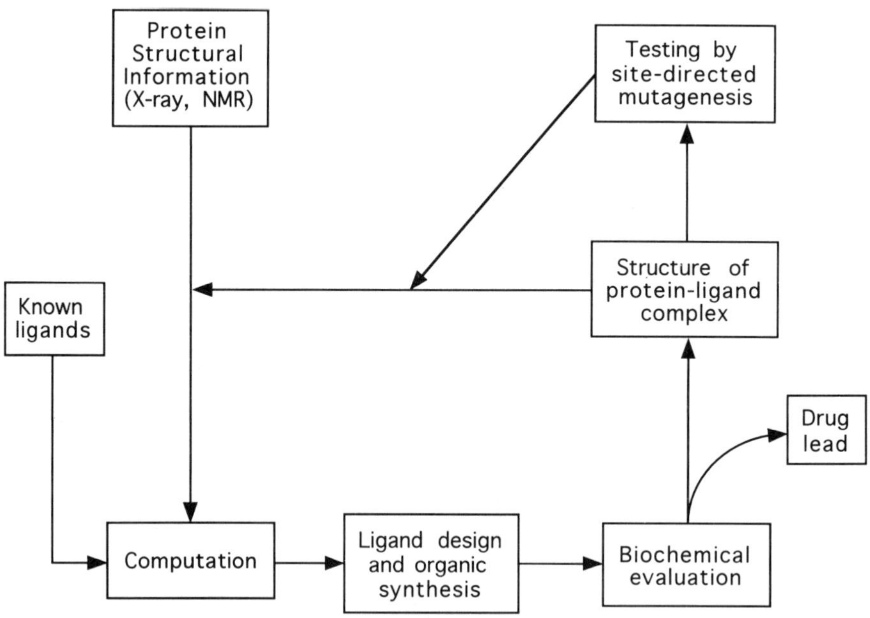

Fig. 5.4. Steps involved in structure-based rational drug design. (Adapted from Appelt *et al.* (1991).)

Recent technological advances

High-resolution structures of hundreds of protein molecules are currently available and many more are being determined with increasing rapidity. This pace of structure determination owes as much to other technological advances as it does to the development of molecular biology, which made unlimited quantities of pure proteins available. Early protein structures were determined using weak X-ray sources and manual scanning of X-ray films. Calculations were performed on computers with inadequate power. Thus, many years were required to determine the structure of even small proteins (Branden and Tooze, 1991).

Currently, instrumentation for the rapid generation, detection and analysis of diffraction patterns, and improved X-ray sources, and synchrotrons which produce X-rays of significantly higher intensity than earlier models, are available. Electronic area detectors capable of detecting and measuring several intensity maxima simultaneously and accurately, interfaced with powerful computers, provide a means for rapid data acquisition and analysis. Computer graphics, unheard of in the earlier days of crystallography, permit rapid three-dimensional visualization of the electron density maps and aid the refinement of structures. New methods for the direct solution of the phase problem by using the computational power of supercomputers are in the early stages, and appear to hold promise for the rapid determination of structures of mid-size and larger molecules, reducing the experimental work and duration in structure determination (Moffat, 1992). In spite of these advances, however, crystallization and the generation of useful heavy-atom derivatives of protein crystals, remain a major bottleneck in the X-ray crystallography of proteins.

NUCLEAR MAGNETIC RESONANCE (NMR)

NMR is a technique whose application to the structure determination of proteins has emerged more recently. This method has been in extensive use for the structure determination of small organic molecules for a number of years (Sanders and Hunter, 1991). Its application to the solution of the three-dimensional structure of larger molecules in recent years has been facilitated by the development of technology for producing highly efficient magnets, electronic monitoring circuits and powerful computers for data analysis. Structure determination is performed by using two-dimensional NMR (2D NMR), and recently 3D and 4D techniques capable of extracting the structural information from larger molecules have been developed (Bax, 1989; Branden and Tooze, 1991; Clore and Gronenborn, 1991).

Principle of NMR

The nuclei of certain atoms have associated with them magnetic moments resulting from a quantum mechanical property known as the spin angular momentum, which is dependent on a quantity called the spin quantum number. Each unpaired proton and each unpaired neutron in the atomic nucleus contributes a value of 1/2 to the total spin quantum number value of a nucleus. Thus, the hydrogen nucleus consisting of a single proton has a spin of 1/2. Whereas the naturally abundant carbon-12 nucleus, composed of six protons and six neutrons, has no net spin, the carbon-13 isotope nucleus has a spin of 1/2 owing to an additional unpaired neutron. Likewise, the abundant phosphorus-31 isotope has a spin of 1/2. Nitrogen-14, with seven protons and seven neutrons, has a spin of 1 resulting from 1/2 each from the unpaired proton and neutron. For a nucleus to be ''visible'' in an NMR experiment it must have a non-zero spin value and for technical reasons, nuclei with a spin value of 1/2 are the ones suited for NMR analysis. Thus, while carbon-12 nuclei, abundant in biomolecules, are useless from the standpoint of NMR, other nuclei naturally found in biological molecules such as hydrogen and phosphorus-31 can produce NMR signals. Samples artificially enriched for the carbon-13 and nitrogen-15 isotopes are capable of producing NMR signals characteristic of these atoms (Cantor and Schimmel, 1980). Substitution of carbon-13 and nitrogen-15 into proteins can easily be achieved during the synthesis of proteins by rDNA methods by growing the expression host cells in the presence of amino acids containing these isotopes.

The NMR technique measures the interactions of the nuclear magnetic moments of the atomic nuclei in the compounds under study with externally applied magnetic fields. The nature and the strength of interaction is determined by the spin value, mass, and charge of the particular nucleus. For instance, nuclei with a spin of 1/2, but differing in mass and/or charge, interact differently with the external magnetic field. Most importantly, the interaction is also influenced by *the local environment of the individual nucleus*, which is determined by factors such as shielding by the electron clouds of the neighboring atoms. Thus, for instance, hydrogen nuclei bonded to different carbon atoms in a molecule interact with the external magnetic field with measurable differences determined by their local environment. It is the measurement of these local environmental effects that gives NMR the power to produce structural information.

Nuclei which contain a non-zero spin can be imagined to be spinning around an axis analogous to a spinning top. This spinning action of the charged nucleus, according to the laws of physics, produces a magnetic moment in the nucleus along the axis of the spin. Thus, these nuclei behave like little magnets. The application of an external magnetic field leads to the alignment of the magnetic moment of a spinning nucleus with respect to the external field as shown in Figs 5.5A and B. Spinning of the nucleus causes the magnetic moment of the nucleus to precess around the external magnetic field. The frequency of precession is determined by the nature of the nucleus and by the net applied magnetic field the nucleus *experiences*. Under these conditions, if an oscillating magnetic field is applied in a direction perpendicular to the aligning, constant field, the nucleus interacts with the oscillating field if the frequency of oscillation is at or near its precession frequency. Such interactions are characterized by the absorption of energy from the oscillating field and energy emission producing a current in the detection system. Different nuclei of the same atomic species present in a molecule experience the constant, aligning magnetic field to different extents determined by the electronic shielding they are under. Therefore, their precession frequencies are measurably different from that of an unshielded nucleus and from those of each other. Consequently, the frequency of the oscillating field at which they absorb and re-emit energy maximally is different. This is the basic principle of NMR spectroscopy.

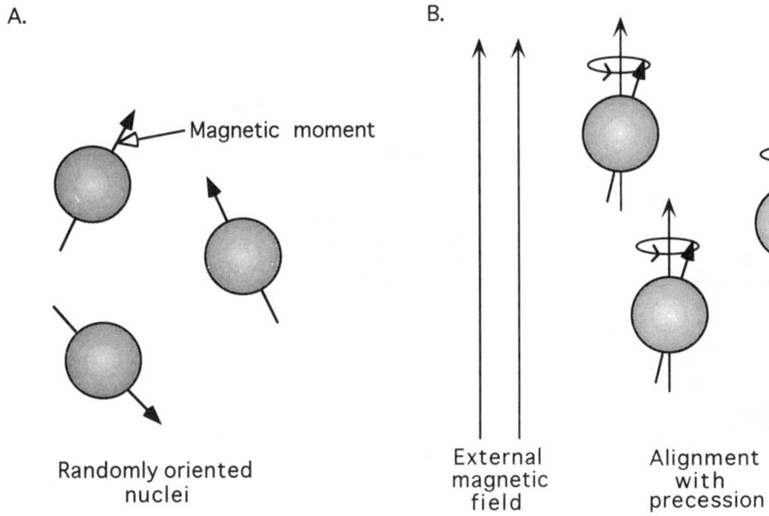

Fig. 5.5. Spinning nuclei as magnets. A. Random orientation in the absence of external magnetic field. B. Alignment and precession in an external constant magnetic field. The arrow along the axis of spin represents the magnetic moment of the nucleus. The circle along the tip of the magnetic moment arrow in panel B represents the path of precession.

The experimental aspect of obtaining an NMR spectrum is shown in Fig. 5.6. A constant magnetic field is applied to the sample to orient the atomic nuclei. An oscillating magnetic field of variable frequency is applied to the sample in a direction perpendicular to the constant magnetic field. A signal detector senses the current generated in a direction perpendicular to both the constant field and the oscillating field. The constant field, the oscillating field, and the detection system are positioned in the *x*-, *y*-, and *z*-axes respectively of the cartesian system. The frequency of the oscillating field or the strength of the constant field is varied continuously (or "swept") so that the precession frequencies of different nuclei in the sample match the oscillating field respectively at their characteristic frequencies or field strengths. This results in energy absorption and emission at specific frequencies or field strengths. An NMR spectrum represents the plot of the oscillating frequency or the strength of the constant magnetic field against the signal current produced in the detection system.

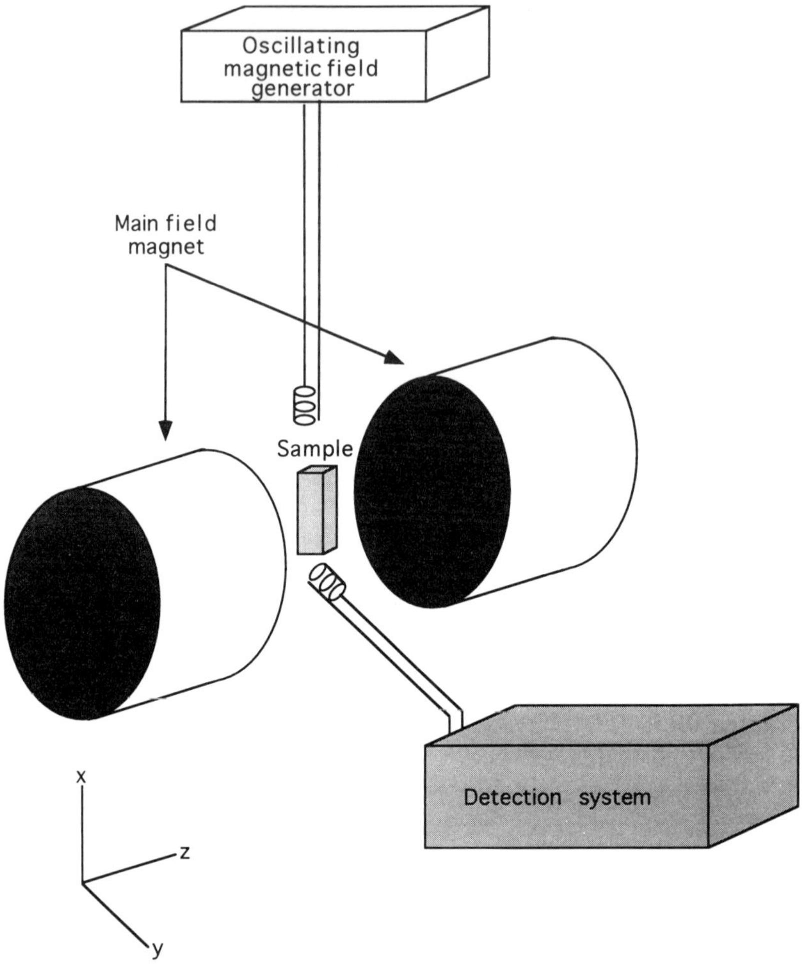

Fig. 5.6. Schematic of a typical experimental set-up for obtaining NMR spectra.

A routinely used, alternative method of obtaining an NMR spectrum is to subject nuclei oriented in the constant field simultaneously to an oscillating field composed of many frequency components. A sharply rising magnetic field pulse can be shown mathematically (by a method known as Fourier analysis) to be composed of oscillating field components of a wide range of frequencies. When such a pulse is applied to the nuclei oriented in a constant magnetic field, each nucleus interacts with the oscillating field component that corresponds to its precession frequency. The composite signal received from different nuclei responding to the different frequency components in the applied pulse is recorded over an interval, and separated into a frequency spectrum by Fourier analysis, yielding the NMR spectrum. This technique is called Fourier transform NMR or FT-NMR.

NMR spectra of small molecules show many well-resolved peaks corresponding to the nuclei in different electronic environments, yielding a "fingerprint" unique to each compound. However, as the size of the molecules increases, the number of responsive nuclei that experience the same or nearly similar electronic environments increases, resulting in many overlapping, unresolvable peaks which provide no useful information. Application of *selected sequences* of multiple magnetic field pulses to such unresolved systems followed by the analysis of the signals emitted over time as a consequence can be used to derive three-dimensional information from larger molecules composed of several hundred nuclei; this is the principle of 2D NMR (Bax, 1989; Wright, 1990; Branden and Tooze, 1991).

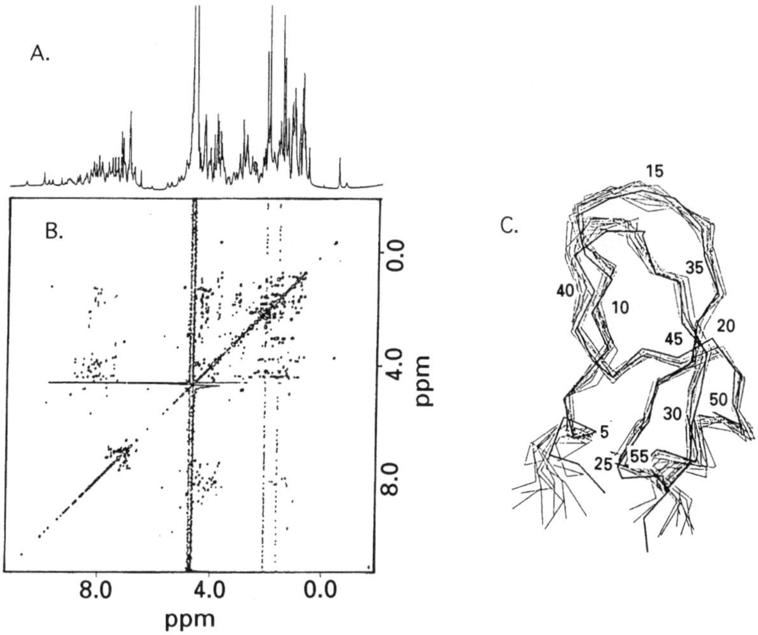

Fig. 5.7. Structure analysis of a 56-amino-acid protease inhibitor peptide by 2D NMR spectroscopy. A. One-dimensional NMR spectrum of the peptide. B. A two-dimensional NMR spectrum of the same peptide. C. Set of possible structures obtained from 2D NMR spectra similar to the one shown in panel B. (Courtesy of Dr Sarah L. Heald, Miles Pharmaceutical Inc. For details see: S. L. Heald *et al.* (1991) *Biochemistry* **30**, 10467–10477.)

Various pulsing schemes using critically timed sets of pulses have been developed to explore the different spatial interactions of nuclei. Nuclei connected to each other through one or a few covalent bonds emit signals which are detected in "correlation spectroscopy" or COSY spectra. The interaction of unlinked pairs of nuclei, through the spatial exchange of magnetization, can result because of physical proximity. The strength of such an interaction, known as the ''nuclear overhauser effect'' (NOE), is dependent on the sixth power of the internuclear distance. NOE interactions are measurable within spatial distances up to 5 Å. Pulsing schemes that detect such interactions are called NOE spectroscopy, and the resultant two-dimensional plot is a NOESY spectrum. Thus, COSY and NOESY spectra yield different spatial information. Using such analysis, three-dimensional structures of proteins up to 100 amino acids in length have been determined. Figs 5.7A and B show respectively a one-dimensional and a two-dimensional NMR spectrum of a 56-amino-acid-long protease inhibitor peptide. The distance information derived from the analysis of the 2D spectrum in Fig 5.7B and others obtained through different pulsing schemes yields a structure for the peptide; the hairpin-like configuration adopted by the protease inhibitor peptide is shown in Fig. 5.7C.

While the 2D NMR techniques described above are adequate for proteins composed of 100 amino acids or less, they are not productive for the structural studies of larger molecules because the number of overlapping peaks in the 2D spectra increases with the number of nuclei. 2D spectra are generally obtained by using the interactions of hydrogen nuclei or protons. Combinations of different 2D NMR spectra and a pulsing scheme measuring the interactions of protons with other nuclei such as carbon-13 (heteronuclear interactions) have been used to design 3D and 4D NMR schemes which permit the structure determination of larger proteins up to 150–300 amino acids (Bax, 1989; Clore and Gronenborn, 1991; Powers *et al.,* 1992).

Analyses of NMR spectral data and the derivation of three-dimensional structures involve complex sets of mathematical calculations. Such analyses yield a set of distance values for each proton or nucleus, describing its placement in the molecule with respect to other nuclei in its vicinity. Here, as in the case of X-ray diffraction, knowledge of the amino acid sequence of the protein is essential for accurate structure assignment. The combination of the spatial constraints of nuclei with the known amino acid sequence produces a set of closely related, equally possible three-dimensional structures. This is because more than one spatial position of a nucleus satisfies the conditions needed to produce a specific NMR peak. All the possible structures obtained are usually drawn superimposed, and, therefore, the molecular structures obtained by NMR appear as if they are a visual blur or like spaghetti, at least in some regions (see Fig. 5.7C). The extents of deviation of the various possible structures from the average structure may not be uniform throughout the length of the molecule. Thus, the structure in some regions may be poorly defined. Nonetheless, the groups of predicted structures are close enough to provide valuable information as has been shown in the case of many proteins (Bax, 1989; Wright, 1990).

Comparison of X-ray crystallographic and NMR methods

Structures determined from NMR spectra are in most cases in agreement with the X-ray structures, and are of comparable quality to 2 to 2.5 Å X-ray structures

(Bax, 1989; Clore and Gronenborn, 1991). Disagreements are attributable in most cases to the fundamental differences in the methodologies (Hodgson, 1993).

X-ray structures are obtained from crystalline samples. Crystallization is a laborious process, and the crystallizability of a protein is unpredictable. Some proteins do not crystallize, and X-ray diffraction is not applicable in these cases. In other cases, heavy atom derivatives needed to solve the "phase problem" may be difficult to obtain. Furthermore, crystals, although highly hydrated, do not represent the structure of the molecule in a true solution. Movements of protein domains are restricted in the crystalline state. NMR methods circumvent some of these difficulties because they are applied to proteins in solution. Therefore, in addition to permitting the determination of structures, the NMR technique is useful for revealing dynamic processes such as protein–protein interactions.

NMR spectroscopy requires concentrated protein solutions of the order of 1 mM. The protein must be pure, soluble and free of aggregates at this concentration. This set of requirements may be difficult to satisfy for many proteins. Further, theoretical considerations limit the size of proteins amenable to NMR analysis to under 40 kD or 400 amino acids. No such size limit has been set for the X-ray diffraction method.

Thus, X-ray diffraction and NMR methods have advantages and disadvantages, but used in conjunction with each other, the methods reveal useful structural information unobtainable by either method alone (Hodgson, 1993). Recently, the joint refinement of structures using crystallographic and NMR data is being explored in order to resolve ambiguities in structures obtained by either method alone (Shaanan *et al.,* 1992). Both techniques are widely used in structural biochemistry laboratories aimed at drug development (Clore and Gronenborn, 1991).

EMPIRICAL, SEMI-EMPIRICAL AND THEORETICAL METHODS

With the advent of rDNA technology, the primary amino acid sequences of thousands of proteins have become available through cloning and DNA sequencing. However, the experimental methods for structure determination described above are labor- and time-intensive, and are also inapplicable to many proteins for technical reasons discussed earlier. Thus, the number of known sequences far exceeds the number of determined three-dimensional structures by a factor of 50. In 1990, whereas the number of proteins for which primary sequence data were available totalled about 25,000, only 300 3D structures with atomic coordinates were available (Bowie *et al.,* 1991). Even under the best circumstances, the availability of the 3D structure information on newly isolated proteins of known primary sequence lags a year or more behind the production and purification of the protein because of the laborious nature of experimental methods. Therefore, there is a great degree of interest in developing methods for the direct prediction of the 3D structures from the amino acid sequence.

The problem of how a primary amino acid sequence dictates the 3D structure or the tertiary structure of a protein has intrigued structural biologists long before the recent sequencing revolution. It is often called the ''folding problem'', and is thought to be governed by a set of poorly understood rules called the ''second genetic code''. Early experiments using the enzyme ribonuclease showed that, under laboratory conditions, completely denatured ribonuclease was capable of refolding and regaining its biological activity. This led to the concept that the amino acid sequence contained all the information needed to determine the three-dimensional structure of a protein, which, in turn, led to the development of approaches for structure prediction (Fasman, 1990; Branden and Tooze, 1991). Since this initial observation, several other proteins have also been shown to be capable of refolding under appropriate laboratory conditions. In fact, this has been the case for a number of proteins of therapeutic interest produced as insoluble aggregates in *E. coli* and other recombinant expression systems as discussed in earlier chapters. It should be noted, however, that the intracellular environment under which most proteins fold is different from the laboratory conditions. Many nascent proteins contain peptide segments known as propeptides, which are removed when the protein matures. These segments influence the folding of the nascent protein in the cell (Baldwin, 1990; Dobson, 1992). In addition, it is becoming increasingly clear that a group of intracellular proteins called ''chaperones'', and enzymatic activities such as disulfide- and proline-isomerases present in cells, guide a nascent protein through its folding pathway expending energy stored in ATP (Ellis, 1992; Ewbank and Creighton, 1992).

Prediction of the completely folded tertiary structure from the amino acid sequence has been addressed through three broad approaches. These are: (1) a comparative method in which the known 3D structure of another protein with sequence homology is used as a guide; (2) prediction of the secondary structures of individual domains followed by packing of these domains into a compact molecule based on energetic and thermodynamic considerations; (3) the use of quantum mechanical and thermodynamic principles *ab initio* to predict secondary and tertiary folding (Fasman, 1989a, 1990; Branden and Tooze, 1991). In practice, combinations of these methods are used to predict and refine the structures. All of these methods rely to varying extents on the high computational capacity of modern computers. Algorithms have been developed to facilitate processes such as sequence comparisons, folding predictions, and thermodynamic and energetic calculations.

The homology method is useful in predicting the structures of members of a family of proteins when experimentally determined atomic coordinates are available for one or a few members (Sali *et al.*, 1990; Branden and Tooze, 1991). Examination of a number of experimentally determined protein structures shows that the framework structures of proteins are composed of a combination of α helices and β sheets (see Chapter 2) with randomly structured loops connecting the helices and sheets. Starting with the known structure, allowances are made for amino acid substitutions, insertions, or deletions in the candidate protein using physicochemical and steric properties of the variant amino acids and the consequent energetic changes. Changes caused by amino acid substitution may be conservative such as an isoleucine to a valine, causing a minimal change between structures. On the extremes, the introduction of glycines (with a hydrogen atom as the side chain) provides added conformational freedom, and the introduction of prolines or disulfide linkages restricts the conformational possibilities (Richardson and Richardson, 1989). With such allowances made, the structure of the protein is inferred by superimposition on the known structure of the related protein. As discussed extensively in earlier chapters, many proteins of similar functions share domains of varying degrees of sequence homologies, suggesting their evolution from a common ancestor (Doolittle, 1990). The homology method therefore can be used to infer structures of such related proteins. Among proteins of pharmaceutical interest, this method was applied to human renin before its crystal structure became available recently. In the period preceding the experimental determination, the structure of human renin inferred from that of a homologous aspartic protease, pepsin, and later from the structure of mouse renin, was used for the development of renin inhibitors (Jansy, 1988; Sielecki *et al.,* 1989; Sali *et al.,* 1990). Similarly, preceding the experimental determination of the X-ray structure, the homology approach was used for the prediction of the dimeric structure of the HIV protease which also belongs to the family of aspartic proteases (Pearl and Taylor, 1987). The HIV protease structure was further refined by using the experimentally determined structure of the related protease from the Rous sarcoma virus, RSV (Blundell and Pearl, 1989; Leis *et al.,* 1990). The overall conclusions regarding the core structures of renin and HIV protease, and the dimeric nature of the HIV protease, were confirmed by subsequent determinations of their crystal structures. However, deviations between the predicted and determined structures were observed to a degree sufficient to affect modeling of the inhibitors (Sielecki *et al.,* 1989; Blundell and Pearl, 1989). Thus, while predicted structures are useful, experimentally determined structures are clearly better, and are often necessary, for the development of inhibitors and other ligands (Appelt *et al.,* 1991; Hodgson, 1991).

The method of predicting protein structures by homology comparison utilizes the sequence homology retained during divergent evolution of proteins from a common ancestor. While sequence homology implies structural similarity, the reverse is not the case. Proteins with similar overall three-dimensional structures or similar domains do not necessarily have amino acid sequence homologies. The ability of unrelated amino acid sequences to form similar structural modules forms the basis for attempts to design novel proteins of desired structure *de novo* in the laboratory (Richardson and Richardson, 1990; Hodgson, 1990; Brandon and Tooze, 1991).

The problem of predicting the 3D structure of a protein with no amino acid sequence homology to another protein of known structure is more complicated. In this case, prediction of the tertiary structure relies on the prediction of the secondary structures of the different regions of the protein followed by the assembly of the individual domains to arrive at an acceptable tertiary structure (Fasman, 1989b, 1990; Branden and Tooze, 1991). Studies of the refolding of isolated proteins in the laboratory support the concept of folding of amino acid stretches within a protein to assume their preferred secondary structures, followed by the formation of a stable tertiary structure involving these individual domains (Dobson, 1992). Thus, several methods have been developed to predict the secondary structure of local regions. These include predictions based on properties such as hydrophobicity, and other physicochemical and steric properties of the individual amino acids. Another data-based approach used widely relies on the environmental preferences or propensities of individual amino acids. This information is derived from experimentally derived protein structures. Examination of known structures has revealed certain amino acids to be preponderant in α-helical regions. Others seem to prefer a β-sheet environment or an unstructured, random coil environment. The occurrence of a run of amino acids of similar structural propensity is taken to suggest the occurrence of that preferred secondary structural motif. While this approach to secondary structure prediction has had some success, it is not always correct for several reasons. Hydrophobicity may not always be a good predictor of the location of particular amino acids. The same stretch of amino acids found in one structural motif in a protein may be found in a different motif in another protein. These discrepancies may be partly due to the short length of a particular motif as well as due to further electrostatic, hydrophobic, and hydrogen-bonding interactions that occur between the domains in a fully folded protein. The energetics of such interactions may override the secondary structure preferences of the individual amino acids and place them in environments of lower preference (Fasman, 1989b,1990; Branden and Tooze, 1991). The secondary structure prediction methods are purported to have between 50 and 75% accuracy (Fasman, 1990). An intense search is underway for methods capable of predicting secondary structures accurately (Thornton and Gardner, 1990; Thornton *et al.,* 1991; Bowie *et al.,* 1991). Techniques such as circular dichroism which measure the relative content of the different secondary structural motifs can also be useful in gross verification of the theoretical and empirical predictions (Neumann and Snatzke, 1990).

Prediction of the tertiary structure from the secondary structure inferred as above is not straightforward. Given a group of secondary structural motifs, it is possible to derive a set of tertiary structures that are all equally possible. Thus, the derivation of tertiary structures by this method has proven to be a "hit-or-miss" proposition with a low degree of success (Fasman, 1990; Branden and Tooze, 1991). Nonetheless, knowledge of the possible secondary structural motifs in themselves has been useful in the understanding of the structure and function of many proteins, notably integral membrane proteins, which are difficult to crystallize in their native state. Transmembrane receptors (discussed extensively in Chapter 4) which traverse the membrane multiple times belong to this class (Popot and Engelman, 1990).

In addition to the above two "knowledge-based" methods which draw upon available experimental data, purely theoretical approaches are also being investigated for the prediction of secondary and tertiary structures of proteins from the amino acid sequence. The guiding principle for this approach is the concept that the stable, fully folded structure of the protein represents a minimum energy state. Methods of quantum mechanics and thermodynamic principles are used to derive the minimum energy conformation of a protein. The nature of the chemical bonds along the polypeptide chain, and the sizes and steric hindrances of the amino acid side chains arising from their bulk and electrical charge, place restrictions on the conformations that a polypeptide chain can assume. The peptide bond that links the individual amino acids has a double-bond character, restricting rotation around this bond. Therefore, free rotation in the main chain can occur only around the two bonds linked to the α-carbon atom, one to the amide nitrogen and the other to the carbonyl carbon atom. However, the steric restrictions imposed by the functional groups linked to the α-carbon atom limit the degree of rotation around these bonds, thus permitting only certain conformations for the main chain (Richardson and Richardson, 1989; Branden and Tooze, 1991). These and other considerations, such as the energy of the interaction with the solvent, are used to derive energy functions. Using highly computer-intensive algorithms, the minimum energy conformation of the protein is sought (Mackay *et al.,* 1989). The success of this approach depends on the ability to formulate appropriate energy functions which include all the relevant variables. Furthermore, many distinct overall conformations may correspond to the same value minimum potential energy. In addition, it is by no means clear if the native conformation of a protein is its thermodynamically most stable, minimum energy state. Because of these difficulties, the success of the *de novo* methods in predicting secondary and tertiary structures has been very limited (Mackay *et al.,* 1989; Fasman, 1989b,1990). Nonetheless, in combination with other experimental and predictive methods, the *de novo* methods of energy minimization are valuable for the analysis of protein structure and the simulation of molecular interactions (Fasman, 1989b; Sielecki, 1991).

Proteins as dynamic entities: molecular dynamics

Protein structures obtained by X-ray crystallography convey the impression of proteins as rigid entities with the positions of atoms fixed with respect to each other. This has led to the comparison of protein–protein and protein–ligand interactions to the close complementarity observed between a lock and its key resulting in a "lock and key" or a "glove and hand" analogy. Over time, this view has been gradually replaced by a view of proteins as dynamic entities. Recent observations favor an "induced-fit" model wherein stabilizing conformational changes occur in the protein and its ligand during binding (Jorgensen, 1991). Experimental and computational approaches have been developed to study the structural transitions and the dynamics of proteins (Wright, 1990; Hajdu *et al.,* 1990; Karplus and McCammon, 1986; Cusak, 1992).

Some segments of a protein must be rigid to maintain the structural features required for its function, but others must move sufficiently to admit substrates and ligands into locales where chemical reactions occur. Thus, a protein must maintain a balance between the degree of rigidity and flexibility in order to execute its function. Experimental methods of structure determination such as conventional X-ray crystallography produce structures which represent the average structure of some 10^{20} molecules present in the crystal. Thus, the movements of segments in individual molecules are difficult to assess by conventional crystallography. However, theoretical calculations and computer simulations have permitted the analysis of the dynamics of proteins in detail. These studies have shown that in some cases the biological activity of a protein would be impossible if the molecule maintained a rigid average structure. For instance, the time taken for the binding and release of oxygen from the protein myoglobin (calculated based on the rigid structure determined by X-ray crystallography) would be many billion years because of the high energy barriers encountered by the oxygen molecule. This clearly is far from the case in actuality. Thus, motion in myoglobin and in many other proteins is vital to their ability to function (Karplus and McCammon, 1986).

Molecular dynamic simulation studies begin with an experimentally derived average structure. The atoms in this structure are subjected to a simulated force which, within the constraints of the model, displaces them from their average position. Their temporal response to this displacement is determined by using the laws of physics. Newton's laws of motion are applied in a manner analogous to the situation of an oscillating pendulum. The motions of relevant segments of the protein molecule as a whole are simulated over very short time periods of the order of 10^{-15} seconds. These structures are projected on a computer screen in a step-wise fashion, allowing the investigator to draw conclusions pertaining to the dynamic properties of the segment. This information is valuable to the understanding of molecular mechanisms which, in-turn, are useful for designing drugs. Molecular dynamic simulations are also frequently used in the refinement of experimentally derived protein structures (Sielecki *et al.,* 1991).

Computers in structure prediction and ligand screening

The power of modern computer technology and its impact on different aspects of molecular structural determination have been discussed earlier. Many of the experimental approaches would be impossible without the high ''number-crunching'' capacity of modern computers. In addition, the prediction methodologies described above, especially those involving *ab initio* structure calculations and molecular dynamic simulations, are also dependent on computer power (Mackay *et al.,* 1989; Dambrot, 1992). However, the impact of advanced computer technology is most visible in the laboratory through the ''on screen'' modeling capabilities. Three-dimensional images of proteins and other macromolecules derived experimentally or through predictive methods are conveniently displayed on monitor screens. These images are amenable to close examination by rotation around the various axes through the molecules. In addition, the binding of natural and synthetic inhibitors, and other ligands can be simulated and displayed instantaneously. Algorithms and software packages that perform these ''docking'' operations on screen have been developed. These programs can be used to study the influence of structural changes in ligands on their binding to the target proteins (Stoddard and Koshland, 1992; Kuntz, 1992). However, as exciting as the on-screen visualization capabilities are, it is essential to approach the computer-drawn images with caution. Often, the computer images lend a false sense of certainty to the particular structure on display, and the uncertainties in the structure due to the limitations of experimental and theoretical methods used to derive it can be easily overlooked. As this is true even for experimentally determined structures, models displayed from empirically derived structures should be approached with a greater recognition of this caveat (Hodgson, 1993).

Computers are powerful tools in the structure-based screening of chemical libraries for drug candidates (Kuntz, 1992). The availability of detailed structures of proteins, and often their complexes with ligands, permits the determination of essential spatial features of the possible binding interactions, and geometric intricacies of the binding site. Thus, a "molecular template" or a "negative surface map" for the binding region of the protein can be defined. Computers can then be used to screen large data bases of compounds for molecules that satisfy the spatial criteria for binding to the template. Several powerful computer programs, emphasizing different search criteria, are commercially available. Various data bases containing the three-dimensional structures of collections of compounds are available for rapid computer screening. These include public-access data bases, and proprietary data bases of pharmaceutical and chemical companies, each containing between 100,000 and 500,000 entries. At current computer capabilities, 100,000 compounds can be screened in less than a week. With the implementation of supercomputers it may be possible to screen 500,000 compounds in a day. This approach is being applied to the development of inhibitors against infectious agents such as viruses and bacteria (Kuntz, 1992).

EXAMPLE APPLICATIONS

The methods described in the preceding sections have been applied to the study of the structures of proteins of various classes and functions. Structural studies have provided valuable information on protein–protein interactions, and on the interaction of proteins with other molecules such as DNA and small cofactors. Examples of application of the structural insights to the modification of proteins by "protein engineering", and to the design of small-molecule inhibitors and ligands, are beginning to emerge at a rapid pace (Hodgson, 1991). Further, the rational design of structure mimetics, based on the structural information obtained through experimental and predictive methods, is also in progress (Saragovi *et al.*, 1992). The following discussion is focused on examples of recently determined protein structures which are useful in the near term in drug development.

HIV enzymes

Infection by the retrovirus HIV leads to the development of AIDS. This disease has acquired epidemic proportions globally, and HIV is a major research target in academic, industrial, and governmental laboratories. The HIV virus encodes a host of enzymatic activities which are required for its replication. Among these, the reverse transcriptase, which converts the RNA genome of the infecting HIV virus into DNA, has been a major target for drug development. In fact, the only FDA-approved AIDS drugs, nucleoside analogs such as AZT, are directed at this enzyme. Reverse transcriptase (RTase) also has another associated enzymatic activity, RNase H, which degrades the viral RNA in the process of its conversion to DNA by RTase. In addition, a viral protease processes the large viral polyprotein encoded by HIV to produce the viral coat proteins and the RTase. The HIV protease is essential for infectivity of the virus.

Structures of the RTase, RNase H, and protease have been determined recently, and these structures are being used in the rational design of AIDS therapeutics. The advances that have occurred with the development of HIV protease inhibitors stand out as a prime example of the power of rational drug design using structural information. HIV protease is a 99-amino-acid protein. From primary sequence information the protease was inferred to belong to the family of aspartic proteases based on three lines of evidence: (1) sequence-relatedness to aspartic proteases; (2) active site motif of asp–thr–gly (DTG, in one-letter code) common to the proteases such as pepsins; (3) weak inhibitory activity of pepstatin, an inhibitor of aspartic proteases. Members of the pepsin family of enzymes have been shown to have a bilobal structure with each half containing a DTG active site motif; the HIV protease had only one DTG motif in its short, 99-amino-acid sequence. Thus, to function as a pepsin-like aspartic protease, the HIV enzyme was predicted to form a homodimer. An initial homodimeric model was proposed by sequence comparison with pepsins (Pearl and Taylor, 1987; Blundell and Pearl, 1989; Sali *et al.*, 1990).

Subsequently, the crystal structures of the protease produced in *E. coli* (Navia *et al.*, 1989; Lapatto *et al.*, 1989) or synthesized chemically (Wlodawer *et al.*, 1989) were determined to resolutions ranging from 2.7 Å to 3 Å. Phase determination involved multiple heavy atom replacements. Molecular replacements based on the known atomic structures of pepsin (Sali *et al.*, 1990) and the protease of Rous sarcoma virus (Leis *et al.*, 1990) were employed to refine the structure. The structures obtained by different groups were shown to be in agreement with each other, and with the structure predicted earlier. These studies showed the HIV protease to be composed of a dimer of the 99-amino-acid monomers associating with each other through their amino and carboxyl termini. This structure is shown in Chapter 2, Fig. 2.3, in different representations. Subsequently, the structure of the protease complexed to a substrate-based inhibitor was determined to 2.3 Å resolution by using molecular replacement based on the newly determined HIV protease structure itself (Miller *et al.*, 1989). These studies also showed that the inhibitor bound the enzyme in a single orientation, and that it interacted extensively with the interface between the two (identical) subunits. In comparison to the unbound protease, the inhibitor-bound form showed substantial changes in structure of both the backbone regions and the flexible ‘‘flap regions’’. This information was used by several laboratories to synthesize new and improved inhibitors, followed by determination of the structures of their complexes with the protease. At least 120 different protease–inhibitor complexes have been examined. A compound, Ro 31-8959, identified as a potent inhibitor of the HIV protease applying this approach, is in phase II clinical trials. Other compounds with similar activities are being developed by using the structural information (Wlodawer, 1992; Krohn *et al.,* 1991). A negative image of the binding site region derived from the structural model of the protease has been used in structure-based computer-assisted searches of chemical libraries (Kuntz, 1992). For instance, screening of the Cambridge Crystallographic Database containing 10,000 molecular structures for steric complementarity to the binding site using the program DOCK led to the identification of bromoperidol, a butyrophenone, as a possible inhibitor. A commercially available antipsychotic, haloperidol, a close relative of bromoperidol, was used in tests of protease inhibition. Haloperidol was found to inhibit the proteolysis weakly (DesJarlais *et al.,* 1990). While haloperidol itself does not appear to be an anti-HIV protease drug candidate, this and other such discoveries serve to illustrate the potential of structure-based rational drug design. In addition, the detailed dimeric structure of HIV protease has revealed the structural basis of subunit interaction. This information can be used for the design of protease inhibitors which act by disrupting the interaction between the subunits (Wlodawer *et al.,* 1989).

Inhibition of the HIV RTase by using nucleoside analogs AZT and ddI is a therapeutic approach currently used in the treatment of AIDS. However, the use of these and other RTase inhibitors is compromised by the development of resistance in the virus population. Thus, the structure of the RTase enzyme has been sought to enable the development of more potent and specific inhibitors (Peliska and Benkovic, 1992). Recently, the crystal structures of the RTase and the associated RNase H have been determined (Davies *et al.,* 1991; Wlodawer, 1992; Arnold *et al.,* 1992; Kohlstaedt *et al.,* 1992).

RTase is a dimer composed of two polypeptide chains of 66 and 51 kilodaltons (kDa). The smaller subunit is identical to the larger, 66 kDa, subunit at the amino terminus, but lacks the 15 kDa segment at the carboxyl terminus of the larger subunit. This 15 kDa segment corresponds to the RNase H activity. Early attempts at the determination of the RTase structure were made difficult by the inability to obtain acceptable protein crystals (Wlodawer, 1992). Crystals capable of producing diffraction data could be obtained only by co-crystallization of RTase with either DNA and an anti-RTase antibody fragment (Arnold *et al.,* 1992), or with a non-nucleoside inhibitor, Nevirapine (Kohlstaedt *et al.,* 1992). These examples illustrate the vagaries involved in protein crystallization, referred to in an earlier section.

The crystal structure of the RNase H that resides at the carboxyl terminus of the 66 kDa RTase subunit was determined by using the 133-amino-acid carboxyl terminal fragment expressed and purified from *E. coli.* Isomorphous replacement using uranium ions was used to solve the phase problem, and further refinement to 2.4 Å resolution was achieved by using the structural information provided by homologous RNase H from *E. coli.* This structure, in addition to providing insights into the mechanism of RNase H activity, provided useful information for the determination of the RTase structure (Davies *et al.,* 1991).

While the structure of the RTase–DNA complex at 7 Å resolution was too crude for use in drug design, the 3.5 Å structure of the RTase inhibitor complex, although not precise enough for drug design, provided crucial structural information (Wlodawer, 1992). Multiple heavy atom replacements with gold, mercury, and platinum combined with the structural information on the RNase H domain was used to solve the structure. One of the key findings was that regardless of the complete homology of the 51 kDa subunit with the amino terminus of the 66 kDa subunit, these subunits of RTase assumed distinctly different structures in the active enzyme. The DNA polymerase and the RNase H activity are resident on the larger subunit, and the non-nucleoside, noncompetitive inhibitor, Nevirapine, binds to the larger subunit. The residues whose mutations result in drug resistance have been approximately located within the structure (Kohlstaedt *et al.,* 1992). This information provides the essential first step towards the application of structure-based rational drug design to HIV RTase.

Development of renin inhibitors

The renin–angiotensin system is involved in the control of blood pressure. Renin, an aspartyl protease, initiates the production of angiotensin I by cleavage of an inactive precursor, angiotensinogen. Angiotensin I is converted by the angiotensin-converting enzyme (ACE) to biologically active angiotensin II, which causes vasoconstriction and an increase in blood pressure. ACE inhibitors such as Captopril and Enalpril are used effectively in the regulation of hypertension (Garrison and Peach, 1990). However, renin, which initiates the production of angiotensin I, shows a high degree of specificity, and has no other known function. Therefore, it has been considered an attractive target for the development of antihypertensives for some time (Repine *et al.,* 1991). Because of the unavailability of the crystal structure of renin, the development of renin inhibitors has relied on the known structures of other homologous aspartic proteases, notably the pepsins (Sali *et al.,* 1990). However, it is generally believed that homology modeling is insufficient to provide a firm base for drug design (Hodgson, 1991).

Human renin, a 340-amino-acid glycoprotein derived from a larger polypeptide, prorenin, is produced and secreted by the juxtaglomerular cells in the kidney. The presence of only low levels of renin in circulation made human renin difficult to obtain in quantities required for drug screens and structural studies. Therefore, the pepsin family of aspartyl proteases was used for the modeling of human renin in drug development (Hodgson, 1991). Subsequently, mouse renin, obtained by conventional and rDNA methods, was used in these studies. However, determination of the crystal structure of mouse renin at desirable resolution was complicated by the inability to obtain suitable crystals. Further, although highly homologous to human renin, mouse renin has subtle structural and functional differences. For instance, mouse renin contains no carbohydrates, and is relatively inactive on human angiotensin. The appearance of rDNA-produced human renin on the scene shifted the structure determination efforts to this molecule.

The first structure of human renin was obtained from prorenin produced by expression of its cDNA in transfected mammalian cells. Prorenin was cleaved in the laboratory to renin using the protease trypsin. Because the carbohydrates in renin are not required for bioactivity, oligosaccharides were removed enzymatically. This process facilitates crystallization in some cases and also removes the contribution of the heterogeneous sugar chains to the diffraction pattern. The structure was determined without the use of heavy-atom derivatives, by application of molecular replacement techniques based on the atomic coordinates of porcine pepsinogen as the model. The molecular dynamic method of refinement was used extensively to arrive at a 2.5 Å resolution structure. However, some of the loop regions were not well resolved in this structure (Sielecki *et al.*, 1989; Sali *et al.*, 1990).

More recently, the X-ray structures of human and mouse renins complexed with their respective inhibitors have been determined to high resolution, providing the structure of fully glycosylated human renin at 1.9 Å and mouse renin at 2.8 Å with *R* factors (see previous section for the definition of *R* factor) between 0.18 and 0.19. Here again, the structures were solved without resorting to heavy-atom replacement by using molecular replacement on the known structures of pepsin (Dhanraj *et al.*, 1992). This study has shown that while mouse and human renins adopt very similar structures, significant regional differences exist between renins and the other aspartic proteases used in their modeling. Subtle differences between the active-site regions of mouse and human renins, sufficient to account for their differing substrate specificities, were noted. The high-resolution structure of human renin, and further definition of the residues involved in its substrate specificity, will undoubtedly lead to vast improvements over the earlier rational searches for renin inhibitors based on homology modeling utilizing the structures of pepsins.

Immunosuppression

Fungal products cyclosporin A (CsA) and FK506, discussed previously in Chapter 4, are potent immunosuppressants that are used in organ transplantation. These agents prevent the activation of T lymphocytes, which are responsible for the rejection of transplants (Chang *et al.*, 1991; Cyert, 1992). At a molecular level, they produce immunosuppression by associating with a family of proteins known as the immunophilins, which are present abundantly in all cell types. The protein that binds CsA is known as cyclophilin. It is different from the protein that binds to FK506, which is known as FK-binding protein or FKBP. No cross-binding has been observed between CsA and FKBP. However, both cyclophilin and FKBP possess an enzymatic activity known as peptidyl prolyl *cis–trans* isomerase, or rotamase, which catalyzes the *cis–trans* isomerization of proline residues in proteins. This activity may aid the folding of nascent, proline-containing proteins during cellular protein synthesis (Ringe, 1991). The prolyl isomerase activity of the immunophilins is inhibited by the binding of their respective ligands, and this was initially thought to be the mechanism of immunosuppression. However, immunophilins are ubiquitous proteins which are present in high levels in all cells, and CsA and FK506 appear to produce their immunosuppressive action at concentrations below the levels needed to bind all the immunophilin present in a cell. This makes the prolyl isomerase inhibition an unlikely target for the specificity of these compounds in the preferential inhibition of T cell activation. Recent studies suggest that the ligand–immunophilin complexes in the cases of CsA and FK506 produce their effect by inhibiting the activity of the protein phosphatase calcineurin. Thus, understanding the mode of binding of CsA and FK506 to immunophilins, and the binding of the complexes to their target, is important to the rational design of more potent immunosuppressants.

Some of the first-identified immunophilins are small proteins of 11 to 17 kDa. Their complete amino acid sequence has been determined. Because of their small size, their structures are amenable for analysis both by NMR in solution and by X-ray crystallography. Recently, solution and crystal structures of FKBP and its complex with FK506 have been determined (Michnick *et al.*, 1991; Van Duyne *et al.*, 1991; Moore *et al.*, 1991). NMR determination used NOE spectroscopy combined with molecular dynamic methods for structure refinement. The X-ray structure was determined by using the multiple heavy atom replacement method. The solution structure is in agreement with the crystal structure. FK506 was shown to bind to a hydrophobic pocket in FKBP. The hydrogen bonds involved in the binding and the interacting amino acids have been identified. Conserved residues that line the hydrophobic pocket were also identified. Binding of FK506 did not produce major changes in the FKBP structure. One key discovery from these studies is the striking change that the structure of FK506 undergoes in binding to FKBP. Similar changes in structure have been observed between the free and cyclophilin-bound forms of CsA, although strict comparison is difficult in this case because of the different solvents used in the two structure determinations (Wuthrich *et al.*, 1991; Jorgensen, 1991). These findings underscore the need for examining the structure of protein–ligand complexes in the process of ligand modification through rational drug design. They also highlight the limitations of drawing structure–activity inferences from the conformation of the uncomplexed ligand (Ringe, 1991).

Immune recognition

Determination of the structures of antigen–antibody complexes is valuable to the remodeling of antibodies (Hodgson, 1990; Co *et al.*, 1991). Three-dimensional structures of the complexes are useful in delineating the contact point of the complementarity-determining regions (CDRs; see Chapter 3) of antibodies with the cognate antigen, and the interaction of the CDRs with the surrounding framework region in the antibody. This information is useful for the creation of effective humanized antibodies as described in Chapter 3. In addition, recent structural studies have also provided insights into the mechanism of cell-mediated immunity involving the histocompatibility proteins (Barinaga, 1992).

Proteins of the major histocompatibility complex (MHC) are cell-surface molecules involved in the presentation of peptide fragments of foreign antigens to lymphocytes. Class I MHC proteins present foreign peptides to a class of immune cells known as cytotoxic T lymphocytes. Class I MHC molecules are expressed on the surfaces of all cells in an animal. Each animal within a species has a unique complement of class I MHC molecules displayed on its cells. If cytotoxic lymphocytes in an animal detect on cell surfaces class I MHC molecules foreign to that animal, as in the case of heterologous transplants, a cytotoxic response leading to the killing of the foreign cells results. In addition, when homologous MHC class I molecules are found associated with foreign peptides, a similar cytotoxic reaction, leading to the death of the presenting cell, is elicited. Normally, the peptides associated with the MHC molecule are derived by degradation of cellular proteins in the cytoplasm; such complexes are ignored as "self" by cytotoxic lymphocytes. In the event where the cell is infected by a virus, fragments of the virus proteins are presented, resulting in a cytotoxic response against the infected cells.

Class II MHC proteins present peptides to a class of lymphocytes known as helper lymphocytes, which stimulate antibody production against the peptides. In this case, the MHC associated peptides are derived by intracellular degradation of extracellular antigens imported into the cell. Association of a peptide foreign to the animal with its class II MHC protein, and recognition of the complex by helper T lymphocytes, initiates a humoral antibody response. Thus, both cell-mediated and humoral immunity are dependent on the formation of peptide–MHC complexes (Golub and Green, 1991). Understanding the nature of the peptide binding sites and the nature of peptides that can be bound to the two classes of MHC molecules have important consequences for the development of strategies for modulating immune recognition in transplantation and in autoimmune disease (Barinaga, 1992). This information may also be useful for the identification and design of highly immunogenic peptide antigens for use as vaccines.

Class I MHC molecules are composed of a single protein that traverses the membrane once. This protein contains all the amino acid variations which confer unique histocompatibility to an individual animal. In addition, it is non-covalently associated on the extracellular side with a highly conserved, small protein called β_2 microglobulin. Foreign peptide fragments are bound to the extracellular domain of the MHC molecule. The crystal structure of the human class I MHC complex was determined a few years ago. Because membrane-spanning proteins are difficult to crystallize, the extracellular, peptide-binding region of the MHC–microglobulin assemblies were released from the cell surface by proteolysis, then crystallized, and subjected to X-ray diffraction analysis. This analysis revealed a peptide-binding region formed by two amino terminal domains in the MHC chain. The peptide-binding pocket is bounded by eight beta strands at the bottom, forming the base, and two alpha helices, forming the sides of the pocket, as shown schematically in Fig. 5.8. However, the structure of the peptide in the pocket could not be visualized because of the diversity of peptides bound to the collection of MHC molecules which were isolated from human cells (Golub and Green, 1991).

Recently, the structure of mouse class I MHC complexed to specific, selected peptides has been determined (Travers and Thorpe, 1992). Previous biochemical studies indicated that peptides bound to MHC were about 8 to 9 amino acids in length. Therefore, two viral peptides, one an octamer and the other a nonamer,

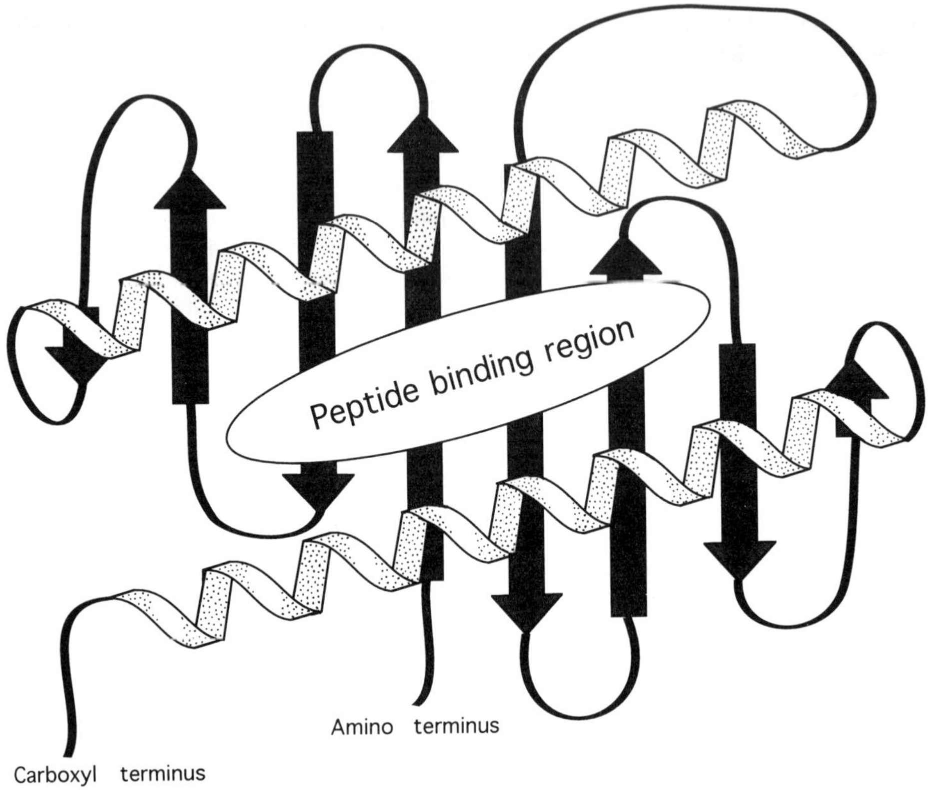

Fig. 5.8. Schematic representation of the structure of the peptide-binding pocket of the MHC class I molecule.

were complexed *in vitro* to soluble mouse MHC protein expressed in *Drosophila* cells, and the structures of the complexes were determined. The peptides appear to bind to the MHC pocket through interactions at their amino and carboxyl terminals, and through a few critical residues within the chain. The critical internal residues belong to a class with specific side chains. The ends of the nonapeptide occupy the same sites in the pockets as those of the octapeptide, with the extra amino acid in the nonapeptide being accommodated by a protrusion along its length. Much of the high affinity of the interaction is generated through hydrogen bonding interactions of the main chain of the peptide as opposed to side-group interactions, which explains the ability of a wide variety of peptides of different sequences to bind to the pocket. These conclusions are corroborated by *in vitro* mutagenesis studies (Barinaga, 1992; Fremont *et al.*, 1992; Matsumura *et al.*, 1992; Latron *et al.*, 1992; Parham, 1992). Class II MHC molecules, which are dimeric transmembrane proteins, also appear to have a similar binding pocket structure, and its structure and peptide-binding properties are currently being determined (Golub and Green, 1991). These and other such studies on immune recognition which are in progress should illuminate the mode of interaction of peptides with MHC proteins, and of this complex with the T cell receptors to produce immune responses, opening new avenues for therapies and drugs (Potera, 1993).

Structures of viruses

Viruses are large macromolecular complexes, composed of protein shells into which the genomic nucleic acid is packaged. In spite of their large sizes, the architecture of many viruses is simple. The protein coat is composed of one or just a few proteins arranged in highly symmetric fashion. The regular arrangement of the coat proteins allows viruses to form crystals which have been useful in the determination of the X-ray structures of whole viruses. However, the determination of such large structures has required the collection and analysis of very large data sets. Thus, the determination of many viral structures at high resolution has become feasible only recently with the advent of advanced data collection techniques and powerful computers. Following these developments, the structure of several plant and animal viruses has been determined (Stubbs, 1989; Hogle *et al.,* 1987; Caspar, 1992). Among these, the poliovirus and the rhinovirus are human pathogens which cause polio and common colds, respectively. Information gained from these studies should permit the identification of key regions of viruses involved in immune recognition by the host, in drug binding, and in the interaction of viruses with cellular receptors, and lead to the development of new strategies to combat viral infections (Edgington, 1992).

Other developments

In addition to the examples discussed above, the structures of many clinically and biologically important proteins have been determined. Some of these are amenable to immediate use in drug discovery efforts. These include enzymes such as dihydrofolate reductase (Jansy, 1988), and thymidilate synthase (Appelt *et al.,* 1991) both of which are involved in the synthesis of DNA precursors. Their inhibition is a target in anticancer chemotherapies. Structures of other proteins such as cAMP-dependent protein kinase, acetylcholinesterase, and the glucocorticoid receptor add to the knowledge base that will open new avenues and targets for drug development (Knighton *et al.,* 1991a,b; Sussman *et al.,* 1991; Luisi *et al.,* 1991; Taylor *et al.,* 1993). Structures of growth factors, peptide hormones, their receptors, and their receptors or antibody complexes are appearing at a rapid rate (Lo, 1992; de Vos *et al.,* 1992; Garcia *et al.,* 1992; Daopin *et al.,* 1992). Structures of independently functioning domains of proteins such as the LDL receptor-binding domain of apolipoprotein E, which is important in atherosclerosis, and others of clinical relevance are also being determined by X-ray and NMR methods (Wilson *et al.,* 1991). This broad data base is expected to pave the way towards rationally designed drugs and mimetics (Saragovi *et al.,* 1992). Although structure-based rational drug design has very few successes in the clinic as yet, powerful drugs based on this approach appear to be around the corner (Hodgson, 1991).

REFERENCES

Alberts, B., Bray, D., Lewis, J., Raff, M., Roberts, K., and Watson, J.D. (1989). *Molecular Biology of the Cell* (New York: Garland Publishing).

Appelt, K., Bacquet, R.J., Bartlett, C.A., Booth, C.L.J., Freer, S.T., Fuhry, M.A.M., *et al.* (1991). Design of enzyme inhibitors using iterative protein crystallographic analysis. *J. Med. Chem.* **34,** 1925-1934.

Arnold, E., Jacobo-Molina, A., Nanni, R.G., Williams, R.L., Lu, X., Ding, J., Clark, Jr., A.D., Zhang, A., Ferris, A.L., Clark, P., Hizi, A., and Hughes, S.H. (1992). Structure of HIV-1 reverse transcriptase/DNA complex at 7 Å resolution showing active site locations. *Nature* **357,** 85–89.

Baldwin, R.L. (1990). How does protein folding get started? In *Proteins: Form and Function.* R.A. Bradshaw and M. Purton, eds. (Cambridge: Elsevier Trends Journals), pp. 125–133.

Barinaga, M. (1992). Getting some backbone: how MHC binds peptides. *Science* **257,** 880–881.

Bax, A. (1989). Two-dimensional NMR and protein structure. *Ann. Rev. Biochem.* **58,** 223–256.

Blundell, T. and Pearl, L. (1989). Retroviral proteinases: a second front against AIDS. *Nature* **337,** 596–597.

Bowie, J.U., Luthy, R., and Eisenberg, D. (1991). A method to identify protein sequences that fold into a known three-dimensional structure. *Science* **253,** 164–170.

Bradshaw, R.A. and Purton, M. (eds.) (1990). *Proteins: Form and Function* (Cambridge: Elsevier Trend Journals).

Branden, C. and Tooze, J. (1991). *Introduction to Protein Structure* (New York: Garland Publishing).

Cantor, C.R. and Schimmel, P.R. (1980). *Biophysical Chemistry: Part II: Techniques for the Study of Biological Structure and Function* (San Francisco: W.H. Freeman).

Caspar, D.L.D. (1992). Virus structure puzzle solved. *Curr. Biol.* **2,** 169–171.

Chang, J.Y., Sehgal, S.N., and Bansbach, C.C. (1991). FK506 and rapamycin: novel pharmacological probes of the immune response. *TiPS* **12,** 218–223.

Clore, G.M. and Gronenborn, A.M. (1991). Structure of larger proteins in solution: three and four dimensional heteronuclear NMR spectroscopy. *Science* **252,** 1390–1399.

Co, M.S., Deschamps, M., Whitley, R.J., and Queen, C. (1991). Humanized antibodies for antiviral therapy. *Proc. Natl. Acad. Sci. USA* **88,** 2869–2873.

Cusak, S. (1992). Frozen stiff. *Curr. Biol.* **2,** 411–413.

Cyert, M.S. (1992). Immunosuppressants hit target. *Curr. Biol.* **2,** 18–19.

Dambrot, S.M. (1992). High performance computers. *Bio/Technology* **10,** 632.

Daopin, S., Piez, K.A., Ogawa, Y., and Davies, D.R. (1992). Crystal structure of transforming growth factor-β_2: an unusual fold for the superfamily. *Science* **257,** 369–373.

Davies, II, J.F., Hostomska, Z., Hostomsky, Z., Jordan, S.R., and Matthews, D.A. (1991). Crystal structure of the ribonuclease H domain of HIV-1 reverse transcriptase. *Science* **252,** 88–95.

de Vos, A.M., Ultsch, M., and Kossiakoff, A.A. (1992). Human growth hormone and extracellular domain of its receptor complex. *Science* **255,** 306–312.

DesJarlais, R.L., Seibel, G.L., Kuntz, I.D., Furth, P.S., Alvarez, J.C., Ortis De Montellano, P.R., DeCamp, D.L., Babe, L.M., and Craik, C.S. (1990). Structure-based design of nonpeptide inhibitors specific for the human immunodeficiency virus 1 protease. *Proc. Natl. Acad. Sci. USA* **87,** 6644–6648.

Dhanraj, V., Dealwis, C.G., Frazo, C., Badasso, M., Sibanda, B.L., Tickle, I.J., and Cooper, J.B. *et al.* (1992). X-ray analysis of peptide-inhibitor complexes define the structural basis of specificity for human and mouse renins. *Nature* **357,** 466–472.

Dobson, C.M. (1992). Resting places in folding pathways. *Curr. Biol.* **2,** 343–345.

Doolittle, R.F. (1990). Similar amino acid sequences revisited. In *Proteins: Form and Function.* R.A. Bradshaw and M. Purton, eds. (Cambridge: Elsevier Trends Journals), pp. 71–74.

Ealick, S.E., Cook, W.J., Vijay-Kumar, S., Carson, M., Nagabhusan, T.L., Trotta, P.P., and Bugg, C.E. (1991). Three-dimensional structure of human interferon-γ. *Science* **252,** 698–702.

Edgington, S.M. (1992). Bauhaus biology: biotechnology and the common cold. *Bio/Technology* **10,** 502–507.

Eisenberg, D. and Hill, C.P. (1990). Protein crystallography: more surprises ahead. In *Proteins: Form and Function.* R.A. Bradshaw and M. Purton, eds. (Cambridge: Elsevier Trends Journals), pp. 75–82.

Ellis, J. (1992). Cytosolic chaperonin confirmed. *Nature* **358,** 191–192.

Ewbank, J.J. and Creighton, T.E. (1992). Protein folding by stages. *Curr. Biol.* **2,** 347–349.

Fasman, G.D. (1989a). The development of the prediction of protein structure. In *Prediction of Protein Structure and the Principles of Protein Conformation.* G.D. Fasman, ed. (New York: Plenum Press), pp. 193–316.

Fasman, G.D. (ed.) (1989b). *Prediction of Protein Structure and the Principles of Protein Conformation* (New York: Plenum Press).

Fasman, G.D. (1990). Protein conformational prediction. In *Proteins: Form and Function.* R.A. Bradshaw and M. Purton, eds. (Cambridge: Elsevier Trends Journals), pp. 135–145.

Fremont, D.H., Matsumura, M., Stura, E.A., Peterson, P.A., and Wilson, I.A. (1992). Crystal structure of two viral peptides in complex with murine MHC class I H-2K^b. *Science* **257,** 919–927.

Garcia, K.C., Ronco, P.M., Verroust, P.J., Brunger, A.T., and Amzel, L.M. (1992). Three-dimensional structure of an angiotensin II–Fab complex at 3 Å: hormone recognition by an anti-idiotypic antibody. *Science* **257,** 502–507.

Garrison, J.C. and Peach, M.J. (1990). Renin and angiotensin. In *The Pharmacological Basis of Therapeutics.* A.G. Gilman, T.W. Rall, A.S. Nies, and P. Taylor, eds. (New York: Pergamon Press), pp. 749–763.

Glusker, J.P. and Trueblood, K.N. (1972). *Crystal Structure Analysis: A Primer* (New York: Oxford University Press).

Golub, E.S. and Green, D.R. (1991). *Immunology: a Synthesis* (Sunderland, Massachusetts: Sinauer Associates).

Hajdu, J., Acharya, K.R., Stuart, D.I., Barford, D., and Johnson, L.N. (1990). Catalysis in enzyme crystals. In *Proteins: Form and Function.* R.A. Bradshaw and M. Purton, eds. (Cambridge: Elsevier Trends Journals), pp. 83–93.

Hodgson, J. (1990). Protein design: rules, empiricism, and nature. *Bio/Technology* **8,** 1245–1247.

Hodgson, J. (1991). Data-directed drug design. *Bio/Technology* **9,** 19–21.

Hodgson, J. (1993). The good, the bad, and the indifferent. *Bio/Technology* **11,** 36–37.

Hogle, J.M., Chow, M., and Filaman, D.J. (1987). The structure of poliovirus. *Sci. Am.* March, 42–49.

Jansy, B. (1988). Exploiting the insights from protein structure. *Science* **240,** 722–723.

Jorgensen, W.L. (1991). Rusting of the lock and key model for protein–ligand binding. *Science* **254,** 954–955.

Karplus, M. and McCammon, J.A. (1986). The dynamics of proteins. *Sci. Am.* April, 42–51.

Knighton, D.R., Zheng, J., Ten Eyck, L.F., Ashford, V.A., Xuong, N-H., Taylor, S.S., and Sowadski, J.M. (1991a). Crystal structure of the catalytic subunit of cyclic adenosine monophosphate-dependent protein kinase. *Science* **253,** 407–414.

Knighton, D.R., Zheng, J., Ten Eyck, L.F., Xuong, N-H., Taylor, S.S., and Sowadski, J.M. (1991b). Structure of a peptide inhibitor bound to the catalytic subunit of cyclic adenosine monophosphate dependent protein kinase. *Science* **253,** 414–420.

Kohlstaedt, L.A., Wang, J., Friedman, J.M., Rice, P.A., and Steitz, T.A. (1992). Crystal structure at 3.5 Å resolution of HIV-1 reverse transcriptase complexed with an inhibitor. *Science* **256,** 1783–1790.

Krohn, A., Redshaw, S., Ritchie, J.C., Graves, B.J., and Matada, M.H. (1991). Novel binding mode of a highly potent HIV–proteinase inhibitor incorporating the (*R*)-hydroxyethylamine isostere. *J. Med. Chem.* **34,** 3340–3342.

Kuntz, I.D. (1992). Structure-based strategies for drug design and discovery. *Science* **257,** 1078–1082.

Lapatto, R., Blundell, T., Hemmings, A., Overington, J., Wilderspin, A., Wood, S., Merson, J.R., Whittle, P.J., Danley, D.E., Geoghegan, K.F., Hawrylik, S.J., Lee, S.E., Scheld, K.G., and Hobart, P.M. (1989). X-ray analysis of HIV-1 proteinase at 2.7 Å resolution confirms structural homology among retroviral enzymes. *Nature* **342,** 299–302.

Larton, F., Pazmany, L., Morrison, J., Moots, R., Saper, M.A., McMichael, A., and Strominger, J.L. (1992). A critical role for conserved residues in the cleft of HLA-A2 in the presentation of a nonapeptide to T cells. *Science* **257,** 964–967.

Leis, J., Weber, I., Wlodawer, A., and Skalka, A.M. (1990). Structure–function analysis of the Rous sarcoma virus-specific proteinase. *ASM News* **56,** 77–81.

Lo, D.C. (1992). NGF takes shape. *Curr. Biol.* **2,** 67–69.

Luisi, B.F., Xu, W.X., Otwinowski, Z., Freedman, L.P., Yamamoto, K.R., and Sigler, P.B. (1991). Crystallographic analysis of the interaction of the glucocorticoid receptor with DNA. *Nature* **352,** 497–505.

Mackay, D.H.J., Cross, A.J., and Hagler, A.T. (1989). The role of energy minimization in simulation strategies of biomolecular systems. In *Prediction of Protein Structure and the Principles of Protein Conformation.* G.D. Fasman, ed. (New York: Plenum Press), pp. 317–358.

Matsumura, M., Fremont, D.H., Peterson, P.A., and Wilson, I.A. (1992). Emerging principles for the recognition of peptide antigens by MHC class I molecules. *Science* **257,** 927–934.

Michnick, S.W., Rosen, M.K., Wandless, T.J., Karplus, M., and Schrieber, S.L. (1991). Solution structure of FKBP, a rotamase enzyme and receptor for FK506 and rapamycin. *Science* **252,** 836–839.

Miller, M., Schneider, J., Sathyanarayana, B.K., Toth, M.V., Marshall, G.R., Clawson, L., Selk, L., Kent, S.B.H., and Wlodawer, A. (1989). Structure of complex of synthetic HIV-1 protease with a substrate-based inhibitor at 2.3 Å resolution. *Science* **246,** 1149–1152.

Moffat, A.S. (1992). New methods make mid-sized molecules easier to solve. *Science* **256,** 309–310.

Moore, J.M., Peattie, D.A., Fitzgibbon, M.J., and Thompson, J.A. (1991). Solution structure of the major binding protein for the immunosuppressant FK506. *Nature* **351,** 248–250.

Navia, M.A., Fitzgerald, P.M.D., McKeever, B.M., Leu, C-T., Heimbach, J.C., Herber, W.K., Sigal, I.S., Drake, P.L., and Springer, J.P. (1989). Three-dimensional structure of aspartyl protease from human immunodeficiency virus HIV-1. *Nature* **337,** 615–620.

Neumann, N. and Snatzke, G. (1990). Circular dichroism of proteins. In *Proteins: Form and Function.* R.A. Bradshaw and M. Purton, eds. (Cambridge: Elsevier Trends Journals), pp. 107–116.

Oldham, R.K. (1985). Interferon: a model for future biologicals. In *Interferons Vol 6.* I. Gresser, ed. (New York: Academic Press), pp. 127–143.

Parham, P. (1992). Deconstructing the MHC. *Nature* **360,** 300–301.

Pearl, L.H. and Taylor, W.R. (1987). A structural model for the retroviral proteases. *Nature* **329,** 351–354.

Peliska, J.A. and Benkovic, S.J. (1992). A handy enzyme for transcription. *Curr. Biol.* **2,** 521–523.

Petsko, G.A. (1992). Fishing in Src-infested waters. *Nature* **352,** 625–626.

Popot, J-L. and Engelman, D.M. (1990). Membrane protein models: possibilities and probabilities. In *Proteins: Form and Function*. R.A. Bradshaw and M. Purton, eds. (Cambridge: Elsevier Trends Journals), pp. 147–151.

Potera, C. (1993). Team from Neurocrine Biosciences/Stanford identifies specific T cells linked to MS. *Genetic Engineering News* **13,** March 15, 1–23.

Powers, R., Garrett, D.S., March, C.J., Frieden, E.A., Gronenborn, A.M., and Clore, G.M. (1992). Three-dimensional solution structure of human interleukin-4 by multidimensional heteronuclear magnetic resonance spectroscopy. *Science* **256,** 1673–1677.

Repine, J.T., Himmelsbach, R.J., Hodges, J.C., Kaltenbronn, J.S., Sircar, I., Skeean, R.W., and Brennan, S.T. *et al.* (1991). Renin inhibitors containing esters at P_2-position. Oral activity in a derivative of methyl aminomalonate. *J. Med. Chem.* **34,** 1935–1943.

Richardson, J.S. and Richardson, D.C. (1989). Principles and patterns of protein conformation. In *Prediction of Protein Structure and the Principles of Protein Conformation*. G.D. Fasman, ed. (New York: Plenum Press), pp. 1–99.

Richardson, J.S. and Richardson, D.C. (1990). The *de novo* design of protein structures. In *Proteins: Form and Function*. R.A. Bradshaw and M. Purton, eds. (Cambridge: Elsevier Trends Journals), pp. 173–182.

Ringe, D. (1991). Binding by design. *Nature* **351,** 185–186.

Sali, A., Overington, J.P., Johnson, M.S., and Blundell, T.L. (1990). From comparison of protein sequences and structures to protein modelling and design. In *Proteins: Form and Function*. R.A. Bradshaw and M. Purton, eds. (Cambridge: Elsevier Trends Journal), pp. 163–171.

Sanders, J.K.M. and Hunter, B.K. (1987). *Modern NMR Spectroscopy: a Guide for Chemists* (New York: Oxford University Press).

Saragovi, H.U., Greene, M.I., Chrusciel, R.A., and Kahn, M. (1992). Loops and secondary structure mimetics: development and applications in basic science and rational drug design. *Bio/Technology* **10,** 773–778.

Shaanan, B., Gronenborn, A.M., Cohen, G.H., Gilliland, G.L., Veerapandian, B., Davies, D.R., and Clore, G.M. (1992). Combining experimental information from crystal and solution studies: joint X-ray and NMR refinement. *Science* **257,** 961–964.

Sielecki, A.R., Hayakawa, K., Fujinaga, M., Murphy, M.E.P., Fraser, M., Muir, A.K., Carilli, C.T., Lewicki, J.A., Baxter, J.D., and James, M.N.G. (1989). Structure of recombinant human renin, a target for cardiovascular-active drugs, at 2.5 Å resolution. *Science* **243,** 1346–1351.

Stoddard, B.L. and Koshland Jr., D.E. (1992). Prediction of the structure of a receptor–protein complex using binary docking method. *Nature* **358,** 774–778.

Stubbs, G. (1989). Virus structure. In *Prediction of Protein Structure and the Principles of Protein Conformation*. G.D. Fasman, ed. (New York: Plenum Press), pp. 117–148.

Sussman, J.L., Harel, M., Frolow, F., Oefner, C., Goldman, A., Toker, L., and Silman, I. (1991). Atomic structure of acetylcholinesterase from *Torpedo californica*: a prototypic acetylcholine-binding protein. *Science* **253,** 872–883.

Taylor, S.S., Kinghton, D.R., Zheng, J., Sowadski, J.M., Gibbs, C.S., and Zoller, M.J. (1993). A template for protein kinase family. *TIBS* **18,** 84–89.

Thornton, J.M., Flores, T.P., Jones, D.T., and Swindells, M.B. (1991). Protein structure: prediction of progress at last. *Nature* **354,** 105–106.

Thornton, J.M. and Gardner, S.P. (1990). Protein motifs and data-base searching. In *Proteins: Form and Function.* R.A. Bradshaw and M. Purton, eds. (Cambridge: Elsevier Trends Journals), pp. 153–161.

Tomasselli, A.G., Heinrickson, R.L., and Watenpaugh, K.D. (1991). Recombinant DNA technology and crystallography: a new alliance in unraveling protein structure–function relationships. In *Purification and Analysis of Recombinant Proteins.* R. Seetharam and S.K. Sharma, eds. (New York: Marcel Dekker), pp. 285–315.

Travers, P.J. and Thorpe, C.J. (1992). Anchored fore and aft. *Curr. Biol.* **2,** 679–681.

Van Duyne, G.D., Standaert, R.F., Karplus, P.A., Schrieber, S.L., and Clardy, J. (1991). Atomic structure of FKBP–FK506, an immunophilin–immunosuppressant complex. *Science* **252,** 839–842.

Wilson, C., Wardell, M.R., Weisgraber, K.H., Mahley, R.W., and Agard, D.A. (1991). Three-dimensional structure of the LDL receptor-binding domain of human apolipoprotein E. *Science* **252,** 1817–1822.

Wlodawer, A. (1992). Another piece of the HIV puzzle falls into place. *Science* **256,** 1766.

Wlodawer, A., Miller, M., Jaskolski, M., Sathyanarayana, B.K., Baldwin, E., Weber, I.T., Selk, L.M., Clawson, L., Schneider, J., and Kent, S.B.H. (1989). Conserved folding in retroviral proteases: crystal structure of a synthetic HIV-1 protease. *Science* **245,** 616–621.

Wright, P.E. (1990). What can two-dimensional NMR tell us about proteins. In *Proteins: Form and Function.* R.A. Bradshaw and M. Purton, eds. (Cambridge: Elsevier Trends Journals), pp. 65–105.

Wuthrich, K. (1989). Protein structure determination in solution by nuclear magnetic resonance spectroscopy. *Science* **243,** 45–50.

Wuthrich, K., Von Freyberg, B., Weber, C., Wider, G., Traber, R., Widmer, H., and Braun, W. (1991). Receptor-induced conformation change of immunosuppressant cyclosporin A. *Science* **254,** 953–954.

6

Nucleic acid therapies

The concept of using nucleic acids, polynucleotides, and oligonucleotides as therapeutics is a unique consequence of the development of rDNA technology. Entire genes or cDNAs, and their segments in DNA or RNA form, are used for the regulation of protein expression that is errant in pathological states, or is therapeutically beneficial. Until this development, drugs were largely believed to produce their action by only altering the rate at which a bodily function proceeds and not by imparting new functions. The introduction of genes, resulting in the long-term production of new proteins, deviates from this long-held pharmacological principle of drug action (Ross, 1990). During the past three to five years many industrial laboratories have been established to exploit the therapeutic and commercial benefits of gene-based therapies (Carey and Hamilton, 1992).

Early development of nucleic acid therapy was aimed at genetic deficiency diseases which were amenable to replacement therapy, or correction by administration of the protein products of the defective genes, as described in Chapter 3. The introduction of the normal counterpart of a defective gene into cells of the patient, resulting in the long-term production of the missing protein, appeared as a desirable alternative to the repeated parenteral administration of purified protein (Verma, 1990; Caskey, 1992). However, the current span of nucleic acid-based therapies far exceeds this limited application conceived initially (Riordan and Martin, 1991; Crooke, 1992a).

As currently defined, nucleic acid therapy approaches fall into three basic categories: *(1) gene therapy:* expression of entire genes producing therapeutic proteins foreign to a cell, increasing the level of a normally expressed protein, or replacing a defective protein; *(2) antisense and triplex technologies:* total suppression or reduction of the expression of undesirable proteins using defined antisense oligonucleotides or nucleic acids which interact with the mRNA or the gene encoding the proteins, by hybridization; *(3) aptamer technology:* inhibition of protein activities by specific, high-affinity binding of oligonucleotides to the proteins.

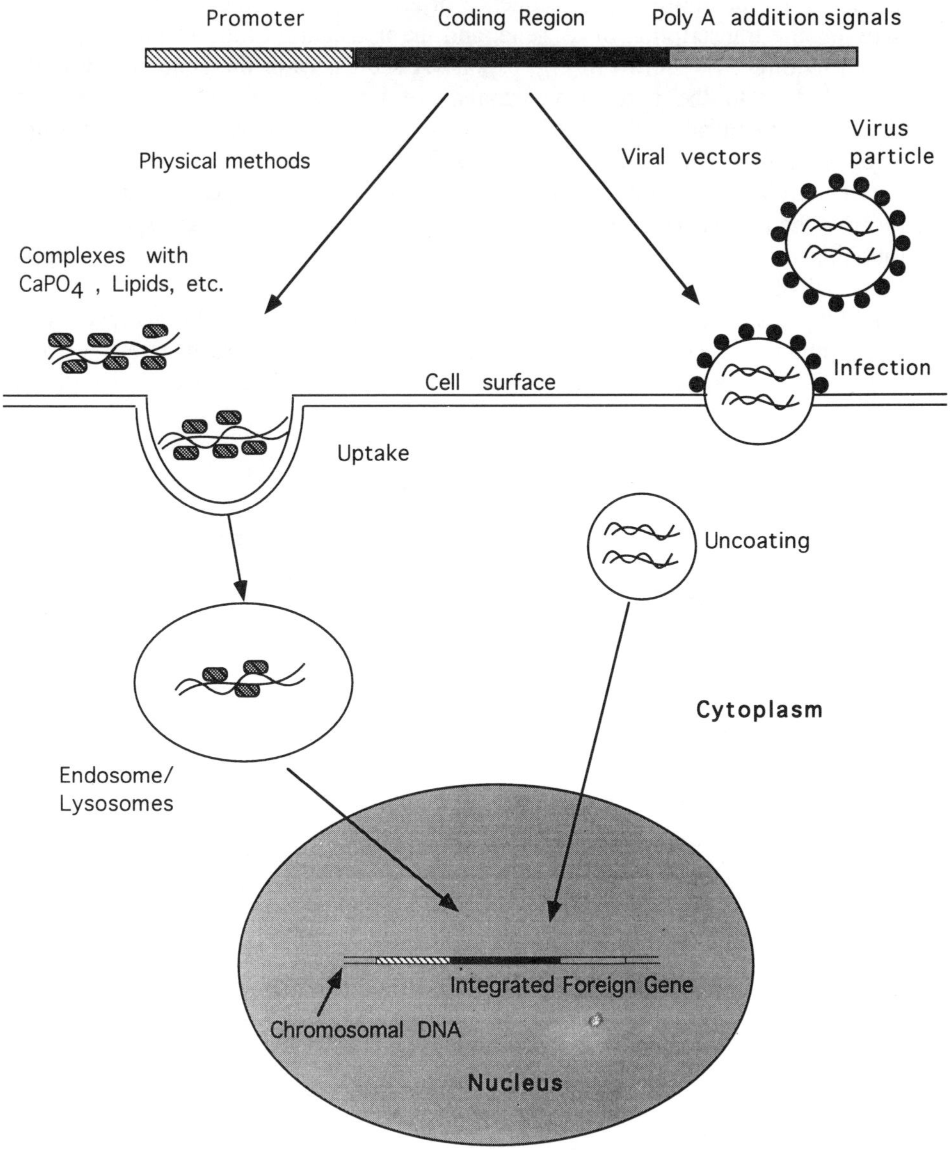

Fig. 6.1. Methods for the introduction of DNA into cells.

The production of therapeutic proteins in cells of an organism by transferring genes or cDNAs for such proteins into cells is referred to as "gene therapy". This approach can be used to correct genetic deficiencies through protein replacement, or for expression of therapeutically beneficial proteins in selected groups of cells. Because the expression of a functional protein is the goal of gene therapy, the introduction of the entire coding sequence of a protein, with appropriate regulatory signals for the transcription of its gene, and the translation of the resulting mRNA, are both required. As shown in Fig. 6.1, DNA sequences or the gene encoding the protein, linked to the regulatory signals, are introduced directly into cells by physical and chemical methods. Alternatively, the gene is delivered with very high efficiency by its encapsidation into viruses. The introduced genes ''integrate'' into the cell's DNA, and provide long-term production of the protein in the cells harboring them. The correction of a genetic deficiency which is responsible for hemophilia by the introduction of a normal factor VIII gene is a typical example of the goal of gene therapy (Verma, 1990; Miller, 1992).

The suppression of gene expression, on the other hand, can be achieved with small segments of DNA or RNA complementary to the messenger RNA for a protein. Single-stranded oligonucleotides of the order of 15–20 bases in length are

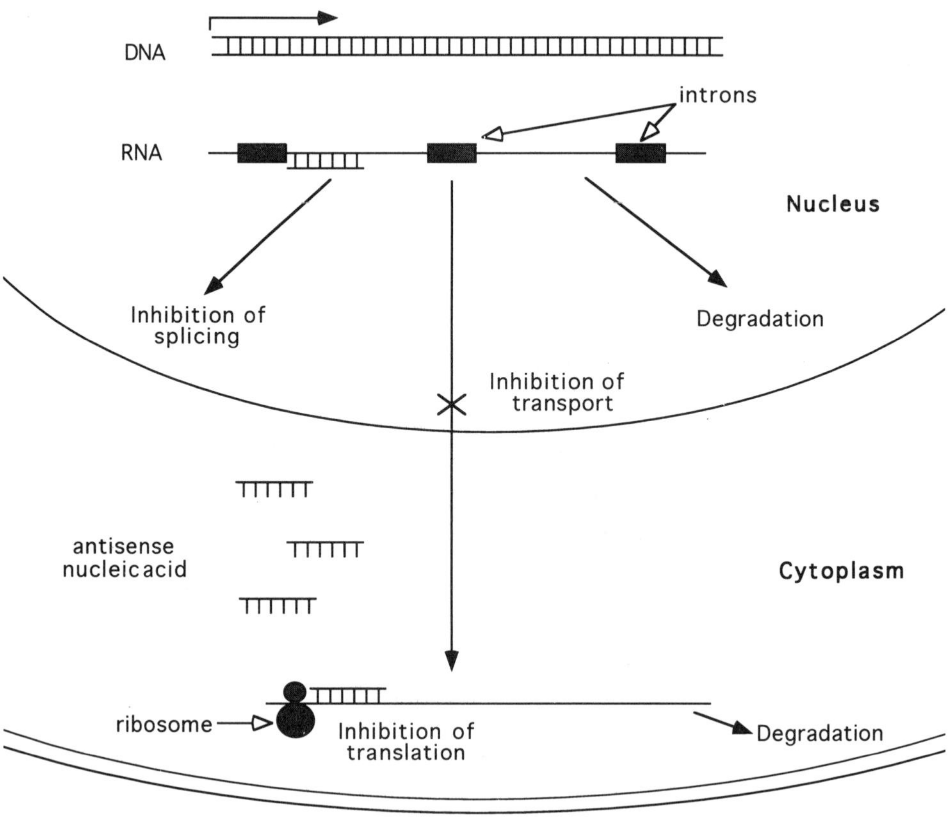

Fig. 6.2. Antisense nucleic acid-mediated inhibition of RNA maturation and function.

capable of binding to the RNA transcript of a gene with great specificity, by complementary base-pairing described in Chapter 2 and in Box 4.1. This binding interferes with maturation of the primary RNA transcript of the gene into a translatable mRNA and/or with translation of the resulting mRNA, as shown in Fig. 6.2. In addition, protein production from the mRNA may also be decreased by making the mRNA susceptible to degradation by nucleases. Small RNAs, known as ribozymes, combine the ability to bind specifically to selected RNA species with the ability to cleave the target RNA enzymatically. The resultant destruction of the mRNA leads to a loss of protein production. These approaches are known as "antisense technologies". Owing to the small size of the oligonucleotides required for therapeutic antisense applications, they can be produced by chemical synthesis. Chemical synthesis also permits the introduction of modifications which increase the stability of the oligonucleotides against degradation by nucleases. Alternatively, antisense RNAs can be produced within a cell by transcription of an antisense expression vector introduced into the cells by the same methods used in gene therapy. This approach is particularly useful in situations where long-term expression of the antisense molecule is desirable. A typical application of the antisense approach is the inhibition of replication of viruses by using antisense RNA or DNA against key RNAs produced by the virus (Murray and Crockett, 1992; Toulme, 1992).

Small oligonucleotides are also capable of binding specifically to predetermined regions of double-stranded DNA to form triple helical structures as shown in Fig. 6.3. This binding can be exploited to inactivate selected genes such as viral genes in infected cells or oncogenes in tumor cells. This aspect of nucleic acid therapy is known as "triplex technology" (Riordan and Martin, 1991; Crooke, 1992a).

Many proteins function by binding to nucleic acids in a sequence-specific manner. These proteins may also bind defined oligonucleotides, and the binding may interfere with their function. It is now possible to screen random pools of oligonucleotides for binding to a protein, and to isolate the ones that bind with high affinity by gene amplification methods. Such oligonucleotides may themselves be useful as therapeutics or may be useful as leads for the development of other active molecules. This approach to therapeutic development is called "aptamer technology" (Riordan and Martin, 1991; Crooke, 1992a). Transcription factors, which bind DNA in a sequence-specific manner, are good examples of proteins amenable to inactivation by this technology.

In discussing gene therapies, a clear distinction needs to be made between somatic and germline therapies. Genes and gene fragments may be introduced into somatic cells of a patient without hereditary consequence to his/her progeny. Genes can also be introduced into germ cells or early embryos, and these genes are passed on to future generations. This is precisely the goal of transgenic animal technologies discussed in Chapter 7. In principle, this approach can be used to correct genetic defects in every cell of an affected individual and his/her progeny. While the application of gene therapy to somatic cells raises mainly new regulatory issues related to risk/benefit, its application to human germ cells or human embryos raises serious ethical questions and theological concerns (Anderson, 1992a; Fox,

1992a). These issues are currently being debated (Anderson, 1992b; Davis 1992). In addition, the possibility of germline manipulation has led to fears and misconceptions associated with "gene therapy" (Pembrey, 1991; Walters, 1991). The following discussion of nucleic acid therapies pertains only to their applications in somatic cells.

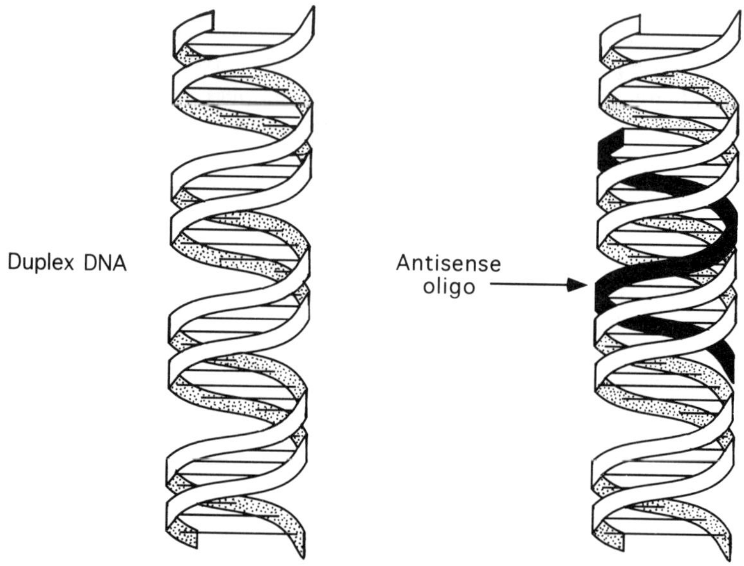

Fig. 6.3. Structure of triple helical DNA. An oligonucleotide bound to a double-stranded DNA molecule.

Somatic nucleic acid therapies may be performed by two methods. Nucleic acids can be delivered into the desired cells by the direct administration of genes or oligonucleotides to the patient in the clinic. This approach is termed *in vivo* gene therapy. Alternatively, genes may be introduced in the laboratory into cells obtained from the patient or from other suitable sources, and the recipient cells selected for desired characteristics may be reintroduced into the patient. This approach is known as *ex vivo* gene therapy.

Among the nucleic acid therapies, gene therapy, having a longer history, is the most advanced. Several clinical trials of gene therapy, ranging from correction of genetic deficiencies to cancer therapy, are in progress. Antisense, triplex and aptamer therapies are at very early stages, and the current research is concerned with establishing their feasibility and efficacy. The molecular biological principles of techniques used in gene therapy, their therapeutic applications and the regulatory issues and concerns are discussed in the following sections.

TECHNOLOGIES AND TECHNIQUES

Introduction of nucleic acids into cells

Nucleic acids are highly charged at biological pH and therefore do not cross biological membranes easily. Thus, a major technological challenge to nucleic acid therapies is the efficient delivery of the therapeutic genes and oligonucleotides to the interior of the cell. A number of physicochemical and biological approaches have been developed for the delivery of DNA into cells. The physicochemical methods rely on the use of free oligonucleotides, or conjugates of oligonucleotides, polynucleotides, and nucleic acids to a variety of agents which facilitate cellular uptake. Efficiency of delivery varies widely depending on the type of nucleic acid and the cell type used. While a number of methods are available for delivery of nucleic acids into cells in culture in a research laboratory, many of these methods are not useful in the clinic. Biological methods of gene delivery rely on packaging the gene of interest into a defective mammalian virus. Viruses deliver their genomes, including the packaged foreign gene, with virtually 100% efficiency.

The introduction of foreign DNA into cells by either of the above methods followed by its random, undirected insertion into the genome of the cells raises the possibility of physical disruption of normal genes, known as "insertional mutagenesis", which could potentially lead to oncogenic transformation. Further, as discussed in the following sections, the effective use of some viral vectors also requires that the recipient cells undergo cell division; many differentiated cells in mammals (such as neurons) do not divide. In addition, the use of viruses as vectors for gene delivery raises serious concern regarding the possibility of generating new viruses by recombination between the viral vector and endogenous or infecting viruses.

Physicochemical methods

Cells are capable of internalizing nucleic acids when presented in the free form. However this process is very inefficient and requires very high concentrations of the nucleic acid. Such high concentrations, often in the range of 50–200 μM (Miller, 1991), are attainable only with small oligonucleotides. Thus only small oligonucleotides can be effectively delivered to cells in a free form. The efficiency of internalization of oligonucleotides and nucleic acids can be further increased by using the methods described below.

A wide range of methods have been developed for the introduction of larger nucleic acids, primarily DNA, into cultured cells. Large fragments of DNA, several kilobases in length, can be introduced into cells by these methods. The methods range from complexation of DNA with cationic polymers, incorporation into lipid vesicles, and precipitation with calcium phosphate to the introduction of free nucleic acids into cells made permeable by a high-voltage electric field, by a method known as electroporation (Felgner and Rhodes, 1991; Chang *et al.*, 1992). Nucleic acids can also be "microinjected" into a wide variety of cells of varying sizes using fine glass pipettes. Microinjection is a very laborious process, and requires sophisticated equipment. Therefore, it is not routinely used with cells in culture, but is central to the production of transgenic animals described in Chapter 7. More recently, ballistic methods, which use accelerated particles of gold and other metals to which DNA is attached, have also been developed successfully as delivery vehicles (Williams *et al.,* 1991; Fitzpatrick-McElligott, 1992). While most of these methods are readily applicable to *ex vivo* gene therapy where isolated cells are used, factors such as stability in blood and tissue fluids, and toxicity limit their use in delivering nucleic acids to cells of patients in *in vivo* therapies.

In vivo gene expression in animals has been obtained after introduction of DNA encapsulated in liposomes, which are lipid vesicles that entrap the DNA. Further, tissue and cell type specificity has been conferred on the liposomes by coupling to cell-type specific antibodies, resulting in "immunoliposomes". In some cases a combination of liposomes and red blood cell membranes has been used for delivery (Felgner and Rhodes, 1991).

Complexes of DNA with cationic lipid reagent, lipofectin, have been used successfully in *in vivo* gene delivery into cells of whole animals. Unlike the liposome delivery systems where the nucleic acids are encapsidated into liposome micelles, many micelles of cationic lipofectin form complexes with the nucleic acids. Intravenous injection of lipofectin complexes has been shown to result in the delivery of a foreign gene to lung tissue. This method has been used to introduce DNA into cells of the arterial wall in the space between the balloons of a double-balloon catheter (Nabel *et al.,* 1990).

DNA co-precipitated with calcium phosphate has been shown to produce *in vivo* expression when injected intraperitoneally into rats (Benvenisty and Reshef, 1986). Further, complexes of DNA with asialoorosomucoid and a positively charged polylysine polymer have been shown to target the liver following intravenous injection (Wu *et al.,* 1989). Here, the targeting is achieved by binding of the asialoorosomucoid to the asialoglycoprotein receptors in the liver. These receptors are normally used for the clearance of glycoproteins whose N-linked glycoprotein chains have lost the terminating sialic acid residues (see Chapter 3). (In this particular method, long-term expression in liver cells required partial hepatectomy, which is unlikely to be desirable in a clinical situation.) Similarly, complexes of DNA with polylysine and transferrin have been used to introduce DNA via the transferrin receptor present in many cell types (Miller, 1992). Furthermore, the efficiency of receptor-mediated uptake has been shown to be enhanced by linking the transferrin–polylysine–DNA complexes to inactivated or defective adenoviral particles (Cotten *et al.,* 1992; Wagner *et al.,* 1992). Such coupling is believed to enhance entry of the complexed DNA by using both the transferrin and the adenovirus receptors. In addition, internalization of the virus particle is thought to cause disruption of the endocytotic vesicles thereby allowing the release of DNA and facilitating its nuclear entry.

While most cells do not take up naked DNA in the absence of the physical or chemical treatments described above, muscle cells appear to be an exception.

Direct injection of free nucleic acids in saline solutions into skeletal and cardiac muscles has been shown to result in prolonged expression (Wolff *et al.*, 1991; Kitsis *et al.*, 1991). By using this method, the 12 kilobase human dystrophin gene, defective in muscular dystrophy patients, has been introduced into the muscle cells of mice (Partridge, 1991; Ascadi *et al.*, 1991).

DNA has been introduced *in vivo* also by using microparticle bombardment. Submicron-sized particles of gold or tungsten absorb DNA spontaneously. Subsequently, they are accelerated onto the surface of cells, resulting in cell penetration. By using this procedure the expression of foreign DNA was observed in a wide variety of tissues such as skin, liver, muscle, intestine, and mammary gland (Felgner and Rhodes, 1991; Williams *et al.*, 1991; Fitzpatrick-McElligott, 1992; Tang *et al.*, 1992). This method of DNA delivery, dubbed the "biolistic process", is likely to find wide-ranging applications (Pecorino and Lo, 1992).

Many cells in culture have been shown to be capable of taking up oligonucleotides added to the culture medium in the absence of serum. Very high concentrations of the free oligonucleotides, in the 50 to 200 μM range, need to be added to the culture medium to produce detectable uptake. The mechanism(s) of this uptake process is not well understood. This uptake is enhanced by chemical modifications of the oligonucleotides, which reduce the negative charges contributed by the phosphate backbone (Miller, 1991). Here again, liposomes and other complexation methods, described above with larger nucleic acids, also appear to enhance uptake (Crooke, 1992a; Akhtar and Juliano, 1992).

Viral vectors

Physicochemical methods of DNA delivery result in stable, long-term expression of the delivered gene in a limited fraction of cells exposed to the nucleic acid. Because viral vectors use the infection mechanisms used naturally by viruses, they are capable of delivering the genes incorporated into them with efficiencies approaching 100%. Further, the replication mechanism of the virus facilitates integration and long-term expression of the gene in the recipient cell.

Infection of a cell by a virus has two outcomes, depending on the nature of the virus and the particular cell type. Some viruses go into a lytic cycle, which results in the replication of the virus and the lysis of the cell. This is the case with viruses such as poliovirus and vaccinia virus, both of which are used in vaccination. The use of live viruses expressing protein antigens in vaccination has been discussed in Chapter 3. In vaccination, the goal is the transient replication of viruses for a period sufficient to raise antibody response. Thus, the use of lytic viruses leading to transient, self-limiting lytic infection is acceptable or even desirable.

Other viruses do not lyse the cell following infection. Their DNA genome integrates into the cell's genome or remains free in the cell nucleus. Although progeny viruses are produced by the infected cell, the cell remains viable. This is the case with retroviruses. Because these viruses do not destroy the cell they infect, they are ideal for introducing foreign genes into cells. Thus, mouse retroviruses, which infect a wide variety of cells including human cells, have received the greatest attention as promising vectors for gene therapy. Alternatively, normally lytic viruses made replication-deficient by deletion of key genes can also be used as gene delivery vectors. This approach has led to the more recent development of adenovirus as a vector for gene therapy (Rosenfeld *et al.,* 1992; Quantin *et al.,* 1992; Lemarchand *et al.,* 1992; Ragot *et al.,* 1993; Le Gal La Salle *et al.,* 1993).

Retroviruses are a class of viruses whose genome is composed of single-stranded RNA. Upon entering a cell, they use the viral enzyme reverse transcriptase to synthesize a double-stranded DNA copy of the RNA known as the "provirus". The DNA copy, or the provirus, integrates into the genome of the infected cell and directs the production of copies of viral RNA which are translated to form the structural proteins and reverse transcriptase. The same RNA is also encapsidated into an infectious viral particle. The infected cell remains viable but viral particles continue to bud off from the cell. While retroviruses such as human immunodeficiency viruses are human pathogens, mouse retroviruses, although capable of infecting human cells, are not known to cause any overt pathology in humans. Therefore, gene therapy vectors currently in development and in use are derived from murine retroviruses (Verma, 1990; Miller, 1992).

The structure of the proviral DNA form of a retrovirus is shown in Fig. 6.4A. Sequences of genes encoding the core proteins (gag), reverse transcriptase, and the envelope glycoprotein are flanked by two identical, directly repeated nucleotide stretches known as "LTRs" (long-terminal repeats). LTRs contain the regulatory regions required for transcription of the viral genome and for the conversion of the viral RNA into proviral DNA. In addition, an important regulatory sequence known as the "psi" sequence, located outside the LTRs, is required for the encapsidation of the viral RNA by viral coat proteins: mutation or deletion of the psi sequence renders the RNA incapable of being packaged into a virus particle (Pembrey, 1991; Caskey, 1992).

The proviral DNA of retroviruses can be isolated and manipulated by standard rDNA methods, and transfected into mammalian cells to generate infectious virus particles. However, simple splicing of therapeutic genes to the retroviral genome, creating a longer viral genome, is not possible because the encapsidation system does not package RNAs larger than the normal viral genome of about 9 kilobases. It is therefore necessary to replace the sequences encoding the viral proteins, but not the regulatory sequences, with foreign genes intended for delivery. Thus, the total foreign DNA that can be incorporated into a retroviral vector is about 7 kilobases long. Some of this available length is required for the inclusion of a drug resistance marker such as the gene for neomycin resistance. Such markers are essential for the selection of vector DNA-transfected cells in the process virus particle production. This further reduces the length of the therapeutic foreign gene that can be incorporated into the vector. Two typical retroviral vectors which have received regulatory approval (Johnston, 1991) are shown in Fig. 6.4B and C. The LTR region of the virus contains a promoter which can be used for transcription of the foreign gene. When more than one gene is contained in the vector, it

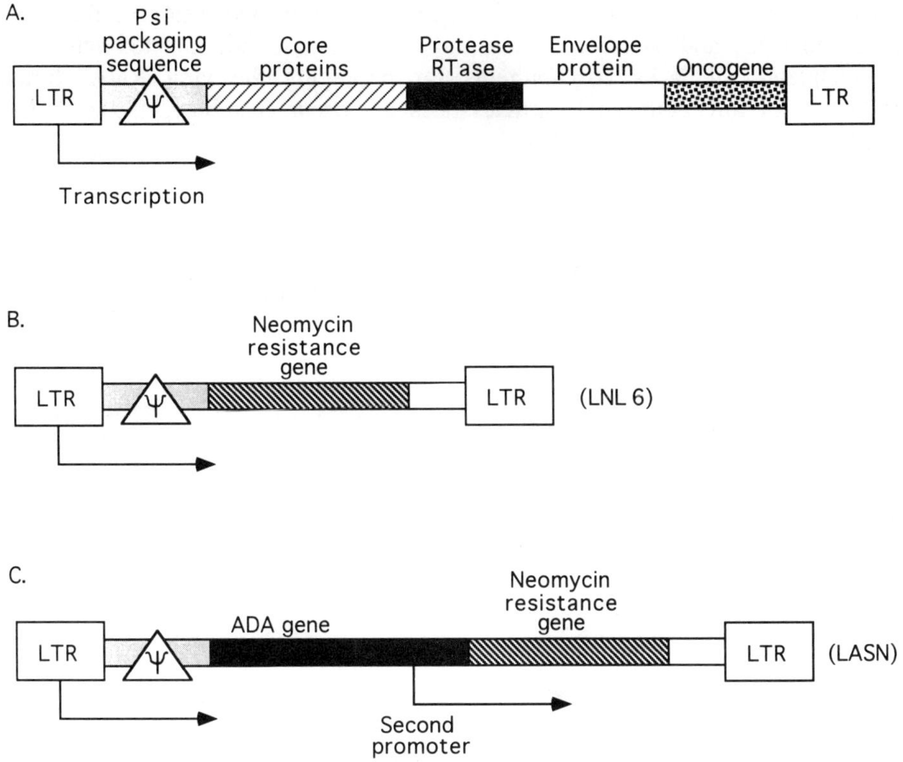

Fig. 6.4. Retroviral vectors. A. Structure of the provirus or the DNA copy of the retroviral genome. B and C. Prototype retroviral vectors approved for use in gene therapy protocols. ADA, adenosine deaminase; LTR, long-terminal repeat; RTase, reverse transcriptase.

necessary to provide an additional promoter for transcription of the second gene (LASN, Fig. 6.4C).

Transfection of the vectors shown in Fig. 6.4B and C into mammalian cells does not result in virus production because the genes encoding the viral coat and envelope proteins are absent. The introduction of the vectors into a cell infected by the parent retrovirus results in the packaging of the vector RNA into infectious viral particles using proteins produced by the parent virus. However, the cell also produces the parental virus, resulting in a mixture of viral particles. Pure virus preparations containing only the vector sequences can be obtained by using ''helper'' cell lines as shown in Fig. 6.5. Helper cell lines contain a version of the parental virus in which the psi sequences have been deleted. The RNA derived from this virus is capable of directing the production of viral proteins but is incapable of being packaged. Transfection of the gene transfer vector into such a helper cell line leads to the encapsidation of only the psi sequence-containing vector RNA into viral particles. The resulting virus preparation, containing only the vector RNAs, is used to infect cells of the patient undergoing gene therapy. This infection leads to conversion of the vector RNA into DNA and its incorporation into the genome of the infected cell. Since the recipient cell lacks coat proteins for packaging the viral RNA, further production of infectious viral particles does not occur (Pembrey, 1991; Caskey, 1992).

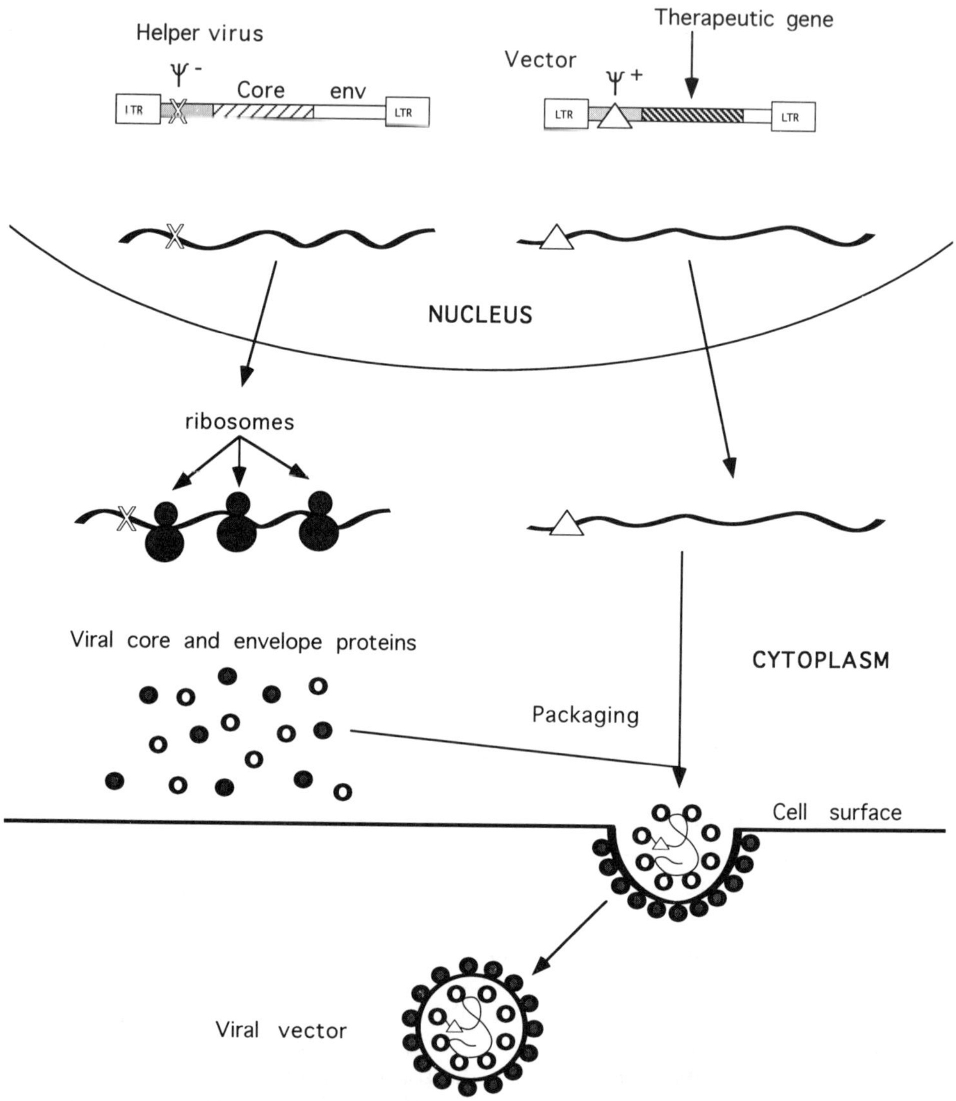

Fig. 6.5. Use of helper cell lines in the production of replication-deficient retroviral vectors for gene therapy.

One of the major drawbacks of retroviral vectors is the limited size of the foreign DNA that can be incorporated into them. With the vectors currently in use this limit is about 7 kilobases. The need to include selectable markers and regulatory sequences further reduces the size of the coding sequences of the therapeutic protein that can be included. Therefore retroviral vectors cannot be used to deliver large genes. Another drawback is that, for a retroviral vector to integrate into the cell DNA, the cell must replicate. Thus, retroviral vectors cannot be used to deliver genes to nondividing cells such as neurons or muscle cells. At present, retroviral vectors are used mainly with hematopoietic cells, which have the capability to divide *in vitro* (Pembrey, 1991; Miller, 1992; Jinnah *et al.*, 1993).

Adenovirus vectors which have received attention recently have some advantages over retroviral vectors. Adenoviruses are pathogens of the human respiratory tract, but are not associated with human malignancies. They have large DNA genomes of nearly 36 kilobases, which is small enough for direct manipulation by standard rDNA methods. Regions of the adenoviral genome dispensable for viral growth have been identified. Foreign genes can be substituted into the viral genome at these locations to create recombinant vectors which are defective in replication. It is possible that adenoviral vectors will permit the incorporation of larger genes than are feasible with retroviral vectors. (Here, similar to the case of the 9 kilobase packaging limit on retroviral vectors, the size of the recombinant viral vector genome that can be packaged is close to 36 kilobases.) The deletion of genes for proteins needed for replication renders the vector defective. However, analogous to the use of helper cell lines for growing retroviral vectors, the defective adenovirus vector stocks can be produced in cell lines expressing the viral protein required for replication and assembly. Adenoviruses infect cells from a wide variety of tissues. A major advantage of adenoviral vectors is that, unlike retroviruses, adenoviruses are capable of stably integrating their genome into the genome of the cell in the absence of cell division. Thus, gene delivery to nondividing cells such as neurons or muscle cell is feasible with adenovirus vectors (Ragot *et al.*, 1993; Le Gal La Salle *et al.*, 1993). Cells of the respiratory tract contain receptors for adenoviruses, and defective adenovirus vectors have been used to deliver the gene defective in cystic fibrosis (CFTR) to cells of the respiratory epithelium of whole animals (Hoffman, 1991a; Rosenfeld *et al.*, 1992; Collins, 1992). Infection by adenovirus vectors shows promise also for the delivery of genes to muscle cells in whole animals and to endothelial cells in isolated human veins (Quantin *et al.*, 1992; Lemarchand *et al.*, 1992). Adenovirus vectors have also been shown to deliver genes to liver cells when injected into the intraportal vein, with expression of the delivered gene detectable for a month (Davies, 1992). Recently, the possible utility of adenovirus vectors in the delivery of genes to neurons and glia in the brain has been demonstrated (Le Gal La Salle *et al.*, 1993). The first human gene therapy trial using a defective adenovirus vector for the treatment of cystic fibrosis has received approval recently (Thompson, 1992c).

Other viruses such as the herpes virus and the adeno-associated virus (AAV) are also being explored as vectors for gene delivery, but these studies are in preliminary stages (Davies, 1992; Collins, 1992). The herpes simplex virus (HSV-1) has a large genome of 150 kilobases and can accommodate up to 30 kilobases of foreign DNA. The vector DNA is maintained stably in a non-integrated form, thereby reducing the probability of insertional mutagenesis. HSV infects many cell types including differentiated cells such as neurons, establishing latent infections. Therefore, HSV vectors are particularly attractive for gene delivery into the nervous system (Jinnah *et al.*, 1993). A provocative approach of using the HIV virus, the pathogenic agent in AIDS, as a vector for gene therapy of AIDS has been proposed. In this case, the HIV virus will be disarmed by deletion of key genes required for replication (Thompson, 1992a).

Chemical modification of nucleic acids

Normal oligonucleotides are susceptible to rapid degradation in body fluids and intracellular compartments by nucleases that are ubiquitous. In addition, the negative charge of the phosphate groups of the sugar–phosphate backbone retards their passage through cell membranes. Both nuclease resistance and cell permeation can be improved by the chemical modification of oligonucleotides. In fact, the success of nucleotide therapies is likely to critically hinge on finding acceptable modifications that improve availability. The phosphodiester backbone can be modified without affecting the base pairing ability of the oligonucleotides, and many of these modifications can be incorporated into the oligonucleotides during chemical synthesis. Fig. 6.6 shows some of the modifications that are currently under investigation.

The negatively charged oxygen atom in the phosphodiester backbone can be replaced by similarly charged sulfur atoms to produce phosphorothioates. The replacement of the oxygen atom with a methyl group results in methylphosphonates which are uncharged. Lack of backbone charge appears to increase the cellular uptake of methylphosphonates. Other groups can also be used to replace the oxygen atom to obtain phosphoramidates and phosphotriesters. Sugar residues can also be modified to affect increased nuclease resistance. Chemical groups which are activated by external agents such as light can be incorporated along the modified backbone. Such groups include psoralen which, when activated by light, can cause cross-linking of the oligonucleotide to the target nucleic acid, thereby increasing its inhibitory potential (Miller, 1991). In addition, chemical groups, called ''pendant groups'', coupled to the ends of the oligonucleotides, increase nuclease resistance. Recently, a new class of antisense polymers known as polyamide nucleic acids (PNAs), containing normal DNA bases, but with the replacement of the entire sugar–phosphate backbone characteristic of an oligonucleotide with a polyamide chain like that of a protein, has been developed. PNAs bind to complementary DNA with higher affinity than conventional oligonucleotides, suggesting their utility in antisense and triplex therapies (Frank-Kamenetskii, 1991). These modifications would confer a high degree of stability to the oligonucleotides against the nucleases in serum, and increased efficacy; for instance, the serum half-life of a normal phosphodiester oligonucleotide was increased from 1 hour to greater than 24 hours by the phosphorothioate substitution (Akhtar and Juliano, 1992, Crooke, 1992a; Murray and Crockett, 1992); a 12-nucleotide-long, psoralen-conjugated methylphosphonate oligonucleotide at a concentration of 5 μM inhibited protein synthesis to the same degree as 100 to 150 μM of the underivatized nucleotide (Miller, 1991). Many of the cell culture studies and the current antisense therapeutics are based on methylphosphonate and phosphorothioate modifications to the backbone, and the

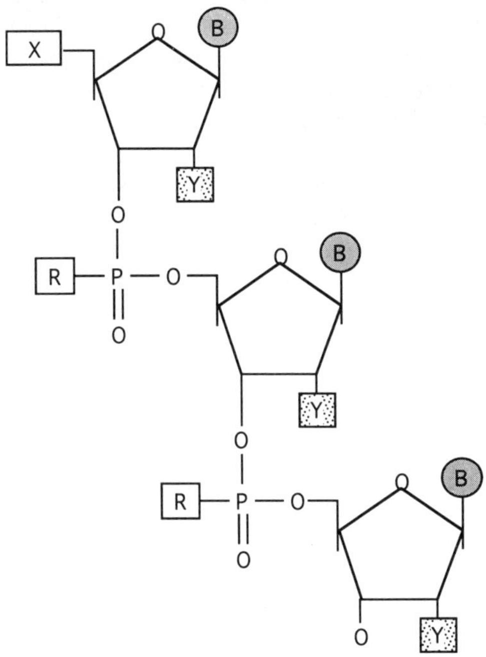

X : Pendant group

R : H (DNA)
S (Phosphorothioate)
CH_3 (Methyl phosphonate)
O-CH_2-CH_3 (Alkyl phosphotriester)

B : Bases A,T,G or C

Y : -H (DNA)
-O-CH_3

Fig. 6.6. Chemical modification of deoxyoligonucleotides aimed at increasing nuclease resistance and cell permeation.

relative superiority of the two modifications is hotly debated (Miller, 1991; Crooke, 1992b; Beardsley, 1992).

MOLECULAR MECHANISMS

Gene therapy

Depending on the nature of the vector used and the method of delivery, a foreign gene may integrate into a chromosome, or may persist autonomously. Integration into the genome of the cell would be expected to be necessary for long-term expression, especially in cells that undergo multiplication. Once in the cell nucleus, the foreign gene is expressed by using the same transcriptional and translational machinery used for the expression of endogenous genes. However, since the integration of exogenous, therapeutic genes into the cell genome occurs at random sites in the chromosomes, the local environment of the integrated gene is different in each independent integration event. Thus the level of transcription of the foreign gene is influenced by the environment in which the gene integrates. Further, the level of translation can also vary with the structure of the engineered mRNA. Promoter elements used for transcribing the gene may influence the level of expression and the long-term expression of the genes, especially *in vivo* (Scharfmann *et al.,* 1991). Regulated expression of the transferred gene becomes a critical issue when the goal of intended gene therapy is to restrict its expression to a specific cell type. In such cases it is necessary to use a promoter element which is transcribed preferentially in the desired tissue or cell type. For example, in correcting the hemoglobin gene defect in thalassemia, it is desirable to restrict the expression of the corrective gene only to progenitors of red blood cells (Pembrey, 1991). The globin gene promoters contain many regulatory elements required for the tissue and developmental stage-specific expression of the genes, and they are the promoters of choice in gene therapies aimed at hemoglobin defects (Dillon *et al.,* 1991).

Antisense inhibition

The finding that antisense RNAs are used normally in nature to regulate gene expression, notably in prokaryotes and probably in eukaryotic cells, supports the use of exogenous antisense nucleic acids in regulating gene expression (Murray and Crockett, 1992). Antisense oligonucleotides or antisense RNAs are believed to inhibit gene expression by interfering with the processing and translation of mRNA, by hybridizing to crucial regions of the RNA. However, the experimental proofs for many of the postulated mechanisms have been difficult to obtain (Crooke, 1992b).

Antisense nucleic-acid-mediated inhibition of gene expression can be obtained either by administering antisense oligonucleotides exogenously or by producing antisense RNA by transcription of an antisense gene from within a cell. In the latter case, an antisense gene is introduced into the cell by the delivery vectors and methods used for gene therapy. The antisense gene is constructed as shown in Fig. 6.7, by placing a segment of the target gene, under the transcriptional control of a promoter, in the direction opposite to the normal transcriptional direction of the target gene. RNA produced from the transcription of the antisense gene is complementary to the normal RNA of the target gene, and inhibits the function of the normal RNA by hybridization to it. Introduction in the form of a transcribable DNA copy is also necessary for the intracellular production of ribozymes, which are catalytically active RNA molecules discussed below.

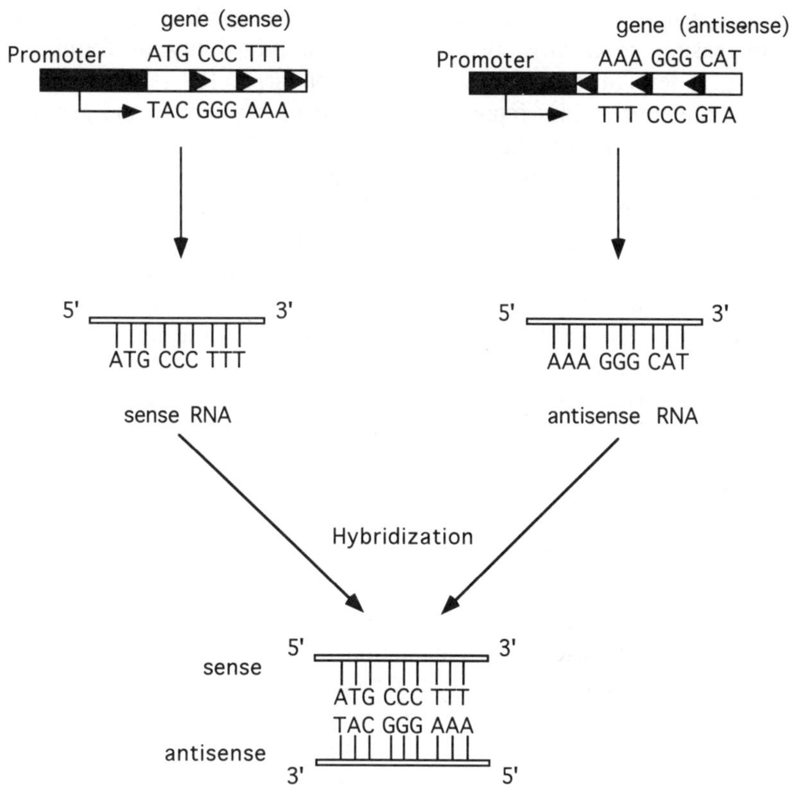

Fig. 6.7. Production and mechanism of action of endogenous antisense RNA.

Once inside the cell, and hybridized to the target RNA, the antisense RNA or oligonucleotides interfere with the maturation of the primary RNA transcript and the translation of the resultant mRNAs. Experimental evidence has been presented for inhibition of biochemical processes at various steps in gene expression. Within the nucleus, hybridization of the antisense nucleic acid to the primary transcript of the gene and to the corresponding region of DNA is believed to inhibit the processes of transcription, splicing-out of introns, and transport of the resulting mRNA to the cytoplasm for translation. In the cytoplasm, antisense sequences hybridized to the mRNA interfere with its translation by ribosomes. In addition to these mechanisms, the hybrid regions have also been suggested to make the RNA susceptible to nucleolytic degradation (Murray and Crockett, 1992; Toulme, 1992; Edgington, 1992a).

The specificity and the binding affinity of antisense nucleic acids are proportional to their length. Oligonucleotides 11 to 15 bases long are thought to be capable of binding specifically to a selected RNA species. By using strategies involving stacking interactions between nearest-neighbor bases, oligonucleotides can be designed to differentiate between a gene and its mutant form containing a single-base change (Crooke, 1992b). Increasing the length of an oligonucleotide, while increasing specificity, also increases the probability of forming hybrids (containing a few mismatches) with other non-target RNAs. Further, antisense RNAs and oligonucleotides represent only a small segment of the genes they are targeted against. Therefore, the choice of the particular region of the gene used to create antisense nucleic acids has been shown to influence the efficiency of inhibition of gene expression. Generally, the splice junction in the primary RNA transcript and the 5′ regions of the mRNA including the initiating AUG codon have been observed to be good target regions. However, antisense nucleic acids directed against other regions of the gene have also been shown to be effective, perhaps resulting from nuclease degradation initiated at the hybridized segments. The effectiveness of an antisense nucleic acid is also dependent on the secondary structure of the target RNA; presence of intramolecular duplexes within the target regions of the RNA may exclude the binding of the antisense strand. Furthermore, there is also cell-type dependence for the effectiveness of antisense nucleic acids depending on the presence of specific nucleases, etc. in a given cell-type. Overall, several variables determine the optimal length and the best target site for antisense design, and therefore *a priori* predictions are difficult. Thus, at the present time, these choices depend on a trial and error approach (Crooke, 1992a,b; Murray and Crockett, 1992).

The extent of antisense-induced inhibition of a gene is also dependent on the intracellular concentration and distribution of the antisense nucleic acid. Generally, a large excess of the antisense nucleic acids over the target RNA appears to be necessary for the successful inhibition of expression of the target gene. Even in cases where such excess is achieved, complete elimination of gene expression has been difficult to obtain, but reductions of one to two orders of magnitude appear possible. However, in many cases, the residual expression of the target gene may be sufficient for cell survival. For instance, small amounts of an enzyme may be sufficient for the cell to retain its normal phenotype. Thus, the antisense inhibition strategy would be expected to be successful only in cases where the phenotype of the cell is proportionally responsive to a decrease in the level of protein produced by the targeted gene. In addition to the stability considerations discussed earlier, the requirement for high intracellular levels of the antisense strand for inhibitory action also contributes to the high concentrations of oligonucleotides required in antisense therapies. One possible approach to reducing the therapeutic concentrations will be the development of ribozymes which act catalytically on the target RNAs (Murray and Crockett, 1992; Crooke, 1992a).

Ribozymes

Ribozymes are catalytic RNA molecules which bind to the target RNA through complementary base pairing, and cleave the target RNA, thereby inactivating it. Ribozymes consist of a stretch of conserved nucleotides required for the catalytic activity flanked by nucleotides that are complementary to the target RNA (Murray and Crockett, 1992; McCall *et al.,* 1992; Edgington, 1992a). There are several types of ribozymes which differ in their secondary structures. The structure of a typical hammerhead ribozyme is shown in Fig. 6.8.

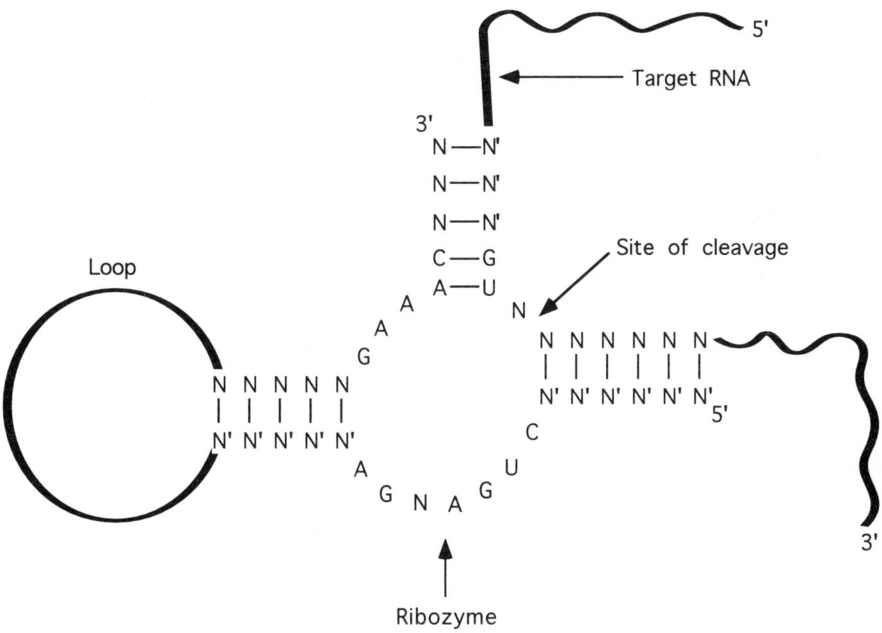

Fig. 6.8. Structure and the cleavage site of a hammerhead ribozyme.

In principle, a ribozyme can be targeted against any RNA molecule by designing flanking nucleotide stretches in the ribozyme to hybridize with the RNA in a manner similar to antisense oligonucleotides. Thus, for instance, it is possible to design a ribozyme directed against HIV viral RNA. While inhibition of RNA function by antisense oligonucleotides requires binding to each target RNA molecule stoichiometrically, ribozyme action being catalytic in mechanism can, in theory, inactivate many RNA molecules complementary to it. However, the general use of ribozymes to inactivate the expression of chosen genes awaits further refinement of the ribozyme design and improvement of catalytic efficiency (Murray and Crockett, 1992; Edgington, 1992a). The recent report of strong inhibition (>95%) of HIV virus protein production in cells in culture by ribozymes delivered through appropriate vectors appears promising for the application of ribozymes in therapy (Thompson, 1992a).

Triplex inhibition of gene expression

Antisense inhibition of RNA function requires the inhibition of thousands of copies of the target RNA present in the cell. However, inhibition of transcription at the level of DNA requires the inactivation of transcription from only one or two active copies of a gene present in the genome; this is the rationale for triplex inhibition of gene expression. Some deoxyoligonucleotides are capable of complexing with double-stranded DNA to form triple helices (Fig. 6.3), resulting in transcriptional inhibition. The phenomenon of triple helix formation *in vitro* in test tubes has been known for over three decades. Recent interest in this area has been rekindled by the possibility of generating specific DNA-cleaving reagents and by possible therapeutic applications (Moffat, 1991; Johnston, 1992).

Deoxyoligonucleotides of lengths over 15 bases can form triple-stranded DNA by binding to the major groove of double-stranded DNA. The bases in the two opposite strands of the target double-stranded DNA remain hydrogen bonded to each other by Crick–Watson base pairing (A with T, and G with C) as in the native state, but the oligonucleotide strand interacts through a different type of base pairing. In this mode, C in the oligonucleotide strand interacts with a G–C base pair of the double-stranded DNA and a T in the oligonucleotide strand interacts with an A–T pair. Further, interaction is only with one of the strands of the double-stranded DNA, requiring that all the purines in the target region occur in the same strand of DNA. Thus, in the most-studied current models, the binding oligonucleotides must be composed of pyrimidines C and T, and all of the purines in the target region must occur in the same strand of the target DNA (Riordan and Martin, 1991; Crooke, 1992a). This requirement places restrictions on the sequences that can be targeted, but further research is expected to help the design of specific oligonucleotides directed at regions that are not so chemically constrained. There is experimental evidence to support the feasibility of this approach in cell culture experiments. For instance, exposure of mammalian cells to a 27-base-long deoxyoligonucleotide designed to bind to the promoter of a gene caused a specific reduction in the levels of mRNA derived from that gene. In this case, the oligonucleotide was composed predominantly of pyrimidines, but a few purines were interspersed along its length (Postel *et al.*, 1991). The triplex inhibition approach is in its infancy, and a significant amount of research on targeting, delivery, and stability of the oligonucleotides remains to be done. The ultimate therapeutic goal of triplex research is to specifically target and turn off the transcription of errant genes such as those of viruses, and those activated in cancers and other diseases.

REGULATORY ISSUES

The use of nucleic acids as therapeutics is an unprecedented concept, and therefore the regulatory guidelines have evolved simultaneously with the technologies, and continue to do so. Because gene therapy using retroviral vectors is the most advanced of the nucleic acid therapies, regulatory issues and concepts are relatively better formulated in this area (Walters, 1991; FDA Report, 1991).

The chief regulatory concerns in using nucleic acids as therapeutics are: (a) toxicity and immunological consequences associated with the introduction of high concentrations of normal and modified oligonucleotides and delivery agents into patients, (b) mutagenic and oncogenic events that occur upon integration of exogenous nucleic acids into the genome, irrespective of the method of delivery, and (c) contaminating infectious viruses and a generation of new viral agents associated with the use of viral vectors.

The first oligonucleotide-based drugs are just around the corner in early clinical trials (Crooke, 1992b; Beardsley, 1992; Sterling, 1992). Some of the intended applications employ topical and intradermal delivery of the oligonucleotides. Further, recently, an antisense 20-mer phosphorothioate oligonucleotide was introduced intravenously into a patient with terminal acute myeloblastic leukemia at a dose rate of 0.5 mg/kg/h to a total dose of 700 mg with no major side-effects. Nonetheless, with the antisense approach being in its early stages of development, the regulatory guidelines are not yet clearly established (Edgington, 1992a). It is clear from early experience that high levels of normal and modified oligonucleotides will be introduced into patients through topical, intradermal and intravenous routes. The pharmacodynamics, pharmacokinetics and the toxicology of oligonucleotides are currently under study and more data are required for the formulation of effective regulatory guidelines (Crooke, 1992a). Very little information exists on the immunological consequences of high levels of oligonucleotides. Although antibodies against DNA are found in some autoimmune diseases, the immunogenic properties of nucleic acids and oligonucleotides are not well understood, and are controversial. However, this is likely to be an important question for regulatory agencies to address (Edgington, 1992b). Similar questions will have to be addressed when the physical methods discussed earlier are used to deliver larger genes or gene complexes. These questions are just beginning to be investigated.

Integration of DNA into the cellular genome can cause interruption of cellular genes, resulting in ''insertional mutagenesis''. Some of these insertions may inactivate important cellular regulatory genes, and others may activate oncogenes or inactivate tumor suppressor genes, thereby initiating early events involved in oncogenic transformation. While the insertions of larger genes delivered through physical methods or viral vectors have high probability of genomic disruption, the mutagenic potential of oligonucleotides has not been studied in sufficient detail (Crooke, 1992a). At this time, most of the questions of insertional mutagenesis and oncogenic potential have been addressed in the context of retroviral vectors, which are currently in human trials; however these considerations also appear to apply to the insertion of genes delivered by other methods.

Retroviruses have been shown to be insertional mutagens in mice, with around 5% of viral integrations causing lethality (Temin, 1990; Rudnicki and Jaenisch, 1991). Therefore, insertional mutagenesis and its consequences are unavoidable. This situation is analogous to the unavoidable trade-offs encountered in cancer chemotherapy where many of the chemotherapeutics themselves have long-term carcinogenic potential. Thus, the regulation of gene therapy should be based on weighing this risk of carcinogenesis against the benefits of the therapy. Based on this reasoning, gene therapy is restricted at this time to life-threatening diseases wherein the benefits far outweigh the risks (Temin, 1990; Cornetta *et al.,* 1991; Culliton, 1991).

The defective retroviral vectors used in gene transfer are capable of integration but are incapable of replication and production of infectious particles. However, one of the major problems encountered with the use of viral vectors is the possibility of introducing pathogenic relatives of the defective vector virus into the patient. This can occur by the production of infectious virus through recombination events occurring in the helper cell between the defective vector and the debilitated helper virus or other silent endogenous viral sequences. Such a virus would then contaminate the viral vector inoculum used in gene therapy. Mouse retroviruses used in vector construction are capable of replication in human cells, leading to the spread of infection. Infectious viruses may also be generated by recombination of the viral vector with endogenous viral sequences present in the genome of the recipient cell, or with viruses that infect the cell subsequently. Exposure of the patient to infectious viruses generated as above can have pathological consequences beyond the patient through the passage of the virus to the patient's progeny via germ cells (Temin, 1990; Cornetta *et al.,* 1991).

Cumulative experience from 106 monkey-years and 23 human-years of retroviral gene therapy had revealed no side-effects or malignancies. Recently, however, three monkeys used in clinical trials developed T cell lymphomas which were traced to a helper virus-contaminated retroviral vector preparation (Anderson, 1992a). Contamination of defective viral vector stocks by infectious viruses produced in helper cells was a serious problem with the early version of the helper cells. New helper cell lines which greatly reduce the probability of virus production have been developed (Miller, 1990). Further, it is also imperative to test the lots of vector virus preparations used in therapy for the presence of other infectious viruses. The probability of generation of infectious viruses in the patient is difficult to estimate but is considered very low. A long-term follow-up of current patients will be necessary to assess this possibility (Temin, 1990; Cornetta *et al.,* 1991). In addition to these considerations of infectious viruses, the exogenous adventitious agents contaminating the cell culture media and sera should also be controlled as with the production of biologicals from mammalian cells.

At this time over two dozen gene therapy protocols have been approved in the US (Johnson, 1992; Anderson, 1992a; Miller, 1992; Thompson, 1992a; Fox, 1992a,b). Similar gene therapy trials have also been initiated in Europe and China (Abbott, 1992; Anderson, 1992a; Thompson, 1992a). All government-funded gene therapy trial protocols in the US approved to date were reviewed for safety and efficacy by the Recombinant DNA Advisory Committee (RAC) of the National Institutes of Health and also by its Human Gene Therapy Subcommittee (Walters, 1991). With a number of protocols already approved, a move to streamline the lengthy approval process, by eliminating the subcommittee, is under consideration (Gershon, 1991; Palca, 1991). In fact, the recent approval of a gene therapy trial, without the involvement of the RAC and the subcommittee, has sparked a serious debate about the role of the RAC and the review process (Thompson, 1992d, 1993). Trials conducted by privately funded organizations, such as industrial laboratories, are exempt from RAC review but require approval by the FDA. In the US, the FDA has the final authority on the approval of all gene therapy trials. Recently, the Center of Biologics Evaluation and Research of the FDA in the US has prepared a guideline document "Points to consider in human somatic cell therapy and gene therapy", which addresses the safety issues and guidelines for vector and cell line preparations (FDA Report, 1991; Epstein, 1991).

APPLICATIONS

The large number of cell culture and animal experiments performed in the 1980s, testing the tools and the concepts involved in the nucleic acid therapies, has brought the field to the threshold of human applications in the 1990s. In keeping with the historic order of emergence, most of the current human trials are in the area of gene therapy (Anderson, 1992a; Miller, 1992), but oligonucleotide therapeutics are fast approaching this phase (Sterling, 1992; Crooke, 1992b; Dutton, 1993). Current activities and the future possibilities in these fields are discussed below.

Gene therapy

Gene therapy clinical trials currently in progress fall into three major categories: (1) gene marking, (2) replacement therapy, (3) cancer therapy (Anderson, 1992a; Miller, 1992). In addition, approaches for AIDS therapy are also under development (Jolly, 1991; Miller, 1992). Almost all of the currently approved gene therapy trials are *ex vivo* experiments, where cells removed from the patient are engineered in the laboratory, in most cases with retroviral vectors, and subsequently returned to the patient.

Gene marking

The very first approved gene therapy trial conducted in 1989 was aimed at the gene marking of lymphocytes in cancer patients, with an easily detectable foreign gene (Anderson, 1992a; Miller, 1992). Being the first, the immediate goals of this experiment were mainly to demonstrate that an exogenous gene could be safely transferred into a patient, and that the cells containing the gene persisted in the patient. This experiment was performed with tumor-infiltrating lymphocytes (TILs), lymphocytes which are found within the malignant tumors. Reinfusion of TILs isolated from the tumors, grown to large numbers in the laboratory, had been previously shown to result in clinical improvement. Thus, the long-range goal of this study was also the optimization of cancer therapy by using TILs, by understanding the homing of the TIL cells to tumor sites and their persistence at these sites.

TILs obtained from tumor biopsies were expanded in the laboratory and infected with a retroviral vector containing the bacterial gene that conferred resistance to neomycin. Cells were reintroduced into the patient. Long-term persistence of the engineered cells was shown by polymerase chain reaction and, in some cases, by isolation of neomycin-resistant cells. This trial showed that a gene could be transferred safely by using retroviral vectors. Since this first study, several gene-marking experiments using TILs and other cells have been designed to determine other parameters that are important in therapies. Marked donor hepatocytes are being used to determine the effectiveness of hepatocyte transplantation to treat acute liver failure. Gene marking is being applied to study HIV–antigen specific T lymphocytes from donors for use in bone marrow transplantation in lymphomas associated with AIDS. Attempts are also in progress to use gene-marked cancer cells to evaluate the efficacy of chemotherapies, and to determine the origin of the tumor cells involved in relapses of leukemias and neuroblastomas. In this case, bone marrow cells obtained from the patient before chemotherapy are purged of cancer cells in the laboratory, gene marked, and reintroduced into the patient after chemotherapy. The marked cells are expected to be helpful in distinguishing between the two possible origins of tumor cells in cases of relapses, as being either from the cell that escaped chemotherapy or from residual tumor cells in the purged autologous bone marrow transfusion.

Replacement therapies

Replacement of defective genes in genetic disorders with their normal counterpart is the goal that led to the conception of gene therapy. A number of genetic disorders are known to be caused by the absence or malfunction of the protein product of a single gene which is altered by mutations. These diseases are usually recessive, with the disease manifesting only in individuals harboring the gene defect in both copies of the gene present in the diploid genome. They are amenable to correction by administration of the protein product of the gene or by enabling the cells in the patient to produce the normal gene product. Table 6.1 shows some of the inherited disorders traced to defects in single genes. These diseases are candidates for gene therapy in all cases where the normal gene is available. There are other inherited disorders where genetic basis is dominant, or multigenic and complex, and such diseases are not amenable to gene-replacement therapy.

Table 6.1. Some current and future targets for gene therapy

Disease	Defective gene
Thalassemias	Hemoglobin
Sickle cell anemia	β-globin
Severe combined immune deficiency (SCID)	Adenosine deaminase
Hemophilia	Factor VIII, factor IX
Gaucher's disease	Glucocerebrosidase
Inherited emphysema	α_1-antitrypsin
Familial hypercholesterolemia	Low-density lipoprotein (LDL) receptor
Cystic fibrosis	Cystic fibrosis transmembrane regulator
Duchenne's muscular dystrophy	Dystrophin

From: Verma (1990); Miller (1992).

Among the diseases listed in Table 6.1, thalassemias resulting from defects in the hemoglobin genes were the first candidates to be considered for gene therapy. Hemoglobin is a protein composed of two protein chains derived from two distinct genes. It became clear, however, that the regulation of the defective hemoglobin gene in a manner to produce the required high levels of hemoglobin in the appropriate cells may be difficult to achieve. Therefore, attention shifted to the gene for adenosine deaminase (ADA), which is defective in patients with "severe combined immunodeficiency" (SCID), leading to elevated levels of adenosine. T lymphocytes of SCID patients are the cells most affected, and hence the immunodeficiency requiring protective isolation of the patients. SCID is treated currently by the administration of polyethylene glycol (PEG)-coupled ADA protein replacement, or by matched bone marrow transplant in which the normal T lymphocytes in the donor marrow contribute predominantly to the therapeutic effect. Therefore, T cells from SCID patients provided an ideal target for gene therapy using ADA gene-containing retroviral vectors.

Clinical trials for SCID patients were initiated in 1990 in ADA-deficient children. T lymphocytes obtained by leukapheresis from the children were induced to grow in plates by the addition of recombinant interleukin-2 (IL-2). Growing T cells were infected with a retrovirus containing the ADA gene and a gene that confers resistance to neomycin (Fig. 6.4C). The cell population was then introduced into the patient. This procedure was repeated several times at a one- to two-month interval. Persistence of the engineered lymphocytes over several months and restoration of the immune function to near-normal levels were achieved through this protocol (Culver *et al.*, 1991). Two children treated by this method for two years have developed functioning immune systems and are no longer in isolation but attend public school. This represents a major breakthrough in the use of gene therapy for the treatment of inherited diseases (Thompson, 1992a).

T lymphocytes have a limited half-life in blood and therefore the gene-corrected lymphocytes are lost from the patient with time. Thus, repeated gene therapy will be required through life to maintain normal immune function in the SCID patient. However, engineering hematopoietic stem cells, the bone marrow progenitor cells which divide to produce T lymphocytes and other hematopoietic cells, may provide a long-term solution. Unfortunately, stem cells have been very difficult to isolate, but progress has been made in enriching the cell populations for stem cells. Gene-replacement trials using the stem-cell-enriched population are currently underway (Thompson, 1992b; Abbott, 1992).

Trials are also in progress for the introduction of the factor IX gene by using retroviral vectors *ex vivo* into skin fibroblasts of patients suffering from hemophilia due to the deficiency of the factor. Similarly, approval has been granted for the introduction of the low-density lipoprotein (LDL) receptor into the hepatocytes of LDL receptor-deficient patients who suffer from hypercholesterolemia (Miller, 1992; Anderson, 1992a). Other protocols for cancer therapies involving antisense inhibition oncogenes, tumor suppressor genes, and lymphokine genes have also been approved recently (Fox, 1992b).

New approaches to gene replacement therapy are also under development. *Ex vivo* gene therapy using myoblasts engineered with retroviral vectors or by direct injection of vector DNA appears promising for gene replacement therapy (Hoffman, 1991b). Advances have also been made in the growth and reimplantation of cells from various tissues (Green, 1991; Van Brunt, 1990, 1991). Encapsidation methods, which may permit the implantation of genetically engineered heterologous cells into patients, are under development (Lacy *et al.*, 1991). These implants offer the option of their removal and/or replacement as necessary. Cells in the implants may be engineered to secrete growth factors such as insulin in response to natural regulatory molecules produced by the patient (Newgard, 1992).

Cancer therapies

The ultimate goal of the TIL lymphocyte study discussed under the gene marking section above was to develop efficient therapies for cancers. Such therapeutic avenues using engineered cells are also in clinical trials (Anderson, 1992a; Miller, 1992). One approach has been to confer upon the TIL the ability to produce certain lymphokines that enhance their anti-tumor potential. With this rationale, the patient's own TIL cells engineered by using retroviral vectors to secrete the tumor necrosis factor (TNF) are being tested in malignant melanoma. Other trials, supported by successful animal studies, are aimed at ''vaccinating'' cancer patients at advanced stages of disease with engineered tumor cells. Cancer cells derived from tumors have been engineered to secrete TNF or IL-2 and reintroduced into the patient with the aim of enhancing the production of anti-tumor TIL cells by the patient's immune system. In these trials, T cells from the lymph nodes proximal to the site of reintroduction of tumor cells will be isolated, grown and expanded in the laboratory, and will be reintroduced into the patient. Other protocols, including one for introducing genes for the foreign histocompatibility proteins into tumor cells directly at the tumor site, with the expectation of stimulating immune rejection, are also in progress. The histocompatibility protocol is notable because it is the first *in vivo* gene introduction, and one that does not use retroviral vectors. Genes will be delivered by using liposome complexes. Retroviral vector-based gene therapy trials, using expression of tumor suppressor genes or antisense inhibition of oncogene protein production, are being considered for lung cancer (Travis, 1992).

In gene therapies using cells secreting foreign proteins, it may be necessary to remove the cells if the treatment leads to toxicity. While this is relatively easy with encapsulated implants, removing direct cell grafts or reinfused circulating cell would be impossible. Therefore vectors containing a ''suicide'' gene have been developed as a means to purge the engineered cells. The thymidine kinase gene of the herpes virus, but not the cellular thymidine kinase gene, is capable of converting the nucleoside analog, gancyclovir, into a cellular toxin. The presence of the herpes thymidine kinase gene in the engineered cells renders them vulnerable to elimination by exposure to gancyclovir (Miller, 1992).

New anticancer gene therapy approaches are in development in animal models. One interesting approach uses a major disadvantage of the retroviral vectors — the inability to productively infect non-dividing cells — to advantage in the therapy of brain tumors. The introduction of suicide gene-containing retroviral vectors into brain tumor sites leads to the preferential infection of the dividing tumor cell by the vector while sparing the non-dividing brain cells. The tumor cells can be eliminated by exposure to agents such as gancyclovir (Culver *et al.,* 1992).

Other applications

Suicide-gene approaches are being developed for the gene therapy of AIDS (Jolly, 1991; Johnson 1992; Thompson, 1992a). The use of a disarmed HIV virus as a delivery vector has been proposed for AIDS gene therapy. In addition, methods for rendering cells resistant to HIV replication by capitalizing on the regulatory mechanisms of HIV are also being developed (Thompson, 1992a). The use of gene transfer for general immunization against various antigens by injecting the genes in lieu of the protein is also an attractive application of gene therapy (Tang *et al.,* 1992; Cohen, 1993). This and other such novel and promising approaches will be tested in the coming years.

Oligonucleotide therapies

Applications of oligonucleotide drugs based on the antisense approach are in the early stages of clinical testing. Two oligonucleotides, OL(1)p53 and G-1128, are in clinical trials in cancer therapy for acute myeloblastic leukemia (AML) and chronic myelogenous leukemia (CML), respectively (Sterling, 1992). OL(1)p53 is an antisense oligonucleotide directed against the p53 tumor suppressor gene (see Chapter 4). Its use is based on the finding of increased levels of p53 protein in

AML leukemic cells. It is not clear how overexpression of a tumor suppressor gene leads to cancer, but the possibility exists that the gene is mutated in cancer cells. The first study was conducted on a single patient, who was infused with the oligonucleotide. The patient succumbed to the disease soon after therapy without a clear demonstration of treatment efficacy. Expanded trials are under consideration.

G-1128 is designed to target the hybrid oncogene present in the CML cancer cells. The hybrid oncogene is produced by a chromosomal translocation occurring between chromosomes 9 and 22, linking the *bcr* oncogene to the *abl* gene. G-1128 targets the mRNA of the hybrid gene at the junction of the two coding sequences and thereby aims to inhibit the production of the hybrid protein without affecting the synthesis of the normal *bcr* and *abl* gene products. G-1128 is currently being tested in *ex vivo* therapy. The rationale of the therapy is to weed out the cancerous cells in the bone marrow and to return the remaining non-cancerous cells to the patient. Bone marrow obtained from patients in chemotherapy is treated in the laboratory to further eliminate the cancer cells by inhibiting their growth through suppression of the hybrid oncogene activity with G-1128. The normal cells that continue to grow are enriched and returned to the patient (Beardsley, 1992; Sterling, 1992).

An antisense oligonucleotide, ISIS 2105, is in clinical trials for the treatment of genital warts caused by the human papilloma virus. ISIS 2105 is designed for subcutaneous injection directly into the wart (Sterling, 1992). Antisense oligonucleotides for antiviral applications against infection by herpes and other viruses are also under development (Crooke, 1992b).

FUTURE PROSPECTS

The field of nucleic acid therapeutics is in its infancy, and many more advances will be required to make this form of therapy a routine commercial venture. The *ex vivo* approaches discussed above rely on the use of specialized technologies, and are expensive. Further, as practiced currently, the advanced scientific and medical expertise required restrict gene therapy treatments to major medical centers (Anderson, 1992a). Several new vectors and gene delivery methods are under development. Among these, the successful development of direct gene delivery methods will free gene therapy from limitation placed by virus-packaging constraints on the size of the therapeutic gene, and from the risks associated with viral vectors. In the long run, the gene should be administrable as easily as a regular biological or chemical drug. Long-term evaluation of the safety of the methods will also be required before gene therapy can be used routinely for treating life-threatening diseases and for its extension to less serious situations. Similarly, the safety, efficacy, delivery, and mechanistic aspects of oligonucleotides will have to be better understood before their widespread use as drugs. These developments are likely to occur as the twenty-first century draws closer.

REFERENCES

Abbott, A. (1992). Italians first to use stem cells. *Nature* **356,** 465.

Akhtar, S. and Juliano, R.L. (1992). Cellular uptake and intracellular fate of antisense oligonucleotides. *Trends in Cell Biol.* **2,** 139–144.

Anderson, W.F. (1992a). Human gene therapy. *Science* **256,** 808–813.

Anderson, W.F. (1992b). Uses and abuses of human gene transfer. *Hum. Gene Ther.* **3,** 1–2.

Ascadi, G., Dickson, G., Love, D.R., Jani, A., Walsh, F.S., Gurusinghe, A., Wolff, J.A., and Davies, K.E. (1991). Human dystrophin expression in mdx mice after intramuscular injection of DNA constructs. *Nature* **352,** 815–818.

Beardsley, T. (1992). Making antisense: drugs that turn off genes are entering human tests. *Sci. Am.* February, 107–108.

Benvenisty, N. and Reshef, L. (1986). Direct introduction of genes into rats and expression of the genes. *Proc. Natl. Acad. Sci. USA* **83,** 9551–9555.

Carey, J. and Hamilton, J. (1992). The gene doctors roll up their sleeves. *Business Wk.* March 30, 78–82.

Caskey, C.T. (1992). DNA-based medicine: prevention and therapy. In *The Code of Codes: Scientific and Social Issues in the Human Genome Project.* D.J. Kevles and L. Hood, eds. (Cambridge, Massachusetts: Harvard University Press), pp. 112–135.

Chang, D.C., Saunders, J.A., Chassy, B.M., and Sowers, A.E. (1992). Overview of electroporation and electrofusion. In *Guide to Electroporation and Electrofusion.* D.C. Chang, B.M. Chassy, J.A. Saunders, and A.E. Sowers, eds. (New York: Academic Press), pp. 1–6.

Cohen, J. (1993). Naked DNA points way to vaccines. *Science* **259,** 1689–1690.

Collins, F.S. (1992). Cystic fibrosis: molecular biology and therapeutic implications. *Science* **256,** 774–779.

Cornetta, K., Morgan, R.A., and Anderson, W.F. (1991). Safety issues related to retroviral-mediated gene transfer in humans. *Hum. Gene Ther.* **2,** 5–14.

Cotten, M., Wagner, E., Zatloukal, K., Phillips, S., Curiel, D.T., and Birnstiel, M.L. (1992). High-efficiency receptor-mediated delivery of small and large (48 kilobase) gene constructs using the endosome-disruption activity of defective or chemically inactivated adenovirus particles. *Proc. Natl. Acad. Sci. USA* **89,** 6094–6098.

Crooke, S.T. (1992a). Therapeutic applications of oligonucleotides. *Annu. Rev. Biochem.* **32,** 329–376.

Crooke, S.T. (1992b). Therapeutic applications of oligonucleotides. *Bio/Technology* **10,** 882–886.

Culliton, B.J. (1991). Gene therapy on the move. *Nature* **354,** 429.

Culver, K.W., Anderson, W.F., and Blaese, R.M. (1991). Lymphocyte gene therapy. *Hum. Gene Ther.* **2,** 107–109.

Culver, K.W., Ram, Z., Wallbridge, S., Ishii, H., Oldfield, E.H., and Blaese, R.M. (1992). *In vivo* gene transfer with retroviral vector-producer cells for treatment of experimental brain tumors. *Science* **256,** 1550–1552.

Davies, K. (1992). Moving straight to the target. *Nature* **358,** 519.

Davis, B.D. (1992). Germ-line therapy: evolutionary and moral considerations. *Hum. Gene Ther.* **3,** 361–363.

Dillon, N., Talbot, D., Philipsen, S., Hanscombe, O., Fraser, P., Pruzina, S., Lindenbaum, M., and Grosveld, F. (1991). The regulation of human β-globin locus. In *Genome Analysis Volume 2: Gene Expression and Its Control.* K.E. Davies and S.M. Tilghman, eds. (New York: Cold Spring Harbor Laboratory Press), pp. 99–118.

Dutton, G. (1993). Gene therapy evolves towards practicable treatment option. *Genetic Engineering News* **13,** January 1, 1–17.

Edgington, S.M. (1992a). Ribozymes: stop making sense. *Bio/Technology* **10,** 256–262.

Edgington, S.M. (1992b). DNA and RNA therapeutics: unsolved riddles. *Bio/Technology* **10,** 993–996.

Epstein, S.L. (1991). Regulatory considerations in human gene therapy. *Hum. Gene Ther.* **2,** 243–249.

FDA Report (1991). Points to consider in human somatic cell therapy and gene therapy. *Hum. Gene Ther.* **2,** 251–256.

Felgner, P.L. and Rhodes, G. (1991). Gene therapeutics. *Nature* **349,** 351–352.

Fitzpatrick-McElligott, S. (1992). Gene transfer to tumor-infiltrating lymphocytes and other mammalian cells by microprojectile bombardment. *Bio/Technology* **10,** 1036–1040.

Fox, J.L. (1992a). Gene therapy policy. *Bio/Technology* **10,** 1408–1409.

Fox, J.L. (1992b). NIHRAC okays more gene therapy. *Bio/Technology* **10,** 1408.

Frank-Kamenetskii, M. (1991). A change of backbone. *Nature* **354,** 505.

Gershon, D. (1991). Cracks in RAC. *Nature* **353,** 591.

Green, H. (1991). Cultured cells for the treatment of disease. *Sci. Am.* November, 96–102.

Hoffman, M. (1991a). New vector delivers genes to lung cells. *Science* **252,** 374.

Hoffman, M. (1991b). Putting new muscle into gene therapy. *Science* **254,** 1455–1456.

Jinnah, H.A., Gage, F.H., and Friedman, T. (1993). Gene therapy and neurological disease. In *Molecular and Genetic Basis of Neurological Disease.* R.N. Rosenberg, S.B. Pruisner, S. DiMauro, R.L. Barchi, and L.M. Kunkel, eds. (Boston: Butterworth-Heinemann), pp. 969–975.

Johnson, R.S. (1992). Recombinant DNA advisory committee passes six gene therapy proposals. *Genetic Engineering News* **12,** March, 2.

Johnston, J. (1991). Gene therapy: after the dream world, the serious science. *J. NIH Res.* **3,** 26–31.

Johnston, J. (1992). Cry threedom! Triple-helix research takes off. *J. NIH Res.* **4,** 36–42.

Jolly, D.J. (1991). HIV infection and gene transfer therapy. *Hum. Gene Ther.* **2,** 111–112.

Kitsis, R.N., Buttrick, P.M., McNally, E.M., Kaplan, M.L., and Leinwand, L.A. (1991). Hormonal modulation of a gene injected into rat heart *in vivo*. *Proc. Natl. Acad. Sci. USA* **88,** 4138–4142.

Lacy, P.E., Hegre, O.D., Gerasimidi-Vazeou, A., Gentile, F.T., and Dionne, K.E. (1991). Maintenance of normoglycemia in diabetic mice by subcutaneous xenograft of encapsulated islets. *Science* **254,** 1782–1784.

Le Gal La Salle, G., Robert, J.J., Berrard, S., Ridoux, V., Stratford-Perricaudet, L.D., Perricaudet, M., and Mallet, J. (1993). An adenovirus vector for gene transfer into neurons and glia in the brain. *Science* **259,** 988–990.

Lemarchand, P., Jaffe, H.A., Danel, C., Cid, M.C., Kleinman, H.K., Stratford-Perricaudet, L.D., Perricaudet, M., Pavirani, A., Lecocq, J-P., and Crystal, R.G. (1992). Adenovirus-mediated transfer of a recombinant human α_1-antitrypsin cDNA to human endothelial cells. *Proc. Natl. Acad. Sci. USA* **89,** 6482–6486.

McCall, M.J., Hendry, P., and Jennings, P.A. (1992). Minimal sequence requirement for ribozyme activity. *Proc. Natl. Acad. Sci. USA* **89,** 5710–5714.

Miller, D.A. (1990). Retrovirus packaging cells. *Hum. Gene Ther.* **1,** 5–14.

Miller, D.A. (1992). Human gene therapy comes of age. *Nature* **357,** 455–460.

Miller, P.S. (1991). Oligonucleotide methylphosphonates as antisense reagents. *Bio/Technology* **9,** 358–362.

Moffat, A.S. (1991). Triplex DNA finally comes of age. *Science* **252,** 1374–1375.

Murray, J.A.H. and Crockett, N. (1992). Antisense techniques: an overview. In *Antisense RNA and DNA.* J.A.H. Murray, ed. (New York: Wiley-Liss), pp. 1–49.

Nabel, E.G., Plautz, G., and Nabel, G.J. (1990). Site-specific gene expression *in vivo* by direct gene transfer into arterial wall. *Science* **249,** 1285–1288.

Newgard, C.B. (1992). Cellular engineering for the treatment of metabolic disorders: prospects for therapy in diabetes. *Bio/Technology* **10,** 1112–1120.

Palca, J. (1991). Changes ahead for gene therapy review process? *Science* **253,** 624–625.

Partridge, T.A. (1991). Muscle transfection made easy. *Nature* **352,** 751–758.

Pecorino, L.T. and Lo, D.C. (1992). Having a blast with gene transfer. *Curr. Biol.* **2,** 30–31.

Pembrey, M. (1991). Prospects for gene insertion therapy in early life. In *Molecular Genetics in Medicine.* D.F. Roberts and R. Chester, eds. (New York: St. Martins Press), pp. 86–96.

Postel, E.H., Flint, S.J., Kessler, D.J., and Hogan, M.E. (1991). Evidence that a triplex-forming oligodeoxyribonucleotide binds to the *c-myc* promoter in HeLa cells, thereby reducing *c-myc* mRNA levels. *Proc. Natl. Acad. Sci. USA* **88,** 8227–8231.

Quantin, B., Perricaudet, L.D., Tajbakhsh, S., and Mandel, J-L. (1992). Adenovirus as an expression vector in muscle cells *in vivo. Proc. Natl. Acad. Sci. USA* **89,** 2581–2584.

Ragot, T., Vincent, N., Chafey, P., Vigne, E., Gilgenkrantz, H., Couton, D., Cartaud, J., Briand, P., Kaplan, J-C., Perricaudet, M., and Kahn, A. (1993). Efficient adenovirus-mediated transfer of a human minidystrophin gene to skeletal muscle of *mdx* mice. *Nature* **361,** 647–650.

Riordan, M.L. and Martin, J.C. (1991). Oligonucleotide-based therapeutics. *Nature* **350,** 442–443.

Rosenfeld, M., Yoshimura, K., Trapnell, B.C., Yoneyama, K., Rosenthal, E.R., Dalemans, W., *et al.* (1992). *In vivo* transfer of the human cystic fibrosis transmembrane conductance regulator gene into airway epithelium. *Cell* **68,** 143–155.

Ross, E.M. (1990). Pharmacodynamics: mechanism of drug action and relationship between drug concentration and effect. In *Pharmacological Basis of Therapeutics.* A.G. Gilman, T.W. Rall, A.S. Nies, and P. Taylor, eds. (New York: Pergamon Press), pp. 33–48.

Rudnicki, M.A. and Jaenisch, R. (1991). Insertional mutagenesis. In *Genome Analysis Volume 2: Gene Expression and its Control.* K.E. Davies and S.M. Tilghman, eds. (New York: Cold Spring Harbor Laboratory Press), pp. 13–40.

Scharfmann, R., Axelrod, J.H., and Verma, I.M. (1991). Long-term *in vivo* expression of retrovirus-mediated gene transfer in mouse fibroblast implants. *Proc. Natl. Acad. Sci. USA* **88,** 4626–4630.

Sterling, J. (1992). Systemic antisense treatment reported. *Genetic Engineering News* **12,** August, 1–28.

Tang, D., DeVit, M., and Johnston, S.A. (1992). Genetic immunization is a simple method for eliciting immune response. *Nature* **356,** 152–154.

Temin, H.M. (1990). Safety considerations in somatic gene therapy on human diseases with retrovirus vectors. *Hum. Gene Ther.* **1,** 111–123.

Thompson, L. (1992a). At age 2, gene therapy enters a growth phase. Researchers test gene therapy against AIDS. *Science* **258,** 744–746.

Thompson, L. (1992b). Stem-cell gene therapy moves towards approval. *Science* **255,** 1072–1073.

Thompson, L. (1992c). Cystic fibrosis trial approved. *Science* **258,** 1728.

Thompson, L. (1992d). Harkin seeks compassionate use of unproven treatments. *Science* **258,** 1728–1729.

Thompson, L. (1993). Healy approves an unproven treatment. *Science* **259,** 172.

Toulme, J-J. (1992). Artificial regulation of gene expression by complementary oligonucleotides — an overview. In *Antisense RNA and DNA.* J.A.H. Murray, ed. (New York: Wiley-Liss), pp. 175–194.

Travis, J. (1992). NIH considers gene therapy for lung cancer. *Science* **257,** 1467.

Van Brunt, J. (1990). Vascular implants' new wave. *Bio/Technology* **8,** 391.

Van Brunt, J. (1991). Artificial organs from culture. *Bio/Technology* **9,** 136–137.

Verma, I.M. (1990). Gene therapy. *Sci. Am.* November, 68–84.

Wagner, E., Zatloukal, K., Cotten, M., Kirlappos, H., Mechtler, K., Curiel, D.T., and Birnstiel, M.L. (1992). Coupling of adenovirus to transferrin–polylysine/DNA complexes greatly enhances receptor-mediated gene delivery and expression of transfected genes. *Proc. Natl. Acad. Sci. USA* **89,** 6099–6103.

Walters, L. (1991). Human gene therapy: ethics and public policy. *Hum. Gene Ther.* **2,** 115–122.

Williams, R.S., Johnston, S.A., Riedy, M., DeVit, M.J., McElligott, S.G., and Sanford, J.C. (1991). Introduction of foreign genes into tissues of living mice by DNA-coated microprojectiles. *Proc. Natl. Acad. Sci. USA* **88,** 2726–2730.

Wolff, J.A., Williams, P., Acsadi, G., Jiao, S., Jani, A., and Chong, W. (1991). Conditions affecting direct gene transfer into rodent muscle *in vivo*. *Biotechniques* **11,** 474–485.

Wu, C.H., Wilson, J.M., and Wu, G.Y. (1989). Targeting genes: delivery and persistent expression of a foreign gene driven by a mammalian regulatory element *in vivo*. *J. Biol. Chem.* **264**, 16985–16987.

7

Transgenic animal models

From the early days of medical science, animal models of human disease have been indispensable to the understanding of the etiologies and progression of diseases, and for the development of therapeutic strategies (Melby, 1987; Kawamata and Melby, 1987; Loew, 1991). Recent advances in cell and molecular biology, and in computer technology, have facilitated the development of cell culture models, mathematical models, and computer simulations, which will undoubtedly be used to replace expensive animal experimentation where possible. However, in spite of these developments and the current societal desire to supplant research animals with cell culture models or computer simulations, animal models continue to remain a necessary and vital component of drug development efforts into the foreseeable future (Trull, 1987; Melby, 1987; Loew, 1991). Currently, progress in the development of treatments for many diseases of considerable societal impact, such as AIDS and Alzheimer's disease, suffers owing to lack of appropriate animal models (Palca, 1992; Joachim and Selkoe, 1992). Animal models are vital in delineating disease mechanisms, in defining intervention targets, in drug screening, and in preclinical drug evaluation.

Until recently, animals used as disease models were naturally occurring genetic variants identified and characterized by observant researchers, or were derived by the treatment of normal animals with physical or chemical agents to produce disease symptoms. For instance, the hypercholesterolemic Watanabe rabbit used in the study of cholesterol metabolism is a naturally occurring variant (Kolberg, 1992). Streptozotocin-induced diabetes in rats has been a valuable model for diabetes research (Tarui *et al.,* 1987). A number of valuable disease models representing a range of diseases have been obtained by these methods. However, their isolation and/or development is laborious, and the process is dependent on chance occurrences, and is hence undirected. Some of the naturally derived models are in large animals, which are expensive to maintain and slow to breed (Kawamata and Melby, 1987; Touchette, 1991; Kolberg, 1992; Davies, 1992; Friend, 1993).

The emergence of rDNA technology and the sophisticated techniques for embryo manipulation have provided the ability to change the genetic composition of mammals by introducing foreign genes into every cell in the animal (First and Haseltine, 1991; Isola and Gordon, 1991). This process, known as "transgenic technology", although not uniformly successful, is already showing promise towards the directed development of animal models for diseases such as cystic fibrosis, where the genetic basis is understood and the gene involved has been isolated (Collins and Wilson, 1992; Kolberg, 1992; Davies, 1992). With the growing pace of elucidation of genetic and cell biological mechanisms of disease processes engendered by molecular biological methods discussed in earlier chapters, further developments of this nature are imminent.

Mice were the first animals in which transgenic technology was demonstrated successfully, and they continue to occupy a central position in transgenic technology (Cuthberton and Klintworth, 1988; Hanahan, 1989). However, although technically more difficult to practice than in mice, transgenic technology has now been applied successfully to rats and larger farm animals such as sheep and cattle (First and Haseltine, 1991). This has opened avenues for the production of proteins of biological interest in the milk of farm animals discussed in Chapter 2 (Bialy, 1991; Spalding, 1992). The laboratory rat has a long history as a research animal in the pharmaceutical industry, and the further development of transgenic rat technology would also be expected to provide valuable animal models (Heideman, 1991). Because most of the transgenic animal model work to date is in mice, the following discussion is focused on transgenic mice.

Since the report of the first transgenic mouse in 1980, scores of transgenic mice have been produced. The goals of creating these mice have not been restricted to disease models. These studies range from those addressing very basic biological questions about animal development, which may have long-term pharmaceutical applications, to the animal models that may be immediately useful in drug development. Transgenic mice provide the methodology to suppress or overexpress a protein in its normal or mutated form, and thus help understand the role of the protein in animal development. Such studies will undoubtedly contribute to human health in the long term. While a major part of the research effort is long term, a good proportion of the ongoing effort is also directed at models for diseases whose genetic mechanisms are defined.

The first patent for a transgenic mouse useful in screening for carcinogens was issued in 1988. However, subsequently, the patentability of transgenic mice as new biological entities has led to controversies at scientific and governmental levels, based on legal, ethical, moral, and animal rights' arguments, particularly in European countries (Raines, 1991; Loew, 1991; Abbott and Klaffke, 1993).

Early transgenic mice were derived by direct injection of the foreign DNA into the nucleus of a fertilized mouse embryo. This method of DNA delivery results in the random integration of one or more copies of the foreign gene into the genome of the injected embryo. Expression of the foreign gene is influenced by several factors, including the site of integration. Thus, the screening of a large number of independently derived transgenic animals is required to identify the ones showing acceptable levels of expression of the "transgene". Further, this approach is applicable only to situations where overexpression of the foreign gene in the normal or mutant form is sufficient to produce a phenotype, as is the case in genetically dominant diseases. This approach has led to a model for sickle cell anemia, and to the correction of the defect in the "shaker mouse" caused by a defect in the gene for myelin basic protein (Greaves *et al.,* 1990; Cuthbertson and Klintworth, 1988; Isola and Gordon, 1991). Unfortunately, many genetic diseases are recessive. This requires that both copies of the mouse homolog of the disease-causing gene in the diploid genome of the mouse be inactivated to produce the disease phenotype. Recent advances in the use of embryonic stem cells (ES cells) for generating transgenic mice have permitted the targeted destruction of mouse genes to produce "knockout" mice in which both copies of a chosen gene have been inactivated (Bradley *et al.,* 1992; Zimmer, 1992). The recent development of models for cystic fibrosis was achieved by using this approach (Collins and Wilson, 1992; Barinaga, 1992b; Dorin *et al.,* 1992). The following discussion is focused on the technical aspects of transgenic technology employing both direct microinjection and ES cells. This is followed by a brief description of some animal models developed successfully through the transgenic route.

TRANSGENIC TECHNOLOGIES

Transgenic mice through DNA microinjection

The majority of the transgenic mice produced to date have been through the microinjection route, which was used for the production of the first transgenic mouse (Isola and Gordon, 1991). In this procedure, fine glass micropipettes are used to introduce extremely small volumes of DNA solutions into the pronucleus of a fertilized, single-cell-stage mouse embryo. Incorporation of the injected gene into the genome of the single-cell-stage embryo makes it a part of the genomes of all the cells derived from the embryo.

The procedure for production of transgenic mice through microinjection is shown in Fig. 7.1. Female mice stimulated to superovulate using fertility hormones (follicle-stimulating hormone/luteinizing hormone, and chorionic gonadotropin) are mated with fertile males. The hormonal treatment increases the number of eggs released from the ovary. The preimplantation embryos are harvested from the oviduct of the mated females 12 hours after fertilization. By using a fine, sharp glass micropipette controlled by a micromanipulator and visualized on a video display microscope, foreign DNA is injected slowly into one of the two pronuclei (usually the more accessible male pronucleus) of the single-cell embryo. The volumes of injected DNA are in the range of 1 to 2 picoliters (picoliter = 10^{-12} liter, or one trillionth of a liter, or a billionth of a milliliter). During injection, the embryo is held in position by gentle suction through a blunt glass pipette. The injected embryos are transplanted into the oviducts of pseudopregnant female mice, which act as surrogate mothers. Pseudopregnancy is induced by mating a female with a vasectomized male. Litters of the implanted females are analyzed for the presence of the injected foreign DNA at about three weeks of age. DNA obtained from the tail tips of the pups is analyzed by using the Southern blot method. Animals positive for the foreign gene, or "the transgene", are tested for the ability to transmit the gene to their offspring.

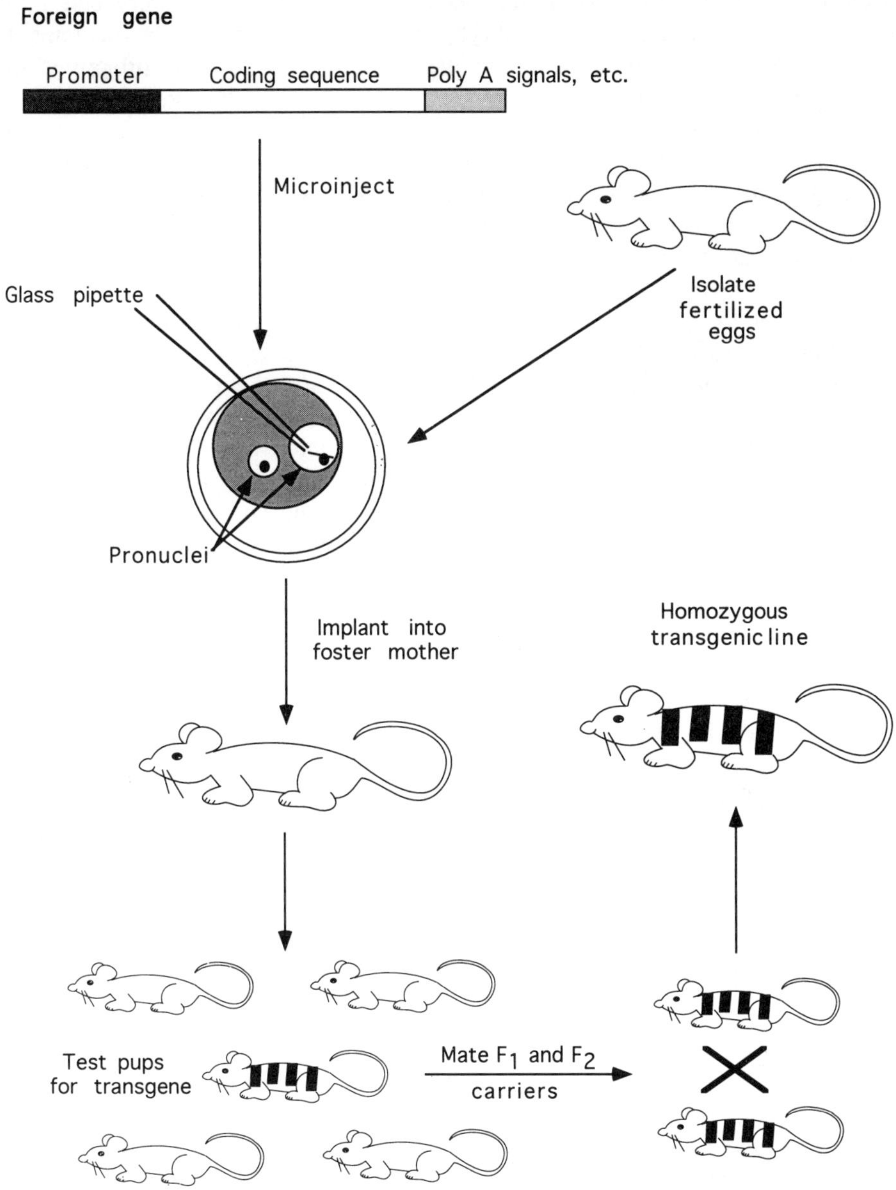

Fig. 7.1. Production of transgenic mice by microinjection of foreign genes.

Microinjected genes have been shown to insert as a tandem array containing 2 to 50 copies, at random locations in the mouse genome (Hanahan, 1990). Mice derived from different injected embryos have the foreign gene integrated at different locations. Thus, each transgenic mouse obtained through microinjection is unique. In a large proportion (~80%) of the injected embryos, the injected DNA integrates immediately at the one-cell stage. Therefore, every cell in the animal derived from such an embryo, including the germ cells, contains the foreign gene. These animals transmit the foreign genes to their offsprings in a Mendelian fashion, and therefore are used as founders of transgenic lines. In 20 to 30% of the cases, integration may occur at the two-cell stage or later. In such cases, only a subset of cells in the resultant animal contains the transgene, resulting in mosaic animals. If the foreign DNA is not present in the progenitors of the germ cells, the mosaic animals are unable to transmit the foreign genes to their offsprings and are hence of no further use.

Once a transgenic line is established, the mice from the line are examined for expression of the gene. Since each line represents a different integration event, and contains a different copy number of the foreign gene, the same foreign gene is expressed to different levels in different lines, and the pattern of expression may also vary among different tissues. Thus, extensive analysis is required to find the line with the desired expression characteristics. The variability of expression makes the generation of transgenic mice by using microinjection highly labor-intensive in terms of both animal breeding and biochemical analysis. The task of analysis becomes simpler if the expression of the gene leads to obvious end-point phenotypes, such as tumors or other altered physical characteristics. Unfortunately, this is not always the case. Because of the time required in the breeding and growth of mice through generations, the production of transgenic animals is also a slow process.

The success rate of production of transgenic mice depends on a number of parameters including the technical skill of the particular laboratory. Typically, 50 to 75% of the microinjected embryos survive, and successful integration occurs in 10 to 40% of the surviving embryos. The success rate of producing transgenic mice is also dependent on the success in inducing pregnancy in embryo-transplanted foster mothers. The strain of the mouse used also appears to influence the success rate (Nomura *et al.*, 1987; Cuthbertson and Klintworth, 1988). In a typical experiment, of the 510 single-cell-stage embryos injected, 348 (68%) surviving the injection were transferred to 27 foster mothers of which 8 became pregnant. Of the 17 pups born, 6 were found to be transgenic. Thus, the success rate of obtaining a transgenic mouse from an injected embryo is low, between 1 and 2%, and is dependent on the dexterity of the injector. Fortunately, it is possible to inject over 200 eggs in a day to offset the low rate of success (Nomura *et al.*, 1987; Hanahan, 1990).

The level and tissue specificity of expression of the transgene is dependent on the chromosomal location that it is integrated into. The nature of the gene construct, particularly the promoter element, can influence the level and tissue specificity of expression. The use of promoters containing appropriate enhancer elements can lead to expression of a gene in a tissue-specific manner. In some (natural) genes, the enhancer elements are located many kilobases away from the promoter, and have to be brought into the proximity of the promoter element in the transgene construct used for injection in order to obtain tissue specificity of expression. By and large, genes constructed with the right control elements yield the anticipated tissue-specific expression pattern, but the expression level is still influenced by the site of integration. However, there are also several instances known where an aberrant expression is observed in tissues in which the promoter element is not known to be active (Cuthbertson and Klintworth, 1988; Isola and Gordon, 1991). Recently, methods for the introduction of large fragments of genomic DNA (greater than 250,000 base pairs) by using yeast artificial chromosomes (YACs) have been developed. Such large fragments of DNA containing the genes and all its regulatory elements should produce a high fidelity of tissue-specific expression of the transgene (Capecchi, 1993). Other methods to improve the levels of expression of the transgenes are under development (Clark *et al.,* 1992).

Tissue-specific promoters can be used to ablate specific cell types which are capable of transcribing the transgene promoter. This is achieved by linking the coding sequence of a toxic protein to the promoter. For example the herpes virus thymidine kinase gene, which converts the nucleoside analog gancyclovir to toxic product, can be linked to a tissue-specific promoter. Exposure of the transgenic mice to gancyclovir at any stage in life leads to the preferential ablation of cells which transcribe and express the thymidine kinase gene. Other cytotoxin genes, such as the diphtheria toxin gene, can be linked to tissue-specific promoters to lead to the ablation of cell lineages during the course of embryonic development, at stages during which the particular promoter becomes active. This approach has been used to ablate exocrine pancreas and lens tissue. Similarly, oncogenes can be linked to tissue-specific promoters to produce tumors in specific tissues (Cuthbertson and Klintworth, 1988; Isola and Gordon, 1991).

Embryonic stem (ES) cell-mediated, directed mutagenesis in transgenic mice

The random nature of integration events in transgenic mice produced through microinjection allows the expression of a foreign gene in the mice, but does not enable the inactivation of genes expressed by the mice. Inactivation of endogenous genes is essential for modeling diseases caused by recessive traits, and for studying the gene's function in the development and maintenance of the animal. In theory, it should be possible to prevent the expression of a gene by expressing an antisense RNA to the gene, as discussed in Chapter 6 (Isola and Gordon, 1991). This approach has shown success in the generation of mice with reduced levels of myelin basic protein (Katsuki *et al.,* 1988), but complete inhibition of the production of a given protein may be difficult for reasons discussed in Chapter 6.

A new approach employing embryonic stem cells (ES cells) permits the targeted destruction of specific genes in transgenic mice as shown in Fig. 7.2 (Capecchi, 1989a,b; Zimmer, 1992; Bradley *et al.,* 1992). ES cells are cells derived from the preimplantation stage embryo (Doetschman, 1991). Under appropriate culture conditions, ES cells multiply in culture and also retain their "totipotency" or "pluripotency", which is the ability to differentiate into any tissue when transplanted into a developing mouse embryo. Thus, the ES cells are amenable to genetic manipulation in the laboratory, and have the ability to colonize all parts of an embryo they are injected into. Colonization of the germ line by the altered ES cells leads to mouse lines that transmit the alteration introduced in the laboratory to their offspring.

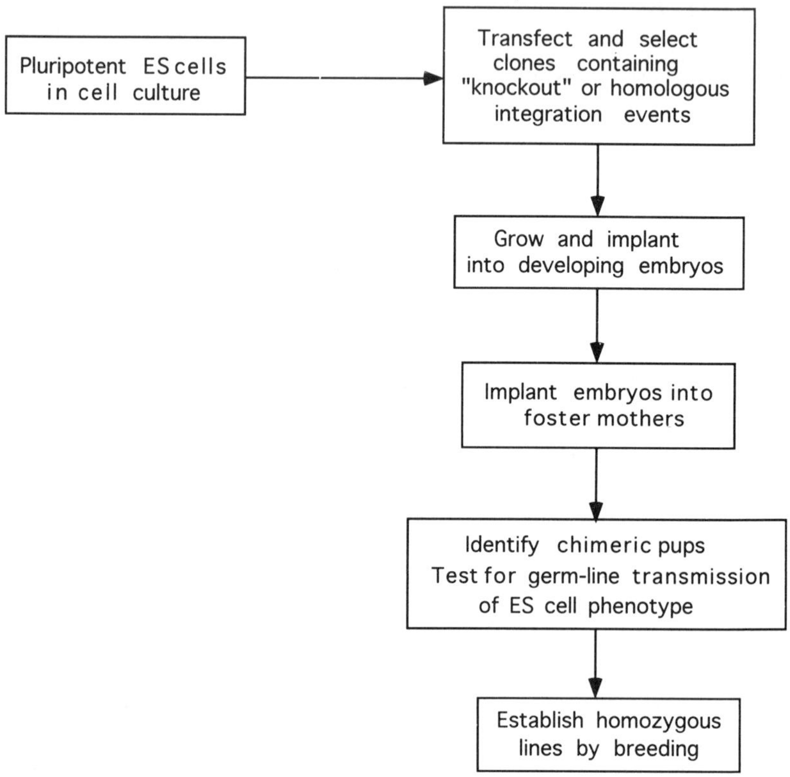

Fig. 7.2. Steps in the production of transgenic mice by using embryonic stem cells.

The techniques and the vectors for disrupting any selected gene have also been developed (Capecchi, 1989a,b; Bradley *et al.*, 1992). As described before, most of the DNA introduced into a mammalian cell by transfection integrates randomly into the cellular DNA by a recombination process that does not require any sequence homology between the foreign DNA and the genomic DNA at the integration site. This type of recombination is termed "nonhomologous" recombination. However, in a small fraction of cells, the foreign DNA integrates into genomic sites which have sequence homology to it. This type of "homologous" recombination targets the foreign gene to its homologous genomic counterpart. Such an event replaces the endogenous gene with the foreign gene as shown in Fig. 7.3. Replacement of the endogenous gene with an interrupted version of the exogenous gene results in

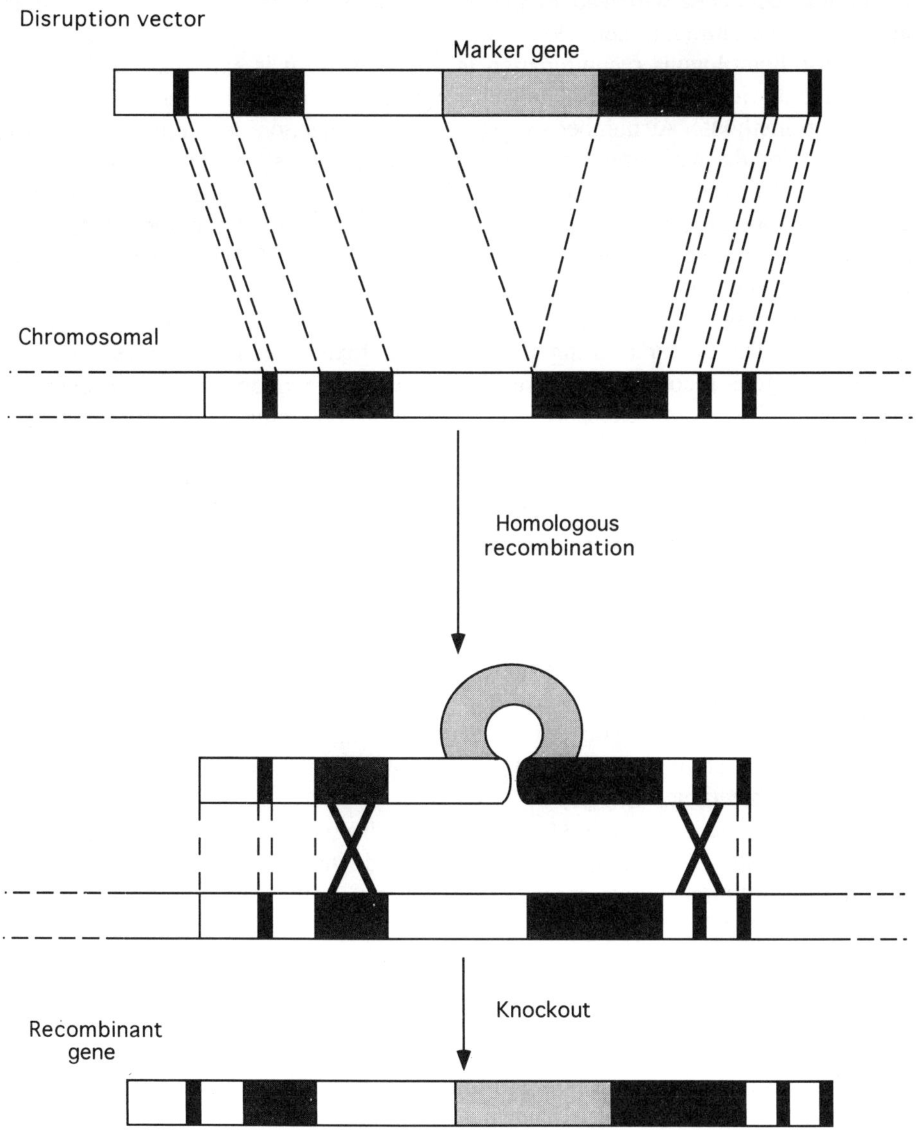

Fig. 7.3. Mechanism of gene knockout resulting from the use of homologous recombination vectors.

a directed disruption or "knockout" of the endogenous gene. The endogenous gene may also be replaced with a copy of the gene containing the desired mutations. The efficiency of homologous recombination increases with the length of the homologies between the endogenous and the exogenous gene. Flanking a nonhomologous sequence stretch (such as marker genes) with long stretches of homologous sequences will lead to the incorporation of the nonhomologous stretch at the targeted site (Zimmer, 1992).

Because homologous recombination is a rare event, it is extremely difficult and forbidding to identify and isolate cells which undergo such events by standard screening methods. A number of vectors and selection techniques have been developed for the enrichment and identification of the cell containing homologous recombination events. ES cells into which vector DNA is introduced generally by electroporation are selected for the presence of the vector by virtue of its ability to confer resistance to antibiotics such as neomycin (G418). The vector also contains a gene such as the herpes virus thymidine kinase, which renders the vector-containing cells susceptible to the toxic effects of the nucleoside analog gancyclovir. The vector is designed so that the toxicity gene in the vector is lost in a homologous recombination event, but not in the random integration events of the vector. Therefore, exposure of the vector-containing cells to gancyclovir results in the elimination of most of the cells containing the random integrations, thus enriching the proportion of cells with homologous recombination events. Individual clones derived from the enriched population are screened by Southern blot analysis and polymerase chain reaction to identify the lines with the desired recombination event. Only one of the two copies of the target gene present in the cell (which is diploid) is disrupted or "knocked out" by the selection process. The second gene can also be disrupted with similar vectors by using different selection markers. However, disruption of both copies is not necessary for the production of homozygous knockout lines because the disrupted and the nondisrupted genes segregate independently during the genesis of haploid germ cells. Therefore, strains of mice with disruption at both copies of the gene can be produced by breeding strategies.

A few pluripotent ES cells (10 to 15 cells) from the clone with disruption or knockout in the desired gene are introduced into the blastocoel cavity of developing preimplantation mouse embryos as shown in Fig. 7.4, and the embryos are implanted into foster mothers. ES cells randomly colonize different organs in the mouse, producing a mosaic mouse containing tissues derived from the natural embryo and the injected ES cells. Mosaic mice are easily recognized based on the coat color. ES cells derived from a mouse of a given coat color are implanted into embryos derived from mice of a different color or from albino mice. The resultant transgenic mice display a mixed, patchy hair coloration. If the germ lines of these mice also happen to be colonized by the ES cells, they are able to transmit the coat color and the disrupted gene to their offspring. Pure strains containing the gene disruption in both copies of the gene can be produced by inbreeding through sibling matings and repeated back-crossing of the founder mouse and its colored offspring.

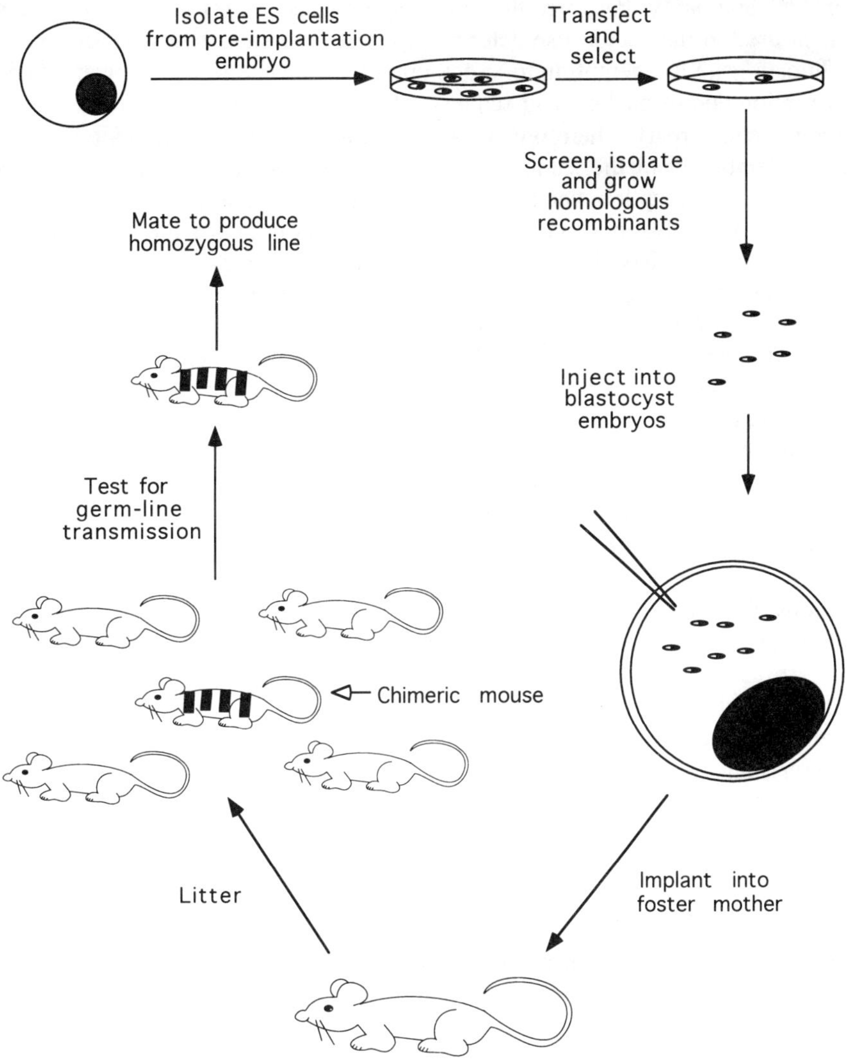

Fig. 7.4. Production of homozygous "knockout" transgenic mice through ES cell technology.

ES cell technology is in its infancy and very few laboratories have the technical competence to practice the methodology. Presently, compared to transgenic mice produced by microinjection, fewer ES cell-derived mice have been made. This situation is rapidly changing as more laboratories and commercial organizations are becoming adept in the use of ES cells. The success rate depends on the strain of mice used, and the culture conditions used for maintaining the ES cells (Bradley *et al.*, 1992). Success of the gene disruption also depends on the particular gene being disrupted and on the type of vectors used in the disruption process. The extent of homology between the endogenous gene and the homologous gene segment used in the vector also determines the success rate. Thus, use of a segment of a human gene in attempting to knock out a mouse gene leads to lower efficiency of disruption due to nucleic acid sequence differences between the human gene and its mouse counterpart. Therefore, it is helpful to isolate the corresponding mouse gene, preferably from the same mouse strain used for the derivation of ES cells, for use in the disruption vector. Transmission of the disrupted gene to progeny depends on the efficiency with which the ES cells colonize the germ line. This efficiency is determined by the source and cell culture history of the ES cell line used in disruption. In cases where disruption of one or both copies of a gene leads to lethality, no offspring carrying the mutation will be produced. Such mutations are called "embryonic lethals". For instance, while heterozygous mice with disruption of the *Rb* tumor suppressor gene in one of the chromosomes show post-natal changes in cancer susceptibilities, loss of both copies in a homozygote results in death of the embryo during gestation. These embryos show defects in neurogenesis and hematopoiesis (Lee *et al.,* 1992; Jacks *et al.,* 1992). Despite such technical difficulties, recent spectacular successes with ES technology underscore the value of this technology to the study of human physiology and diseases (Travis, 1992; Barinaga, 1992a,b). In addition to the application in creating "knockout" mutations, ES cells have been used recently to create transgenic mice incorporating large fragments of foreign DNA (larger than 250,000 base pairs) introduced via yeast artificial chromosomes (YACs). In this application, which is closer in principle to microinjection, yeast cells harboring the YACs are fused directly with ES cells, and the cells are used to generate mice as described above. It is interesting and surprising that the yeast genomic DNA introduced into the ES cell along with the YAC in the fusion process seems to have had no adverse effect on the ability of the ES cells to yield transgenic mice (Capecchi, 1993).

APPLICATIONS

Since the emergence of transgenic technology in 1980, scores of transgenic mice engineered with a wide variety of genes have been developed. These mice have been used to address critical questions in several areas of biology such as developmental biology, immunology, virology, intermediary metabolism, oncogenesis, and neurobiology (Cuthbertson and Klintworth, 1988; Hanahan, 1989, 1990; Adams and Cory, 1991). Attempts have been made at modeling several disease states, with varying degrees of success. A large number of these attempts have been focused on cancers because of the ease of assaying the malignant phenotype which leads to visible tumors. Some examples of models that are useful in cancer research are shown in Table 7.1. In addition, gene replacement therapy approaches using naturally occurring animal mutants as recipients for the normal gene have been attempted in some cases. Some examples of these and other models, including the more recent additions through the ES cell technology, are also shown in Table 7.1. (Also see Appendix.) A few of the promising models are discussed below. While spectacular successes have been obtained in modeling some diseases (especially through ES cell technology), some attempts have failed unexpectedly, and some models do not reproduce the characteristic human pathologies in fine detail. For example, although HPRT enzyme deficiency in humans leads to Lesch–Nyhan syndrome, mice deficient in the HPRT, disappointingly, were normal. Less extreme deviations have been noted in other models discussed below. These differences between mice and humans may arise owing to genetic, anatomical and pathophysiological factors (Davies, 1992; Collins and Wilson, 1992).

Table 7.1. Examples of transgenic disease models developed

Disease model	Gene	Ref.
Cancers		
Oncogenes in a variety of tissues	Oncogenes linked to specific promoters	1, 2, 3, 8, 19–22
Multidrug-resistant cancers	P glycoprotein	9
Suppressor gene deletion	p53 gene (knockout)	10
Gene therapies		
Myelin basic protein defect	Myelin basic protein	2
Dwarfism	Growth hormone	2
Thalassemia	Human β globin gene	1
Fertility	Gonadotropin-releasing hormone	1
Hypercholesterolemia	LDL receptor	1, 2, 3
Virology		
Hepatitis	Hepatitis B virus surface antigen	1, 2
Demyelinating disease	JC virus early region	1, 2
	Antisense to myelin basic protein	1
Kaposi sarcoma	HIV *tat* gene	3
Neurofibromatosis	HTLV-1 *tat* gene	1, 2, 3
Spongiform encephalopathies	Prion protein (PrP)	4
Immunology		
Immunodeficiency	RAG-1 and RAG-2 genes (knockout)	5, 6
Autoimmunity	Histocompatibility antigens	7
Immune development	Antibody genes	1
Multifocal inflammatory disease	Transforming growth factor-β_1	24
Other disease models		
Sickle cell anemia	Human β-globin mutant	11, 12
Cystic fibrosis	CFTR gene (knockout)	13, 14
Lesch–Nyhan syndrome	HPRT gene (knockout)	1, 2
Gaucher's disease	Glucocerebrosidase (knockout)	15
Learning and memory	Protein kinases (knockout)	16, 25
Multiple sclerosis (?)	Histocompatibility gene	17
Polycythemia	Erythropoietin gene	18
Atherosclerosis	Apolipoprotein E (knockout)	23
	Apolipoprotein(a) expression	26

References: 1. Isola and Gordon (1991); 2. Cuthbertson and Klintworth (1988); 3. Hanahan (1989); 4. Chesebro (1992); 5. Travis (1992); 6. Thompson (1992); 7. Hanahan (1990); 8. Wang (1992); 9. Mickish *et al.* (1991); 10. Donehower *et al.* (1992); 11. Greaves *et al.* (1990); 12. Weatherall (1990); 13. Barinaga (1992a); 14. Collins and Wilson (1992); 15. Tybulewicz *et al.* (1992); 16. Barinaga (1992b); 17. Parham (1991); 18. Semenza *et al.* (1989); 19. Sinn *et al.* (1987); 20. Leder *et al.* (1990); 21. Schmidt *et al.* (1988); 22. Adams and Cory (1991); 23. Plump *et al.* (1992); 24. Shull *et al.* (1992); 25. Grant *et al.* (1992); 26. Lawn *et al.* (1992).

Cancer models

Transgenic mice expressing a number of oncogenes under the control of various promoters have been created to serve as models for carcinogenesis (Adams and Cory, 1991). Many of these are commercially available under the generic name "oncomouse", and serve as models and screening systems for oncogenesis.

Transgenic mice engineered with the *ras* oncogene of the Harvey murine sarcoma virus (H-*ras*) under the transcriptional control of the steroid-inducible promoter of the mouse mammary tumor virus (MMTV) show the development of spontaneous mammary adenocarcinomas at 3–6 months of age. Mammary adenocarcinomas also develop in transgenic mouse strains bearing the c-*myc* oncogene (cellular counterpart of the viral *myc* oncogene) linked to the MMTV promoter. Crosses between the *ras* and the *myc* oncogene strains above result in progeny with an increased rate of development of the same tumors (Sinn *et al.*, 1987). Similarly, the expression of a mutationally activated cellular *neu* oncogene in transgenic mice resulted in strains showing high incidence of mammary adenocarcinomas (Muller *et al.*, 1988). These models are useful for the studies of the development and therapy of mammary carcinomas.

Mice bearing the H-*ras* oncogene under the control of the embryonic globin gene, serendipitously, yielded mice that develop papillomas in response to abrasion. Papillomas are also produced in response to tumor promoters such as phorbol esters, and some of these developed into squamous cell carcinomas and sarcomas. Treatment with retinoic acid, an antagonist of tumor promotion by phorbol esters, resulted in the delayed and reduced incidence of papillomas. This strain of transgenics provides a model system for screening tumor promoters and agents that block their action. In addition, it may be a good screen for mutagens and carcinogens (Leder *et al.*, 1990). Transgenic mice engineered to express the c-*myc* oncogene under the influence of the immunoglobulin transcriptional enhancer develop a narrow spectrum of pre-B-cell lymphomas (Schmidt *et al.*, 1988). Models for other cancers using other oncogenes are also under development (Adams and Cory, 1991; Wang, 1992).

Atherosclerosis models

The circulating level of cholesterol has been established as a risk factor in the development of atherosclerosis, resulting in myocardial infarction in humans. The metabolism of cholesterol involves a set of apolipoproteins involved in transporting cholesterol in vesicular complexes and the low-density lipoprotein (LDL) receptors on cells (Brown and Goldstein, 1990).

Overexpression of the LDL receptor under the control of a heavy metal-inducible transcriptional promoter in transgenic mice resulted in the increased clearance of circulating cholesterol (Hoffmann *et al.*, 1988). Transgenic mice expressing the human apolipoprotein apoA-1 gene were shown to have increased levels of the high-density lipoprotein (HDL). ApoA-1 is an abundant lipoprotein present in human HDL whose levels are negatively correlated with incidence of coronary heart disease (Walsh *et al.*, 1989). Recently, transgenic mice with the gene for apolipoprotein apoE knocked out through ES cell technology have been shown to suffer severe hypercholesterolemia (Plump *et al.*, 1992). ApoE is a ligand for the LDL receptor, and is involved in the clearance of several classes of cholesterol-containing particles. Loss of apoE by knockout results in over 10-fold increases in the levels of plasma cholesterol. By ten weeks after birth these mice develop atherosclerotic lesions in the aorta, and coronary and pulmonary arteries.

Elevated plasma levels of lipoprotein Lp(a) increase the risk of atherosclerosis in humans. Apolipoprotein(a), a constituent of Lp(a), is not found in most species other than primates. Transgenic mice expressing the human apolipoprotein(a) gene, placed on an atherogenic diet, show increased susceptibility to the development of lipid-containing lesions in the aorta (Lawn *et al.*, 1992; Scott, 1992).

These transgenic mice are potentially promising models for the study of atherosclerosis and cardiovascular disease, and also for the development and testing of cholesterol-lowering drugs.

Sickle cell anemia

Sickle cell anemia is the result of a single amino acid mutation in the sixth position of the human β-globin gene. Upon deoxygenation, the hemoglobin (an α, β heterodimer) containing the mutant subunit polymerizes, deforming the red cells into a characteristic "sickle" shape. Painful crises and life-threatening conditions result from the sickling of red cells in small vessels (Weatherall, 1990). A transgenic model for sickle cell disorder was produced by preferential expression of a normal human α-globin gene and the sickle cell version of the human β-globin gene in red cells of mice (Greaves *et al.*, 1990). The human genes expressed under the transcriptional regulation of globin control regions produced sickle cell hemoglobin levels ranging from 10 to 80% of the total hemoglobin. Red cells from these mice sickled when deoxygenated, reproducing the human phenotype at a cellular level, and irreversibly sickled cells were also found in circulation. However, although promising, these mice do not show many of the pathological sequelae of sickling, such as anemia. Development of pathologies may require higher levels of expression of the sickle cell hemoglobin, or may be unobtainable owing to structural differences between human and mouse red cells. Nonetheless, these mice will be useful for the development of antisickling agents (Greaves, 1990; Weatherall, 1990).

Gaucher's disease

Mutation in the gene encoding the enzyme glucocerebrosidase responsible for degrading the sphingolipid cerebroside is the cause of Gaucher's disease. This is a relatively common lysosomal storage disorder leading to accumulation of glucocerebroside in lysosomes, the degradative organelles of cells. Cells of the reticuloendothelial system are the most affected, and show morphological changes due to accumulation of glucocerebroside. Increases in glucocerebroside can be 50 to 100 times the normal value in affected tissues of patients. Clinical manifestations involve pathological changes in the spleen, the liver and bones, and neurological symptoms. An acute form of neuropathic disease becomes evident by three months of age and is fatal within three years (Fredrickson, 1979; Brady *et al.,* 1993). Because Gaucher's disease stems from the lack of an enzyme, it has been a candidate for protein replacement therapy and for gene therapy (Chapter 6).

A transgenic mouse model for Gaucher's disease has been developed through ES cell technology by knocking out the endogenous glucocerebrosidase gene by using a vector containing an interrupted copy of the same mouse gene, the neomycin-resistance gene, and herpes virus thymidine kinase genes (Tybulewicz *et al.,* 1992). A stably transformed ES cell with the disruptive homologous recombination event was estimated to occur at a frequency of about 1 in 236 of total transformants isolated. Four such lines were injccted into mouse embryos, and a chimeric (mosaic) male derived from one of the cell lines transmitted the mutation to offsprings, resulting in mice heterozygous for the Gaucher gene. Further inbreeding of the offsprings resulted in a homozygous mutant.

The activity of glucocerebrosidase was reduced to about 45% of wild-type levels in heterozygous mice, and to less than 4% in homozygous mutants. Homozygous mutants, unlike their heterozygous counterparts, died within 24 hours after birth, and showed pathological changes characteristic of the disease in humans, although no single cause of the early death was identified. Because the short life of this model mice places restrictions on their use, other mutant lines with less deleterious mutations will be required for protracted experimentation. These mutant mice and others developed along these lines will bc useful in studying the pathological changes and therapeutic approaches to Gaucher's disease (Tybulewicz *et al.,* 1992; Davies, 1992).

Cystic fibrosis

Cystic fibrosis (CF) is a recessive genetic disorder resulting from mutations in both copies of the CFTR gene (cystic fibrosis transmembrane conductance regulator: Chapter 4). Product of the CFTR gene is a chloride channel, whose loss leads to an imbalance in chloride and water flux across cell membranes, resulting in the dehydration of secretions. The increased viscosity of the secretions leads to obstructive damage in the organs involved and to bacterial infections in the respiratory system (Collins and Wilson, 1992; Barinaga, 1992b).

Two laboratories have independently created transgenic mouse strains in which both copies of the CFTR gene were knocked out through ES cell technology (Snouwaert *et al.,* 1992; Dorin *et al.,* 1992). Both these mouse strains show the expected channel defect and the basic CF pathology. However the progression and manifestation of pathology were different between the two strains. In one case, all the mice died within 40 days after birth owing to intestinal blockage, a complication that occurs in about 10% of the CF patients. They showed no lung or gonadal pathology which is observed in the majority of the CF patients (Collins and Wilson, 1992; Barinaga, 1992b). The second strain appeared to be viable for longer periods and developed lung and gonadal changes similar to those in CF patients (Dorin *et al.,* 1992).

Different vectors and disruption strategies were used in the two cases. Also, the genetic background and the mating schemes used in deriving homozygous knockout mice were different in the two cases. The difference in phenotypes could be attributed possibly to the complete loss of CFTR activity in the first case, resulting in acute intestinal effects and early death, compared to the leaky, low-level production of CFTR in the second case, leading to longer-lived mice which grow to develop symptoms involving the lungs and gonads (Dorin *et al.*, 1992). The phenotypic difference may also have been caused by genetic differences between the mouse strains, which were from their differing genetic backgrounds. The phenotypic differences in the two independently derived transgenic knockout lines with the same gene disrupted highlight the variety of factors that affect the production of animal models even in cases where changes are made through homologous recombination.

The CFTR-negative mice should provide excellent models for understanding the pathology of CF, and for the testing of traditional drugs and gene therapy approaches to the treatment of CF. They should provide powerful alternatives and adjuncts to current clinical trials, which are expensive and lengthy, and reduce the long-term risks involved in testing drug candidates in children (Barinaga, 1992b; Hyde *et al.*, 1993).

FUTURE PROSPECTS

The successes discussed above underscore the power of transgenic technology in developing useful animal models. The combined power of the microinjection and ES cell approaches should permit the development of suitable animal models for other diseases. The development of therapies for many major human diseases such as Alzheimer's disease, Parkinson's disease and AIDS stands to benefit immensely from convenient animal models. Application of transgenic technology requires a clear understanding of the genetic basis of the disease being modeled, and cloning of the gene(s) involved in the disease. With the current advances in these areas, there is good reason to be optimistic about the development of animal models for other major diseases.

REFERENCES

Abbott, A. and Klaffke, O. (1993). Europeans protest against patent for Harvard mouse. *Nature* **361,** 574.

Adams, J.M. and Cory, S. (1991). Transgenic models of tumor development. *Science* **254,** 1161–1167.

Barinaga, M. (1992a). Knockouts shed light on learning. *Science* **257,** 162–163.

Barinaga, M. (1992b). Knockout mice offer first animal model for CF. *Science* **257,** 1046–1047.

Bialy, H. (1991). Transgenic pharming comes of age. *Bio/Technology* **9,** 786–788.

Bradley, A., Hasty, P., Davis, A., and Ramirez-Solis, R. (1992). Modifying the mouse: design and desire. *Bio/Technology* **10,** 534–539.

Brady, R.O., O'Neill, R.R., and Barton, N.W. (1993). Glucosylceramide lipidosis: Gaucher's disease. In *The Molecular and Genetic Basis of Neurological Disease.* R.N. Rosenberg, S.B. Pruisner, S. DiMauro, R.L. Barchi, and L.M. Kunkel, eds. (Boston: Butterworth-Heinemann), pp. 467–484.

Brown, M.S. and Goldstein, J.L. (1990). Drugs used in the treatment of hyperlipoproteinemias. In *The Pharmacological Basis of Therapeutics.* A.G. Gilman, T.W. Rall, A.S. Nies, and P. Taylor, eds. (New York: Pergamon Press), pp. 874–896.

Capecchi, M.R. (1989a). Altering the genome by homologous recombination. *Science* **244,** 1288–1292.

Capecchi, M.R. (1989b). The new mouse genetics: altering the genome by gene targeting. *TIG* **5,** 70–76.

Capecchi, M.R. (1993). Mouse genetics: YACs to the rescue. *Nature* **362,** 205–206.

Chesebro, B. (1992). PrP and the scrapie agent. *Nature* **356,** 560–561.

Clark, A.J., Cowper, A., Wallace, R., Wright, G., and Simons, J.P. (1992). Rescuing transgene expression by co-integration. *Bio/Technology* **10,** 1450–1454.

Collins, F.S. and Wilson, J.M. (1992). A welcome animal model. *Nature* **358,** 708–709.

Cuthbertson, R.A. and Klintworth, G.K. (1988). Biology of disease: transgenic mice — a gold mine for furthering knowledge in pathobiology. *Lab. Invest.* **58,** 484–502.

Davies, K. (1992). Mulling over mouse models. *Nature* **359,** 86.

Doetschman, T.C. (1991). Gene targeting in embryonic stem cells. In *Transgenic Animals.* N.L. First and F.P. Haseltine, eds. (New York: Butterworth-Heinemann), pp. 89–101.

Donehower, L.A., Harvey, M., Slagle, B.L., McArthur, M.J., Montgomery Jr., C.A., Butel, J.S., and Bradley, A. (1992). Mice deficient for p53 are developmentally normal but susceptible to spontaneous tumors. *Nature* **356,** 215–221.

Dorin, J.R., Dickinson, P., Alton, E.W.F.W., Smith, N., Geddes, D.M., Stevenson, B.J., Kimber, W.L., Fleming, S., Clarke, A.R., Hooper, M.L., Anderson, L., Beddington, R.S.P., and Porteous, D.J. (1992). Cystic fibrosis in the mouse by targeted insertional mutagenesis. *Nature* **359,** 211–215.

First, N.L. and Haseltine, F.P. (Eds) (1991). *Transgenic Animals* (New York: Butterworth-Heinemann).

Fredrickson, D.S. (1979). Gaucher's disease (glucosyl ceramide lipidosis). In *Cecil Textbook of Medicine.* P.B. Beeson, W. McDermott, and J.B. Wyngaarden, eds. (London: W.B. Saunders), pp. 2012–2014.

Friend, S.H. (1993). Genetic models for studying cancer susceptibility. *Science* **259,** 774–775.

Grant, S.G.N., O'Dell, T.J., Karl, K.A., Stein, P.L., Soriano, P., and Kandel, E.R. (1992). Impaired long-term potentiation, spatial learning, and hippocampal development in *fyn* mutant mice. *Science* **258,** 1903–1910.

Greaves, D.R., Fraser, P., Vidal, M.A., Hedges, M.J., Ropers, D., Luzzato, L., and Grosveld, F. (1990). A transgenic mouse model of sickle cell disorder. *Nature* **343,** 183–185.

Hanahan, D. (1989). Transgenic mice as probes into complex systems. *Science* **246,** 1265–1275.

Hanahan, D. (1990). Transgenic mouse models of self-tolerance and autoreactivity by the immune system. *Ann. Rev. Cell Biol.* **6,** 493–537.

Heideman, J. (1991). Transgenic rats: a discussion. In *Transgenic Animals.* N.L. First and F.P. Haseltine, eds. (New York: Butterworth-Heinemann), pp. 325–332.

Hoffmann, S.L., Russell, D.W., Brown, M.S., Goldstein, J.L., and Hammer, R.E. (1988). Overexpression of low density lipoprotein (LDL) receptor eliminates LDL from plasma in transgenic mice. *Science* **239,** 1277–1281.

Hyde, S.C., Gill, D.R., Higgins, C.F., Trezise, A.E.O., MacVinish, L.J., Cuthbert, A.W., Ratcliff, R., Evans, M.J., and Colledge, W.H. (1993). Correction of ion transport in cystic fibrosis transgenic mice by gene therapy. *Nature* **362,** 250–255.

Isola, L.M. and Gordon, J.W. (1991). Transgenic animals: a new era in developmental biology and medicine. In *Transgenic Animals.* N.L. First and F.P. Haseltine, eds. (Boston: Butterworth-Heinemann), pp. 3–20.

Jacks, T., Fazeli, A., Schmitt, E.M., Bronson, R.T., Goodell, M.A., and Weinberg, R.A. (1992). Effect of an *Rb* mutation on mouse. *Nature* **359,** 295–300.

Joachim, C.L. and Selkoe, D.J. (1992). The seminal role of β-amyloid in the pathogenesis of Alzheimer's disease. *Alzheimer Disease and Ass. Disorders* **6,** 7–34.

Katsuki, M., Sato, M., Kimura, M., Yokoyama, M., Kobayashi, K., and Nomura, T. (1988). Conversion of normal behavior to shiverer mice by myelin basic protein antisense cDNA in transgenic mice. *Science* **241,** 593–595.

Kawamata, J. and Melby, E.C. (Eds) (1987). *Animal Models: Assessing the Scope of Their Use in Biomedical Research: Progress in Clinical and Biological Research,* Vol. 229 (New York: Alan R. Liss).

Kolberg, R. (1992). Animal models point the way to human clinical trials. *Science* **256,** 772–773.

Lawn, R.M., Wade, W.P., Hammer, R.E., Chiesa, G., Verstuyft, J.G., and Rubin, E.M. (1992). Atherogenesis in transgenic mice expressing human apolipoprotein(a). *Nature* **360,** 670–672.

Leder, A., Kuo, A., Cardiff, R.D., Sinn, E., and Leder, P. (1990). v-HA-*ras* transgene abrogates the initiation step in mouse skin tumorigenesis: effects of phorbol esters and retinoic acid. *Proc. Natl. Acad. Sci. USA* **87,** 9178–9182.

Lee, E.Y.-H.P., Chang, C.-Y., Hu, N., Wang, J.Y.-C., Lai, C.-C., Herrup, K., Lee, W.-H., and Bradley, A. (1992). Mice deficient in Rb are nonviable and show defects in neurogenesis and hematopoiesis. *Nature* **359,** 288–294.

Loew, F.M. (1991). Animal agriculture. In *The Genetic Revolution: Scientific Prospects and Public Perceptions.* B.D. Davis, ed. (Baltimore: The Johns Hopkins University Press), pp. 118–131.

Melby, Jr., E.C. (1987). Overview of the state of the art of development and utilization of animal models in the U.S.A. In *Animal Models: Progress in Clinical and Biological Research,* Vol. 229. J. Kawamata and E.C. Melby, eds. (New York: Alan R. Liss), pp. 1–10.

Mickish, G.H., Merlino, G.T., Galski, H., Gottesman, M.M., and Pastan, I. (1991). Transgenic mice that express the human multidrug-resistance gene in bone marrow enable rapid identification of agents that reverse drug resistance. *Proc. Natl. Acad. Sci. USA* **88,** 547–551.

Muller, W.J., Sinn, E., Pattengale, P.K., Wallace, R., and Leder, P. (1988). Single-step induction of mammary adenocarcinoma in transgenic mice bearing activated c-*neu* oncogene. *Cell* **54,** 105–115.

Nomura, T., Katsuki, M., Yokoyama, M., and Tajima, Y. (1987). Future perspectives in the development of new animal models. In *Animal Models: Progress in Clinical and Biological Research,* Vol. 229. J. Kawamata and E.C. Melby, eds. (New York: Alan R. Liss), pp. 337–354.

Palca, J. (1992). A surprise model for AIDS. *Science* **256,** 1630–1631.

Parham, P. (1991). The case of the wonky mouse. *Nature* **353,** 503–505.

Plump, A.S., Smith, J.D., Hayek, T., Aalto-Setala, K., Walsh, A., Verstuyft, J.G., Rubin, E.M., and Breslow, J. (1992). Severe hypercholesterolemia and atherosclerosis in apolipoprotein E-deficient mice created by homologous recombination in ES cells. *Cell* **71,** 343–353.

Raines, L.J. (1991). The mouse that roared. In *Transgenic Animals.* N.L. First and F.P. Haseltine, eds. (New York: Butterworth-Heinemann), pp. 335–345.

Schmidt, E.V., Pattengale, P.K., Weir, L., and Leder, P. (1988). Transgenic mice bearing the human c-*myc* gene activated by an immunoglobulin enhancer: a pre-B cell lymphoma model. *Proc. Natl. Acad. Sci. USA* **85,** 6407–6451.

Scott, J. (1992). Arterial hardening in mice. *Nature* **360,** 631–632.

Semenza, G.L., Traystman, M.D., Gearhart, J.D., and Antonarakis, S.E. (1989). Polycythemia in transgenic mice expressing the human erythropoietin gene. *Proc. Natl. Acad. Sci. USA* **86,** 2301–2305.

Shull, M.M., Ormsby, I., Kier, A.B., Pawlowski, S., Diebold, R.J., Yin, M., Allen, R., Sidman, C., Proetzel, G., Calvin, D., Annunziata, N., and Doetschman, T. (1992). Targeted disruption of the mouse transforming growth factor-β_1 gene results in multifocal inflammatory disease. *Nature* **359,** 693–699.

Sinn, E., Muller, W., Pattengale, P., Tepler, I., Wallace, R., and Leder, P. (1987). Coexpression of MMTV/v-Ha-*ras* and MMTV/c-*myc* genes in transgenic mice: synergistic action of oncogenes in vivo. *Cell* **49,** 465–475.

Snouwaert, J.N., Brigman, K.K., Latour, A.M., Malouf, N.N., Boucher, R.C., Smithies, O., and Koller, B.H. (1992). An animal model for cystic fibrosis made by gene targeting. *Science* **257,** 1083–1088.

Spalding, B.J. (1992). Transgenic pharming advances. *Bio/Technology* **10,** 498–499.

Tarui, S., Yamada, K., and Hanafusa, T. (1987). Animal models used in the research of diabetes mellitus — with special reference to insulitis-associated diabetes. In *Animal Models: Progress in Clinical and Biological Research,* Vol. 229. J. Kawamata and E.C. Melby, eds. (New York: Alan R. Liss), pp. 211–224.

Thompson, C.B. (1992). RAG knockouts deliver a one/two punch. *Curr. Biol.* **2,** 180–181.

Touchette, N. (1991). Send in the murines: new mouse model mimics human immune system. *J. NIH Res.* **3,** 21–23.

Travis, J. (1992). Scoring knockout in mice. *Science* **256,** 1392–1394.

Trull, F.L. (1987). Animal "rights" vs animal research: a worldwide movement challenges biomedical science. In *Animal Models: Progress in Clinical and Biologi-*

cal Research, Vol. 229. J. Kawamata and E.C. Melby, eds. (New York: Alan R. Liss), pp. 327–336.

Tybulewicz, V.L.J., Tremblay, M.L., LaMarca, M.E., Willemsen, R., Zablocka, B., Sidransky, E., Martin, B.M., Huang, S.P., Mintzer, K.A., Westphal, H., Mulligan, R.C., and Ginns, E.I. (1992). Animal model for Gaucher's disease from targeted disruption of the mouse glucocerebrosidase gene. *Nature* **357**, 407–410.

Walsh, A., Ito, Y., and Breslow, J. (1989). High levels of human apolipoprotein A-I in transgenic mice result in increased plasma levels of small high density lipoprotein (HDL) particles comparable to human HDL_3. *J. Biol. Chem.* **264,** 6488–6494.

Wang, J.Y.J. (1992). Modelling chronic myelogenous leukemia. *Curr. Biol.* **2,** 70–71.

Weatherall, D.J. (1990). Mice, men and sickle cells. *Nature* **343,** 121.

Zimmer, A. (1992). Manipulating the genome by homologous recombination in embryonic stem cells. *Ann. Rev. Neurosci.* **15,** 115–137.

8

Diagnostic applications of biotechnology

Rapid, accurate and reliable diagnostic tests are vital aids to the routine practice of medicine, in the conclusive diagnosis of diseases and for monitoring the progress of therapy. They are also valuable to drug development in the clinical evaluation of the efficacy of putative drug candidates. In addition to the major therapeutic advances described in the previous chapters, developments in biotechnology have also impacted on the diagnostic arena by improving established test methods, and by opening new avenues for rapid diagnostics (Hoffman and Rosenberg, 1992). Because diagnostic capabilities impact on the development of therapeutics, the aim of this chapter is to highlight the biotechnological advances resulting in the development of diagnostics. The advent of monoclonal antibodies (Mabs) has improved and expanded the range of tests based previously on the use of polyclonal antibodies. In addition, the ability to produce most proteins in unlimited quantities, and in pure form, through rDNA methods, has provided the antigens needed for the design of serological tests for diseases such as AIDS (George and Schochetman, 1992; Schochetman, 1992; Luciw and Steimer, 1989), and for the standardization of new diagnostic tests (Ghrayeb *et al.,* 1989; Petteway *et al.,* 1989; Decker and Dawson, 1989). Nucleic acid probes have added a new dimension to diagnostic medicine by providing sensitive and specific tests for infectious diseases, cancer, and genetic diseases (Caskey, 1987; Allen, 1991; Diller, 1992). Combined with the amplification techniques of polymerase chain reaction (PCR) and ligase chain reaction (LCR), nucleic acid probes provide unprecedented levels of sensitivity in detecting pathogens and errant genes (Eisenstein, 1990; Erlich *et al.,* 1991; Engleberg, 1991; Weiss, 1991). By one estimate, the market size of biotechnology-based human *in vitro* diagnostics involving Mabs and nucleic acid methods is projected to exceed a billion dollars by 1997 (Hoffman and Rosenberg, 1992).

From a broader perspective of the diagnostics products, the impact of biotechnology has been limited to a few areas that represent small segments of the overall *in vitro* diagnostic market. Clinical chemistry involving the chemical measurement of metabolites, and classical hematology involving microscopic examination of cells, which form 50% to 70% of the total diagnostic tests, have been affected marginally or not at all by the advances in biotechnology. In comparison, immunology, serology, microbiology, and histology and cytology, which together form a smaller segment of the diagnostic market, have been influenced by the new reagents and techniques produced by biotechnology (Hoffman and Rosenberg, 1992). However, further developments such as biosensor technology utilizing enzymes and antibodies produced through the biotechnology route will undoubtedly expand the influence of biotechnology to areas like clinical chemistry (Campbell, 1991).

The accuracy and rapidity of many of the established immunological tests have been improved by the use of Mabs, and new tests have been made possible by the higher specificity afforded by Mabs. The improved properties of Mabs have led to the development of many new immunological diagnostic assays. Further, unlimited supplies of desired Mabs obviate the need for repeated characterization and standardization of antibody preparations used in earlier tests based on polyclonal antibodies. This advantage of Mabs, combined with the availability of pure antigens produced by rDNA methods, has improved the reliability of immunoassays while reducing their cost (Scott and Fleischman, 1991). These improvements are particularly valuable when mass screening and surveillance efforts for diseases such as AIDS are contemplated (Bloom and Glied, 1991; George and Schochetman, 1992; Schochetman, 1992).

The availability of appropriately labeled synthetic oligonucleotides and gene segments has provided a new method based on nucleic acid hybridization for the detection of foreign nucleic acid of pathogens in tissues, and for the detection of diseases caused by defined genetic mutations (Caskey, 1987; Allen, 1991; Caskey, 1992). Further, enzymatic amplification methods of PCR and LCR extend the limit of detection of specific nucleic acid sequences to very low levels (Erlich *et al.,* 1991; Weiss, 1991). For instance, a single HIV genome in 10,000 cells (Kwok *et al.,* 1989), or a single cell expressing HIV RNA among a million nonexpressing cells, can be detected by PCR (Schochetman and Sninsky, 1992). This enhanced sensitivity is valuable to the early detection of genomes of pathogens such as the AIDS virus which is present in low levels in the initial stages of an infection.

The ability to determine the genetic predisposition to a variety of diseases has raised serious moral, ethical and economic issues relating to the use of the information derived through the powerful nucleic acid tests. Combined with the techniques of amniocentesis or with chorionic villus sampling techniques of obtaining fetal cells (Lilford, 1991; Laurence, 1991), nucleic acid probes permit the early detection of a variety of genetic disorders in the developing embryo. Many such diseases are amenable to diagnosis, but lack known therapeutic avenues. However, the ambiguous nature of the negative test results themselves, combined with the societal position on abortion, leads to complex moral and ethical questions (Cowan, 1992; Wexler, 1992; Bluestone, 1992). In a similar context, the availability of information regarding the genetic predisposition of individuals to diseases, obtained through post-natal genetic tests, opens the possibility of discrimination by employers, and health and life insurance discrimination by insurance companies who aim to reduce risks among the insured (Greely, 1992; Kevles and Hood, 1992; Bluestone, 1992). These problems are further compounded by the documented lack of competence among the general public in comprehending the meaning and consequences of the results of genetic tests. The situation is further aggravated by the lack of qualified personnel, physicians as well as genetic counsellors, in sufficient numbers for interpretation of test results and for counselling (Bluestone, 1992; Roberts, 1993). How these factors are addressed will determine the desirability and the widespread use of genetic testing.

The following discussion is focused on *in vitro* applications of monoclonal antibodies and nucleic acid probes as diagnostic reagents. The principles of production and characteristics of Mabs are described in Chapter 2. Their use as *in vivo* diagnostic imaging agents has been discussed in Chapter 3 in the context of therapeutic applications, and is not discussed further here. The principles of PCR and nucleic acid hybridization have been discussed in Chapter 2 and Chapter 4, respectively.

MONOCLONAL ANTIBODY-BASED DIAGNOSTIC TESTS

Antibody-based immunological tests were in vogue before the development of monoclonal antibodies. For example, earlier pregnancy tests were based on the detection of fertility hormones by using polyclonal antisera. To a large extent, this and other such tests now use monoclonal antibodies, and occupy a large segment of the commercial immunoassay market (Campbell, 1991; Scott and Fleischman, 1991; Hoffman and Rosenberg, 1992).

Polyclonal antiserum raised against an antigen is a mixture of several classes of antibodies directed to different regions of the antigen (see Chapter 2). The composition of a polyclonal antiserum varies from animal to animal, and with each bleeding of the same immunized animal. The volume of each lot of antiserum and the total amount available from one animal vary with size of the animal species used in antiserum production. In addition to the antibodies directed at the immunizing antigen, the polyclonal antiserum contains variable levels of antibodies directed against other immunogens that the animal is naturally exposed to; some of these antibodies cross-react with an undefined component of the samples under analysis, leading to high background readings. These factors contribute to the need for extensive quality control of each batch of polyclonal antiserum used to manufacture diagnostic kits.

The constancy of Mab preparations with respect to composition, reactivity and purity, together with the unlimited availability, renders them better suited for use in diagnostic kits. Since Mab-producing clones are separated and individually tested during the production procedure, the antigen preparation used in Mab production does not have to be purified extensively. Mabs are easy to purify from cell-culture supernatants or from ascites fluids. Unlimited availability permits the use of high levels of antibody where necessary, and assures reproducibility. When chosen correctly, Mabs are highly specific, and therefore, are insensitive to contaminating proteins or other reactive materials present in the test sample. Mabs with the desired assay characteristics can be obtained by using screening assays designed to respond to the desired degrees of antigen affinity demanded by the assay.

While there are great advantages to Mab reagents, their use has some problems as well. The initial identification of the correct antibody is a labor-intensive and expensive process. Many of the monoclonal antibodies produced are of lower antigen affinity, and may therefore cross-react with unrelated epitopes. Proper design of screening assays is crucial for the identification of Mabs with high antigen affinity. High-affinity antibodies which are too specific to their epitope may also pose problems in assays by their inability to recognize small variations in the antigen as is often the case within families of pathogens such as bacteria and viruses. The monospecificity of Mabs, reacting with only one epitope on the antigen, renders them unsuitable for use in agglutination reactions, and in nephelometric assays which rely on the formation of antigen–antibody networks. Each antigen molecule binds to only one of the two binding sites in the antibody, resulting in two antigen molecules bound to the antibody. The antigen does not interact with another antibody to form networks, as is the case with polyclonal antisera which contain sets of antibodies to different epitopes on the antigen. However, this limitation can be overcome by using a defined mixture of two Mabs that recognize non-overlapping epitopes in the antigen.

Mabs are used in diagnosis in different assay formats, and utility in each assay format is determined by the characteristics of the antibody and the sensitivity desired. The basic principle of these assays is shown in Fig. 8.1. Radioimmunoassay and other competitive assay formats (depicted in Fig. 8.1A) use the competition between purified labeled antigen and the same antigen or analyte in the sample, resulting in the decrease of labeled antigen bound to the antibody. High-affinity antibodies are required in this assay format, and the detection limits are generally in the range of 10^{-9}–10^{-11} M of antigen. Non-competitive assay formats, where the amount of antigen bound is detected directly, offer greater sensitivity of about two orders of magnitude over the competitive assays and also a broader detection range. Therefore, they are used increasingly in diagnostic applications. These assays often use a sandwich format in which an antibody to the antigen is attached to a solid support such as plastic. Antigen in the clinical sample binds to the attached antibody, and is detected by the binding of a second antibody directed against a different epitope in the test antigen. Thus, the antigen is "sandwiched" between the two antibodies. The second antibody has an enzyme (or other detection label) covalently linked to it. Hydrolysis of an appropriate substrate by the linked enzyme leads to production of a colored reaction product in proportion to the amount of second antibody retained by the assay matrix. This format requires the antigen to be large enough to accommodate the binding to two antibody molecules, and, therefore, is not useful in the detection of small molecules such as drugs. In addition, Mabs are also useful in immunocytochemical analysis of pathological specimens, and for studies of cell populations using fluorescence-activated cell sorting (FACS) aimed at the enumeration of cells expressing specific cell-surface protein markers (Campbell, 1991; Scott and Fleischman, 1991).

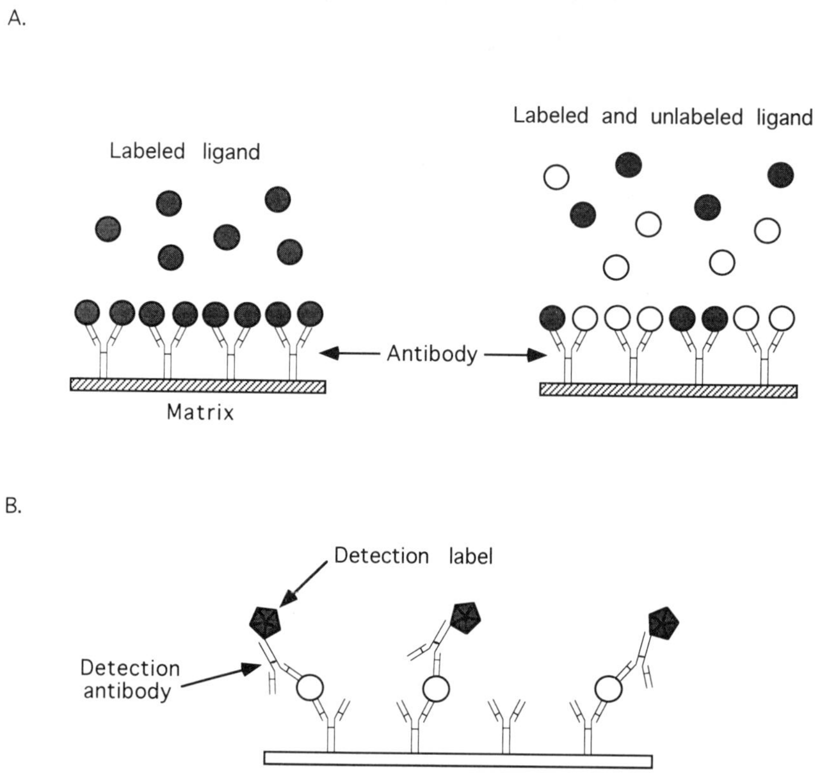

Fig. 8.1. Immunoassays using antibodies. A. Competitive assay. B. Non-competitive ''sandwich'' assay.

Mab-based immunoassays have found application in a number of clinical areas (Scott and Fleischman, 1991). In the infectious disease area, Mab-based assays have been useful in the diagnosis of *Chlamydia, Legionella,* and other bacterial agents. Also, assays have been developed for the detection of herpes, hepatitis B, and HIV viruses. Assays for a number of polypeptide hormones such as the human growth hormone, and for IgE antibodies involved in allergies, have been developed. Mab-based immunoassays have found application in blood-group typing as well as in the detection of small-molecule therapeutic drugs such as theophylline, and metabolites such as vitamins. Mab kits for the detection of tumor markers characteristic of many cancer cells have been developed for application in oncology. Mabs have paved the way for the identification of a large number (about 100) of cell-surface markers on human hematopoietic cells known as differentiation antigens. These markers, known as "CD" (cluster determination) markers, permit the identification of the lineage and the subclass of the leukocytes and their differentiation stage. CD marker-based classification, which has been valuable to research in immunology and to clinical situations involving the immune system, would have been impossible without the development of Mab technology (Campbell, 1991). For instance, the antigen CD4, present predominantly on helper T lymphocytes, is the receptor for the AIDS virus HIV. Helper T cells are depleted in AIDS patients owing to HIV-induced killing, and monitoring the number of CD4-bearing cells is used as an index in AIDS monitoring and therapy (Landay and Ohlsson-Wilhelm, 1992; Horsburgh, 1992). Many more Mab-based diagnostic immunoassays will undoubtedly be developed as a greater understanding of the molecular basis of diseases is gained through the advances in molecular and cell biology described in previous chapters.

NUCLEIC ACID-BASED DIAGNOSTICS

The high specificity of nucleic acid hybridization reaction (Chapter 2), combined with the uniqueness of sequences found in the genomes of different organisms, provides the basis for the use of nucleic acid probes as diagnostic reagents. The critical diagnostic question addressed by the nucleic acid-based diagnostic techniques is whether a particular sequence stretch is present in a DNA or an RNA sample. The ability to answer this question permits the application of nucleic acid technologies discussed below to diagnostic situations ranging from those in clinics to forensic laboratories. Thus, genomes of foreign organisms such as bacterial and viral pathogens can be detected with great specificity and sensitivity. Nucleic acid probes can also be used to detect mutations that cause inherited diseases, as these result in changes in the normal sequence of the gene (Caskey, 1987; Allen, 1991).

Nucleic acid probes are synthetic oligonucleotides 20 to 80 bases in length, or fragments of cloned genes. They are labeled in a variety of ways to permit their detection after they are bound to the target sequences. The use of radioisotopes such as phosphorus-32 as labels permits detection by counting the radioactive emissions or by exposure to photographic film. While this method is used extensively in research laboratories, because of the safety hazards, governmental regulations, and the loss of isotope activity due to radioactive decay, it is not well suited for use in small clinical laboratories and doctors' offices. Various chemical detection labels have been developed to replace the radioactive labels. For instance, probes can be labeled without affecting their hybridization properties by incorporation of a biotinylated analog of thymidine. The bound probe is visualized through binding of biotin to its high-affinity ligand avidin to which an enzyme is linked. The hydrolysis of an appropriate colorless substrate to a colored product by the avidin-linked enzyme permits the detection of the bound probe. Alternatively, chemiluminescent compounds, such as acridinium ester, are linked to the oligonucleotide probe (Allen, 1991). Exposure to high temperature results in the hydrolysis of the chemiluminescent label from the unhybridized probe while it is retained by the hybridized probe. The amount of light emitted, measured using a luminometer, is proportional to the amount of probe bound (Engleberg, 1991). Fluorescent labels can also be attached to the oligonucleotides. Labeled oligonucleotides and larger gene segments are particularly useful for visualizing the localization of the probe in the cytological specimen and in chromosome preparations, and provide a desirable replacement for radioactive probes (Busch *et al.,* 1989; Diller, 1992; Sasavage, 1992). The use of fluorescent labels with different emission wavelengths to tag different oligonucleotide probes permits the simultaneous visualization of hybridization of multiple probes.

Oligonucleotide probes have been used in the infectious disease area to detect the presence of DNA or RNA of bacterial and viral pathogens. In the case of bacteria, unique sequences in the genome or specific genes, such as those for toxins, provide the target for the probes. Unique regions of ribosomal RNA which is found in thousands of copies in the cells also provide sensitive targets for detection. Picogram (10^{-12} gram) amounts of target DNA corresponding to as few as 1–5 million bacteria in the clinical sample can be detected by using oligonucleotide probes. In these tests, the total DNA in a clinical sample is attached to a solid matrix such as a nylon membrane or filter paper, denatured to separate the two strands, and hybridized with the labeled probe. Alternatively, nucleic acid probes can also be applied to tissue sections, cells, and chromosome spreads, where the architecture of the specimen is preserved (Busch *et al.,* 1989; Diller, 1992). The degree of progress of an infection can be assessed by the proportion of infected cells detected by this ''*in situ*'' hybridization procedure. By using these approaches, tests have been developed for the detection of microbial pathogens such as *Mycoplasma, Chlamydia,* tuberculosis bacterium, and for gram-negative bacteria such as *E. coli* and *Salmonella* species. Tests have also been developed to detect viruses that cause rabies, hepatitis, herpes, papilloma, and polio (Allen, 1991; Engleberg, 1991). The sensitivity of nucleic acid probe tests provides rapid diagnosis, especially in the case of slow-growing organisms, which require several weeks of growth in culture for detection.

While nucleic acid probes offer great promise, they have not yet gained wide use in the diagnostic laboratories because of cost, need for expertise, and lack of broad clinical acceptance (Hoffman and Rosenberg, 1992). Further, although the tests provide high-sensitivity detection of sequences, the clinical consequence of the presence of the target sequences at such low levels is not always clear. In this regard, the sensitivity of the nucleic acid-based diagnostic tests, especially those involving amplification techniques such as PCR, have often outstripped the clinical limits (Schmeichel, 1991).

DNA probes are also useful for screening for genetic mutations that lead to diseases. Allele-specific oligonucleotides (ASOs) permit the screening for mutations which, in previous studies, have been shown to cause diseases such as sickle cell anemia, thalassemias, and cystic fibrosis (Caskey, 1987; Allen, 1991). Mutations may be detected by the hybridization of an oligonucleotide whose sequence incorporates the mutation. An alternative method relies on detecting the restriction length polymorphism (RFLP) associated with the mutation (Caskey, 1987; Davies, 1991). Often, the disease-causing mutation in the DNA may create or destroy the cleavage site for a specific restriction endonuclease, thereby changing the length of the restriction fragment containing the gene, generated by the endonuclease. This change in fragment length can be detected by Southern blot analysis of the restriction enzyme-digested DNA, by using a gene-specific nucleic acid probe.

In the simplest cases amenable to RFLP analysis, the disease-causing mutation itself creates or destroys the restriction site. However, inconsequential "silent" base changes that occur within the disease gene itself, or in sequences proximal to the disease gene, also lead to RFLPs (Caskey, 1987; Davies, 1991). Genomes of individuals within a population show many silent base changes resulting in RFLP patterns characteristic of individuals, which are shared with related individuals in the population. It is the individualistic character of RFLPs which is used in excluding (but not identifying with certainty) the accused in paternity lawsuits and in forensic medicine (Allen, 1991; Lander, 1992). The analysis of RFLP patterns of families with a prevalence of inherited diseases has led to the identification of RFLP patterns that are associated with the high probability of disease occurrence, even in cases where the disease gene itself is unidentified (Tsui and Estivill, 1991; Lehrach and Bates, 1991). Because of the relative proximity of the RFLP-generating base change to the defective gene, these two remain associated tightly during the gene-shuffling process that is associated with the meiotic cell division preceding the generation of germ cells, only rarely being separated; the closer the physical proximity between the two on the chromosome, the tighter the association during gametogenesis. The identification of RFLP markers with tight linkages to a disease, coupled with the powerful techniques of molecular biology, has been used to identify and isolate disease genes. For instance, RFLP analysis has led to the identification and isolation of the CFTR gene which is defective in cystic fibrosis (Tsui and Estivill, 1991). By using RFLP analysis, the gene mutation involved in Huntington's disease has been localized to the short arm of a human chromosome 4, although the sequence, the function, or even the exact position of the gene itself is unknown (Wexler, 1992; Roberts, 1992). Similarly, two genes involved in familial forms of Alzheimer's disease have been localized to human chromosomes 14 and 21, and there may be others yet to be identified (Marx, 1992a). RFLP analysis of genetic diseases is a laborious and sometimes frustrating process requiring the analysis of DNA from large numbers of affected and unaffected individuals in groups that show incidence of the genetic disease. In the early stages, genomic DNA obtained from each individual is analyzed for hybridization with several probes distributed over the whole genome. Clearly, genetic analysis of this nature, while fruitful with single-gene diseases, can be very complicated when applied to diseases such as schizophrenia, which appear to be influenced by multiple genes.

Because probes are designed from known sequences, screening of putative carriers of a disease mutation with nucleic acid probes is capable of detecting only previously known mutations. In situations where a disease is caused in all cases by a single or a few documented mutations, the tests have a high predictive capability. In cases where each of several distinct mutations, many unknown, causes a disease, the test lacks predictive accuracy. For instance, nucleic acid probe tests are good predictors of sickle cell anemia which is caused by the same mutation in all known cases, but do not offer the same degree of certainty in the case of cystic fibrosis where over a hundred different mutations have been identified, and others may yet be discovered (Caskey, 1987; Tsui and Estivill, 1991). Several mutations, often previously unknown, have also been found to be associated with other inherited diseases such as muscular dystrophies (Caskey, 1987; Roberts *et al.,* 1992). In such cases, while nucleic acid probes offer a means of determining the carrier status of the members of a family in which the disease is caused by a known mutation, screening at a population level may not provide adequate accuracy (Davies, 1992).

As discussed in Chapter 4, many cancers are associated with mutations in specific oncogenes. Nucleic acid probes can be used to detect specific mutated oncogenes in tumors. This approach shows promise for the early detection of colorectal cancers in which a high incidence of *ras* oncogene mutations has been observed, and may also be applicable to other malignancies such as breast cancer (Marx, 1992b; King, 1992; Roberts, 1993). Knowledge of the specific oncogene that is errant in a tumor may provide the rationale for the selection and optimization of a therapeutic modality, and for monitoring the effectiveness of therapy. In addition, nucleic acid probes, combined with the amplification methods discussed below, can be used in prenatal sex determination, and HLA analysis and tissue typing required for organ transplants (Eisenstein, 1990).

The sensitivity of nucleic acid-based detection methods has been increased many orders of magnitude by gene amplification techniques, notably polymerase chain reaction (PCR). The principle of PCR has been described in Chapter 2. By using PCR and other amplification methods, a single copy of a candidate gene present in a large excess of unrelated DNA in a sample can be identified. The technology of PCR, using heat-stable DNA polymerase and repeated cycles of heat denaturation and synthesis, has been fully automated. Nonetheless, because of the expertise and equipment required, PCR and other amplification methods are far from being tools in routine clinical testing laboratories (Lewis, 1992; Hoffman and Rosenberg, 1992).

Among the gene amplification technologies, PCR was the first to be discovered, and to date dominates the amplification methods used in diagnosis (Erlich *et al.,* 1991; Eisenstein, 1990). However, the proprietary nature of PCR has precluded its general commercial use, and this has led to the development of a number of novel amplification techniques, many of which have similar sensitivity (*ASM News,* 1991; Lewis, 1992; Aldhous, 1992). PCR-based tests for the detection of a number of bacterial and viral pathogens are under development. For example, PCR-based assays are being used for the early detection of infectious agents such as HIV in latent stages, where only a small fraction of cells harbor or express the viral genome (Kwok *et al.,* 1989; Schochetman and Sninsky, 1992).

The most recent addition to the amplification techniques is the ligase chain reaction, LCR, which differs from all the other amplification techniques, which are based on the use of DNA or RNA polymerizing enzymes. In contrast, LCR uses the ability of DNA ligase to join two synthetic DNA oligonucleotides contiguously juxtaposed by binding to a continuous stretch of target DNA (Weiss, 1991; Engleberg, 1991; Lewis, 1992). The principle of LCR is described in Box 8.1.

Box 8.1. Ligase chain reaction (LCR)

Ligation of two oligonucleotides bound to a continuous strand of DNA requires the bases at, and very close to, the ligation point to be perfectly base-paired to the template or target DNA strand. The failure to satisfy this condition, resulting from base mismatches caused by mutations in the template DNA, prevents the ligation of the two oligonucleotides. Successful ligation of this pair of oligonucleotides is the first cycle in LCR. Each strand of a double-stranded DNA can catalyze the ligation of a pair of oligonucleotides. Members of the pair of oligonucleotides that hybridize to one of the template DNA strands are also complementary to the oligonucleotides that hybridize to the other DNA strand. But their hybridization does not lead to ligation because of the lack of continuity. The process of LCR amplification is shown in Fig. 8.2.

Upon heat denaturation, each DNA template strand can participate in the ligation of another pair of similar oligonucleotides. The two continuous oligonucleotides generated by the ligation in the first cycle can also serve as the template for the ligation of a pair of oligonucleotides complementary to them, resulting in four ligated oligonucleotides. Each further cycle of heating and ligation results in the doubling of ligated oligonucleotides, leading to an exponential increase in the ligation product. The process of LCR has been facilitated by the discovery of a thermostable ligase analogous to the thermostable DNA polymerase used in PCR. The use of this ligase obviates the need for repeated ligase enzyme addition after each heat-denaturation step.

Failure to obtain the ligation product in an LCR reaction reflects the absence of an appropriate template DNA to initiate ligation, or a base change in the template DNA caused by mutation. The use of oligonucleotides corresponding to a mutated version of the gene produces positive LCR results with DNA from individuals harboring the mutation. One of the advantages of LCR is that it can detect mutations present in only one of the two copies of the gene present in a diploid genome, thereby permitting the screening of carriers of recessive mutations.

Although polymerase-based amplification techniques such as PCR appear to be more sensitive than LCR, they do not yield information on the sequence of the amplified DNA fragment unless followed by DNA sequencing, or probing with

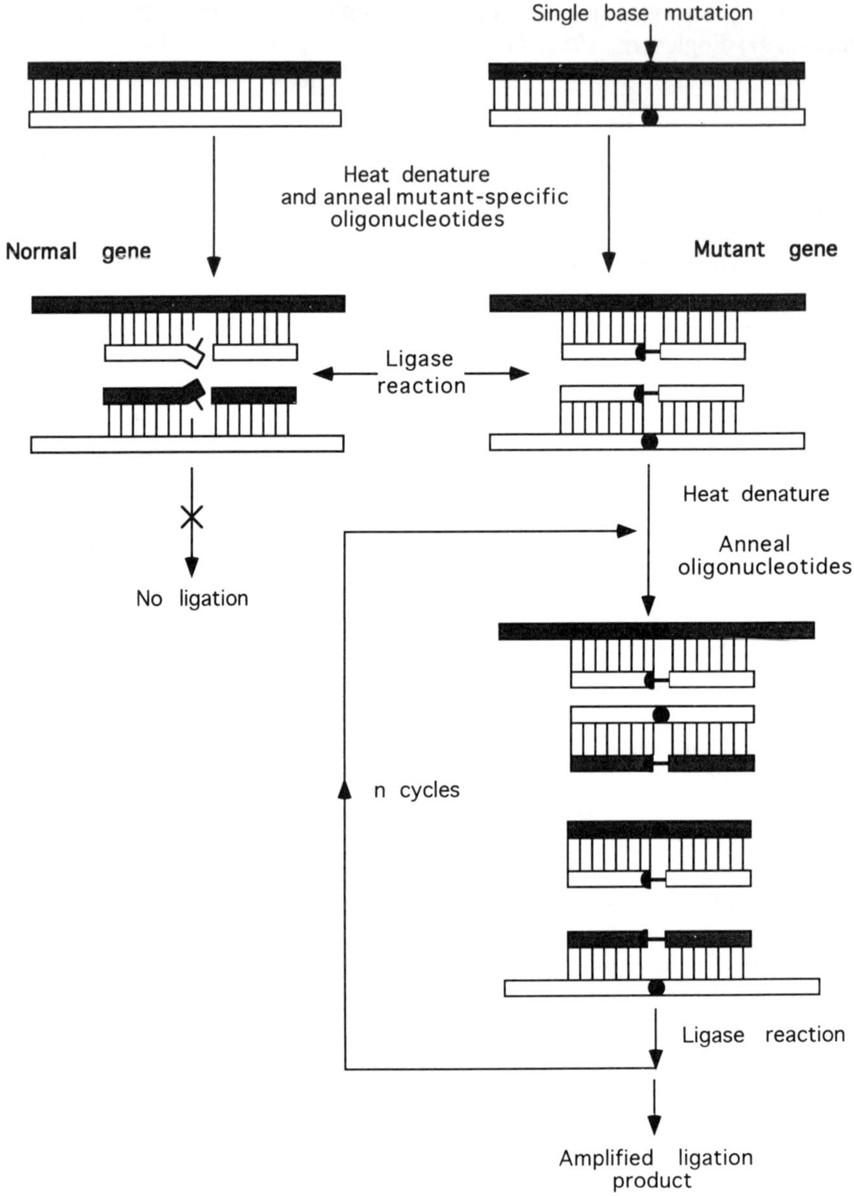

Fig. 8.2. Principle of ligase chain reaction (LCR).

allele-specific oligonucleotides. However, sequence information is the ultimate goal of screens for disease-causing mutations. By contrast, LCR assures the presence of the exact sequence being screened for. Therefore LCR is valuable in screening for genetic mutations and for virulent variants of bacterial and virus strains. The LCR technique is being adapted to the simultaneous testing of multiple sites in a gene for mutations, and for detecting virulent variant viruses arising in vaccine strains of the polio virus. It is also being used to detect mutations associated with oncogenes in many cancers. Further, the combination of the higher sensitivity of PCR with the specificity of LCR is expected to result in the development of rapid, sensitive and specific diagnostic tests. However, LCR is in its early stages of development, and all of the factors affecting the specificity of the ligation reaction remain to be determined (Weiss, 1991; Lewis, 1992).

Nucleic acid probe methods which rely on the specificity of nucleic acid hybridization reaction, combined with the powerful methods of nucleic acid amplification, are expected to spawn many new diagnostic tests which may be useful in the detection and treatment of infectious diseases, cancer, and inherited disorders. The impact of development and applications of diagnostic tests based on nucleic acid probes and on Mab technology will be felt increasingly as deeper understanding of diseases at a molecular level is gained.

REFERENCES

Aldhous, P. (1992). Roche gets tough on illicit sales of PCR reagents. *Science* **258,** 1572–1573.

Allen, R.W. (1991). DNA probes informative for diagnosis and identification. In *Recombinant DNA Technology and Applications.* A. Prokop, R.K. Bajpai, and C. Ho, eds. (New York: McGraw-Hill), pp. 232–254.

ASM News (1991). PCR diagnostics: ownership, technology are changing. *ASM News* **57,** 503–504.

Bloom, D.E. and Glied, S. (1991). Benefits and costs of HIV testing. *Science* **252,** 1798–1804.

Bluestone, M. (1992). Pitfalls of genetic testing: genetic counsellors face delicate task: ignorance about genetic testing. *Bio/Technology* **10,** 1394–1398.

Busch, M.P., Beckstead, J.H., Hollander, H., and Vyas, G.N. (1989). *In situ* hybridization: a histomolecular approach to the detection and the study of human immunodeficiency virus infection. In *HIV Detection by Genetic Engineering Methods.* P.A. Luciw and K.S. Steimer, eds. (New York: Marcel Dekker), pp. 209–242.

Campbell, A.M. (1991). *Monoclonal Antibody and Immunosensor Technology* (New York: Elsevier).

Caskey, C.T. (1987). Disease diagnosis by recombinant DNA methods. *Science* **236,** 1223–1229.

Caskey, C.T. (1992). DNA-based medicine: prevention and therapy. In *The Code of Codes: Scientific and Social Issues in the Human Genome Project.* D.J. Kevles and L. Hood, eds. (Cambridge, MA: Harvard University Press), pp. 112–135.

Cowan, R.C. (1992). Genetic technology and reproductive choice: an ethics for autonomy. In *Scientific and Social Issues in the Human Genome Project.* D.J. Kevles and L. Hood, eds. (Cambridge, MA: Harvard University Press), pp. 244–263.

Davies, K. (1992). Genetic screening for cystic fibrosis. *Nature* **357,** 425.

Davies, K.E. (1991). The DNA map. In *Molecular Genetics in Medicine: Advances, Applications and Ethical Implications.* D.F. Roberts and R. Chester, eds. (New York: St. Martin's Press), pp. 25–33.

Decker, R.H. and Dawson, G.J. (1989). Recombinant antigens as diagnostic and screening reagents for HIV infections: experience with a commercial test. In *HIV Detection by Genetic Engineering Methods.* P.A. Luciw and K.S. Steimer, eds. (New York: Marcel Dekker), pp. 77–98.

Diller, W. (1992). Products for sepsis diagnosis may aid therapeutic use. *Genetic Engineering News* November 1, 1–21.

Eisenstein, B.I. (1990). The polymerase chain reaction: a new method of using molecular genetics for medical diagnosis. *New England J. Med.* **322,** 178–183.

Engleberg, N.C. (1991). Nucleic acid probe tests for clinical diagnosis — where do we stand? *ASM News* **57,** 183–186.

Erlich, H.A., Gelfand, D., and Sninsky, J.J. (1991). Recent advances in the polymerase chain reaction. *Science* **252,** 1643–1650.

George, J.R. and Schochetman, G. (1992). Serologic testing for the detection of human immunodeficiency virus infection. In *AIDS Testing: Methodology and Management Issues.* G. Schochetman and J.R. George, eds. (New York: Springer-Verlag), pp. 48–78.

Ghrayeb, J., Kaplan, P.M., Mueller, W.T., and Putney, S.D. (1989). Detection of HIV antibodies using recombinant envelope and core proteins. In *HIV Detection by Genetic Engineering Methods.* P.A. Luciw and K.S. Steimer, eds. (New York: Marcel Dekker), pp. 41–58.

Greely, H.T. (1992). Health insurance, employment discrimination, and the genetics revolution. In *Scientific and Social Issues in the Human Genome Project.* D.J. Kevles and L. Hood, eds. (Cambridge, MA: Harvard University Press), pp. 264–280.

Hoffman, D.C. and Rosenberg, S.B. (1992). The impact of biotechnology on the in-vitro diagnostic medical market. *Genetic Engineering News* June 15, 8–9.

Horsburgh, C.R. (1992). Prognostic indicators for progression of human immunodeficiency virus disease. In *AIDS Testing: Methodology and Management Issues.* G. Schochetman and J.R. George, eds. (New York: Springer-Verlag), pp. 143–151.

Kevles, D.J. and Hood, L. (Eds) (1992). *The Code of Codes: Scientific and Social Issues in the Human Genome Project* (Cambridge, MA: Harvard University Press).

King, M-C. (1992). Breast cancer genes: how many, where and who are they? *Nature Genetics* **2,** 89–90.

Kwok, S., Mack, D.H., Sninsky, J.J., Erlich, G.D., Poiesz, B.J., Dock, N.L., Alter, H.J., Mildvan, D., and Grieco, M.H. (1989). Diagnosis of human immunodeficiency virus in seropositive individual: enzymatic amplification of HIV viral sequences in peripheral blood mononuclear cells. In *HIV Detection by Genetic Engineering Methods*. P.A. Luciw and K.S. Steimer, eds. (New York: Marcel Dekker), pp. 243–256.

Landay, A.L. and Ohlsson-Wilhelm, B.M. (1992). Use of flow cytometry to monitor HIV disease. In *AIDS Testing: Methodology and Management Issues*. G. Schochetman and J.R. George, eds. (New York: Springer-Verlag), pp. 123–142.

Lander, E. (1992). DNA fingerprinting: science, law, and the ultimate identifier. In *The Code of Codes: Scientific and Social Issues in the Human Genome Project*. D.J. Kevles and L. Hood, eds. (Cambridge, MA: Harvard University Press), pp. 191–210.

Laurence, K.M. (1991). Fetal diagnosis and the need for support. In *Molecular Genetics in Medicine: Advances, Applications and Ethical Implications*. D.F. Roberts and R. Chester, eds. (New York: St. Martins Press), pp. 73–85.

Lehrach, H. and Bates, G. (1991). Molecular techniques in the analysis of genetic disease. In *Molecular Genetic Approaches to Neuropsychiatric Diseases*. J. Brosius and R.T. Fremeau, eds. (New York: Academic Press), pp. 3–17.

Lewis, R. (1992). PCR's competitors are alive and well and moving rapidly towards commercialization. *Genetic Engineering News* **12,** June 1, 1–9.

Lilford, R.J. (1991). Fetal tissue sampling. In *Molecular Genetics in Medicine: Advances, Applications and Ethical Implications*. D.F. Roberts and R. Chester, eds. (New York: St. Martins Press), pp. 51–72.

Luciw, P.A. and Steimer, K.S. (Eds) (1989). *HIV Detection by Genetic Engineering Methods* (New York: Marcel Dekker).

Marx, J. (1992a). Familial Alzheimer's linked to chromosome 14 gene. *Science* **258,** 550.

Marx, J. (1992b). Test could yield improved colon cancer detection. *Science* **256,** 32.

Petteway, Jr., S.R., Reed, D.L., Tribe, D.E., and Kennedy, W.R. (1989). HIV recombinant proteins: immunological analysis and applications as reagents for serological tests. In *HIV Detection by Genetic Engineering Methods*. P.A. Luciw and K.S. Steimer, eds. (New York: Marcel Dekker), pp. 59–76.

Roberts, L. (1992). The Huntington's gene quest goes on. *Science* **258,** 740–741.

Roberts, L. (1993). Genetic counselling: a preview of what's in store. *Science* **259,** 624.

Roberts, R.G., Bobrow, M., and Bently, D.R. (1992). Point mutations in the dystrophin gene. *Proc. Natl. Acad. Sci. USA* **89,** 2331–2335.

Sasavage, N. (1992). Painting by the chromosome numbers. *J. NIH Res.* **4,** 44–46.

Schmeichel, C.J. (1991). Molecular medicine: too much, too soon? *Bio/Technology* **9,** 1063–1065.

Schochetman, G. (1992). Testing for AIDS and other human retroviruses. In *AIDS Testing: Methodology and Management Issues*. G. Schochetman and J.R. George, eds. (New York: Springer-Verlag), pp. 1–5.

Schochetman, G. and Sninsky, J.J. (1992). Direct detection of human immunodeficiency virus infection using polymerase chain reaction. In *AIDS Testing: Methodology and Management Issues*. G. Schochetman and J.R. George, eds. (New York: Springer-Verlag), pp. 90–110.

Scott, M.G. and Fleischman, J.B. (1991). Monoclonal antibodies in diagnostic medicine. In *Recombinant DNA Technology and Applications.* A. Prokop, R.K. Bajpai, and C. Ho, eds. (New York: McGraw-Hill), pp. 255–282.

Tsui, L-C. and Estivill, X. (1991). Identification of disease genes on the basis of chromosomal localization. In *Genome Analysis Volume 3: Genes and Phenotypes.* K.E. Davies and S.M. Tilghman, eds. (New York: Cold Spring Harbor Laboratory Press), pp. 1–36.

Weiss, R. (1991). Hot prospect for new gene amplifier. *Science* **254,** 1292–1293.

Wexler, N. (1992). Clairvoyance and caution: repercussions from the human genome project. In *Scientific and Social Issues in the Human Genome Project.* D.J. Kevles and L. Hood, eds. (Cambridge, MA: Harvard University Press), pp. 211–243.

9

Future prospects

Previous chapters described the molecular biological and biotechnological concepts and developments that are currently leading to, or that are closely targeted on, drug development. The goal of this last chapter is to describe briefly some of the newer techniques and technologies under development. These range from advances in molecular biological techniques and instrumentation to the ambitious international effort aimed at sequencing the entire human genome. Some of these technologies have arisen through developments within molecular biology, while others combine the advances in computer and electronic-sensing technologies with developments in biotechnology. These developments will contribute new tools and/or facilitate the application of existing techniques to drug development. The examples described below also serve as indicators of other future developments that will undoubtedly occur.

ANTIBODIES WITHOUT ANIMALS

As described in Chapter 3 , antibodies are valuable reagents in therapeutic and *in vitro* imaging applications. Human antibodies, which are free of the immunogenic complications associated with the use of antibodies from non-human species, are the most appropriate for use in clinical situations. Methods for the "humanization" of rodent monoclonal antibodies (Mabs) permit the reduction of their immunogenicity, but are not always successful. Further, as described in Chapters 2 and 3, the current methods for the direct production of human Mabs are limited by technical problems and ethical difficulties in immunizing humans. The method of generating useful human antibodies bypassing the use of humans or animals holds promise for the development of human antibodies for therapeutic applications (Lerner *et al.,* 1992; French, 1992).

The molecular and cellular mechanisms involved in the generation of antibodies are described in Chapter 2. Essentially, each chain of an antibody is assembled by randomly combining variable region sequences from two pools of variable regions (one coding for the heavy chains and the other for the light chains) with a limited number of constant regions for each chain. One heavy and one light chain assembled in each immunoglobulin-producing B lymphocyte combine to produce an antibody characteristic of that B cell. Exposure to an antigen results in the proliferation of cells expressing antibodies capable of binding the antigen. Thus, the generation of antibodies involves a combinatorial process followed by antigen-directed selection. This process can be simulated in the laboratory provided all the members of the variable regions of both the chains can be isolated, combined in random pairs, and assayed for binding to a given antigen. This rationale has been tested in the laboratory in the past few years, and appears to have the potential for generating antibodies without the use of animals (Lerner *et al.,* 1992; French, 1992).

The light and heavy chain variable region sequences are isolated from human blood cells by using polymerase chain reaction (PCR: see Chapter 2), and are cloned into suitable phage or phage–plasmid (phagemid) expression vector. Each expression vector contains the coding sequence for a light and a heavy chain drawn randomly from the PCR-generated sequence pools. Infection of bacterial cells with such vectors results in the expression of the individual chains and their combination to form Fab antibodies. In the most widely used expression system, called phage display, the Fab antibody encoded by the phagemid is expressed as fusion to a phage protein, and is, therefore, displayed on the surface of the phage particles. This allows the isolation and enrichment of phages that bind antigen by ''panning'' on antigen-coated plates. Infected cells or phages are probed for the ability to bind to the desired antigen. Isolation and growth of the antigen-specific expression vector phage or phagemid permits the isolation of the variable sequences which, when combined, generate the antibody of desired binding specificity. Antibodies to some proteins and small haptens have been produced by using this approach. The Fab antibodies can be converted to complete antibodies by joining the variable region coding sequences to desired constant region sequences.

In addition to the random combination of heavy and light chain variable regions, further antibody diversity in animals is generated by somatic mutations that occur during and after the recombination events involved in the assembly of genes for the individual chains. This process is involved in the generation of antibodies of higher affinity, or ''affinity maturation'', in the immunized animal. The affinity maturation process has been simulated in the laboratory by introducing random mutations in the variable region sequences of the initial antibody gene isolate in the phagemid, followed by screening of the phage population for increased binding affinity as described above. To date, combinatorial libraries have been made from light and heavy chain sequences obtained from immunized and non-immunized animals. Immunization or ''education'' of the immune system permits the biasing of the sequences in the library towards the immunizing antigen. Efforts are also in progress to generate combinatorial expression libraries containing large numbers of random coding sequences generated by using random oligonucleotides introduced into the hypervariable CDR regions found within the variable regions (see Chapter 3). While early studies using combinatorial libraries have demonstrated great potential, the extent of their utility is only beginning to be explored. The ability to synthesize a large collection of random sequences, combined with the feasibility of performing *in vitro* binding assays under harsher conditions than those occurring within an animal, should permit the isolation of antibodies useful in therapy, diagnostics and in catalysis (Lerner *et al.,* 1992; Brown, 1992).

DIRECTED EVOLUTION

In a manner analogous to their use in the affinity maturation of antibodies, the phage display system described above, and other similar genetic selection systems, can also be used for the development and selection of protein and peptide ligands with improved receptor-binding characteristics. In this approach, a peptide ligand known to bind to a receptor is displayed on phage surfaces by using a phagemid vector. Random mutations resulting in amino acid substitutions are introduced into the sequence of the ligand, and the resultant phages with higher binding affinities for the ligand are selected by preferential binding to receptor-coated plates. A number of protein ligands and receptors, including antibodies and hormones, have been displayed successfully on phage surfaces, permitting the application of directed evolution to any such proteins (Dower, 1992). For example, the well-studied trypsin inhibitor, BPTI, has been remodeled using this approach to bind with high affinity to human neutrophil elastase (HNE), which is involved in a number of respiratory diseases including cystic fibrosis (Roberts *et al.,* 1992; Birenbaum, 1992). Similarly, this approach has been applied to the screening of galactose-binding mutants of the B chain of ricin, for use in the construction of immunotoxins (Swimmer *et al.,* 1992). This approach can also be used to select and improve the affinity of nucleic acid binding proteins. A similar approach can be applied for the selection of nucleic acids and oligonucleotides with binding affinity for specific proteins (Brown, 1992).

RAPID-SCREENING TECHNOLOGIES

While the development of ligands with therapeutic potential by the rational route is a central goal of molecular biological approaches, improved mass-screening technologies are also being developed to identify potential ligands to receptors (Brown, 1992). Although these approaches are applicable in principle to the synthesis and screening of large numbers of variant compounds of different chemical structures, most of the current efforts are focused on peptides. This is because many of the natural ligands are peptides, and because of the chemical diversity easily attainable via the chemical synthesis of peptides. For example, given the twenty possible natural L-amino acids, $20^2 = 400$ dimers, $20^3 = 8000$ trimers, and $20^6 = 64$ million hexamers are possible. It is not difficult to chemically synthesize such hexamers or even longer peptides, or synthesize them biologically by using corresponding gene segments. However, unlike biological systems which utilize only L-amino acids, with chemical synthesis it is possible also to incorporate unnatural amino acids such as D-amino acids and other variants of interest, thereby increasing the complexity of the random pool of peptides of a given length.

The random pools of peptides can be exposed to receptor preparations to allow binding. Knowing the sequence of the bound species provides the starting point for the development of other peptide and non-peptide ligands. Since the amounts of bound ligand can be low, and since multiple peptides may bind the receptor, identification of the bound ligand by direct peptide sequencing can be difficult. It is therefore necessary to have ''address tags'' on each unique species so that the sequences of the peptides binding the receptor may be ascertained. Many methods have been developed to tag each member of the random peptide pool with a unique label. Some methods use multiple partially defined pools followed by iterative screening to ''home-in'' on the receptor-binding peptide species (Houghten *et al.*, 1991). Others use a single pool in which each unique species has a recognition address attached by different methods. These range from the localization of unique sequences at specified locations in a small grid through light-directed synthesis (Fodor *et al.*, 1991), synthesizing all members with a given sequence attached to one macroscopic bead that can be physically isolated upon receptor binding (Lam *et al.*, 1991), and attaching PCR-amplifiable nucleic acid tags to each unique species during synthesis (Brenner and Lerner, 1992; Amato, 1992), to biologically amplifiable screening systems such as bacteriophage where each peptide is displayed on a different phage particle (Brown, 1992). Other novel biological ''tags'' using nucleic acid binding protein fusions have also been developed (Cull *et al.*, 1992). In all these cases, the sequences of the peptides that bind to the receptor can be easily determined. This approach should allow simultaneous screening of millions of peptide sequences for binding to the receptor of choice, and pave the way for development of novel ligands with possible therapeutic applications. It is also possible to extend this technology to other classes of random polymeric compounds such as polynucleotides (Brown, 1992).

BIOSENSORS AND OTHER INSTRUMENTATION

Advances in microelectronic technology, combined with the specificity of interactions of biological molecules such as antibodies and receptors, have led to the development of biosensors where the signal generated by the molecular interaction is transduced into electronic signals. Biosensors have applications in diagnostics where predefined molecular interactions are measured. They can also be valuable in the research laboratory for the characterization of rates of biomolecular interactions. Biosensors based on electrochemical, piezoelectric, and optical phenomena are under development. Optical transduction methods are based on diverse phenomena such as fluorescence, chemiluminescence, bioluminescence, and internal reflection spectroscopy (see Chapter 12 in Campbell (1991)). The following discussion is focused on some examples which are relatively new developments. The ultimate utility of these techniques will only be determined in the coming years.

An instrument based on the internal reflection phenomenon known as surface plasmon resonance (SPR), introduced in the market recently, is a good example of the new biosensor instrumentation capabilities that are under development. This instrument permits real-time monitoring of biological interactions without the attachment of chemical or radioactive labels to the interacting molecules under study. A beam of light passing from a medium of higher refractive index to one of lower refractive index is reflected back from the interface of the two media if the angle of incidence of the light beam is below a critical value, resulting in internal reflection. SPR spectroscopy is based on the loss of intensity of the internally reflected, polarized light occurring at a certain angle (known as the resonance angle) when a thin metal film of gold or silver is introduced at the reflecting interface. The resonance angle is influenced by the refractive index of the region immediately adjacent (about 300 nm) to the metal film. The instrument designed to measure SPR, the BIAcore, exploits the change in refractive index caused by the binding of a ligand to a receptor which is coupled to the surface of the metal film. The change in refractive index is proportional to the mass of protein ligand bound, and is independent of the amino acid composition. For instance, the binding of a protein ligand, or whole microorganisms, to an antibody immobilized on the metal film causes shifts in the resonance angle. Such changes can be measured in real-time, allowing the visualization of the binding kinetics over very short periods of the order of minutes. Thus, kinetic constants, concentrations, specificity, binding patterns, and complex formations involving multiple components can all be measured. The SPR technique has applications in the study of protein–protein, nucleic acid–protein, drug–protein, and other receptor–ligand interactions. This method has been proven to be effective in the study of antigen–antibody interactions involved in the production of vaccines and immunotherapeutics, in that of receptor–ligand interactions in signal transduction and cell-adhesion, and for the study of nucleic acid binding proteins. A kinetic comparison of the interactions of natural proteins with that of their mutant counterparts is also possible through SPR. Many chemistries are available for the immobilization of biomolecules to the metal surface. The SPR method, including the coupling process, is fully automated and offers sensitivity in the picomolar to nanomolar range in small sample volumes. Samples of 1 to 50 μL flow past the immobilized biomolecule. However, because mass increments less than 5000 Da are difficult to measure, the method is restricted to molecules larger than a medium-sized peptide of about 50 amino acids in length (Granzow and Reed, 1992; Malmqvist, 1993; Publications of Pharmacia Biosensor AB, Piscataway, New Jersey).

By using the power of silicon and electronic technologies, an instrument known as a microphysiometer (or as Cytosenor commercially) capable of measuring the minute changes in the pH caused by the action of exogenously applied agents on intact cells has been developed recently (McConnell *et al.*, 1992; Brown, 1992). Live cells are held in a microchamber whose base is composed of a pH-sensitive insulator overlaid on a silicon chip. Illumination of the silicon chip with light flashes results in the flow of current. The threshold voltage required for the generation of the photocurrent is determined by the pH in the vicinity of the insulating material. It has been shown that exposure of mammalian and other cells to exogenous stimuli results in metabolic changes that are reflected by pH changes in the extracellular medium of the cells. Different agents induce pH changes whose rates and final extents are characteristic of the agent and its dose. These changes occur over a time scale of minutes, and the same cells can be challenged repeatedly, unless prolonged stimulation leads to an alteration in the receptor's response due to phenomena such as down-regulation. The system is automated and computer-interfaced to allow rapid screening and characterization of bioactive molecules. Measurable signals can be obtained from 10^4 to 10^6 cells. The microphysiometer has been used in studies of receptor–ligand interactions, modulation of second messenger pathways, and the course of viral infections. The use of this approach holds promise for the identification and characterization of the activities of "orphan" receptors and ligands (receptors and ligands with no known function), discovered using the gene isolation techniques described below. The microphysiometer should facilitate the screening of many putative drugs (McConnell *et al.,* 1992; Brown, 1992). However, the manufacturer's claims of the utility of this instrument in the wide range of applications discussed above remain to be generally validated in the field.

The technique of mass spectrometry has been extended to the determination of molecular weights of proteins to a high degree of precision. This degree of precision is unattainable through current analytical methods, chiefly gel electrophoresis (Chait and Kent, 1992). The crucial facilitating technical development in this area is the methods suitable for the ionization of large protein molecules by using laser desorption or electrospray ionization. Typically, proteins released into vapor phase by using laser desorption or electrospray techniques of ionization are permitted to travel to the detector under the influence of a constant electric field. The time of travel of the ionized molecules in a constant electric field is proportional to the mass to charge (m/z) ratio. Mass spectrometry permits the determination of molecular weights to an accuracy of 1 part in 10,000. Proteins of molecular masses greater than 100 kDa are amenable to analysis by mass spectrometry. The ability to determine molecular weights with high precision has applications in the characterization of proteins derived from defined cDNAs. Often, because of post-translational modifications such as proteolysis, glycosylation and phosphorylation, the observed molecular weights differ from those predicted from the cDNA sequence. Thus, the new mass spectrometry techniques permit the accurate determination of protein molecular weights, and, therefore, the probable post-translational modifications in proteins.

The techniques described above, and others in development, will facilitate the applications of molecular biology to drug development by providing new, high-precision analytical tools with high throughputs.

EXPRESSED cDNAs: A ROUTE TO NOVEL PROTEINS

The power of gene isolation and sequencing technologies has advanced to a point where mass isolation and automated sequencing of genes from various tissues can be performed rapidly. These methods have been applied to the isolation and sequencing of cDNA fragments from tissues such as the brain, which is believed to express scores of proteins that are yet to be discovered. Comparison of the sequences of the newly isolated cDNA fragments with those deposited in the worldwide gene data bases has permitted the identification of unique cDNA fragments, known as expressed sequence tags (ESTs), that had not yet been identified by other more routine means (Adams *et al.,* 1991, 1992). The nature and the function of proteins encoded by the full-length counterparts of such cDNA fragments are unknown. An attempt to patent such novel cDNA fragment sequences has led to a major controversy relating to the patentability of the cDNA fragments whose existence is obvious but whose function and benefits are unknown (Bluestone, 1991; Strimpel, 1992). In the opinion of many legal experts, the issuance of a patent appears unlikely in this case because of the general detrimental effect such exclusive rights would have on the research efforts in biotechnology (Adler, 1992; Kiley, 1992; Roberts, 1992a).

The novel cDNA fragments will serve as useful landmarks known as sequence-tagged sites (STSs) along the different human chromosomal locations they are derived from, and will aid in the human genome project discussed below (Adams *et al.,* 1991). In addition, the unique ESTs will aid isolation of the corresponding full-length cDNAs, and identification of novel proteins, some of which may have therapeutic properties. Although assigning functions to orphan proteins is an extremely difficult task, use of database comparisons to identify functional domains may lead to the identification of a putative function. Efforts towards commercial development of protein corresponding to the ESTs have begun on the premise that success in a very few cases, as small as five, should make the effort commercially successful, even in the absence of patent protection for the ESTs themselves (Roberts, 1992a).

THE HUMAN GENOME PROJECT

With the fundamental developments in molecular biology in the past decade, the exciting possibility of determination of the sequence of the entire human genome of 3 billion base pairs became technically feasible (Judson, 1992). An international co-operative effort to sequence the human genome and those of other model organisms such as the mouse, fruit fly (*Drosophila melanogaster*), plant (*Arabidopsis thaliana*), yeast (*Saccharomyces cerevisiae*), the nematode (*Caenorhabditis elegans*), and bacteria (*Escherichia coli* and *Bacillus subtilis*) has been initiated (Yager *et al.,* 1991; Hood, 1992; Hodgson, 1992). The model organisms chosen have been studied extensively at the genetic level, and are amenable to manipulations such as controlled breeding. Parallel analysis of their genomes is expected to contribute to the understanding of the structure of the human genome and the details of its function.

The goal of the human genome project (HGP) is to create a reference information base by integrating the resources of the international scientific community, and by harnessing various scientific and by engineering disciplines together (Yager *et al.,*

1991). A genetic map, a physical map, and the complete nucleotide sequence of the human genome are the three key goals of the project. A genetic map is obtained through analysis of large numbers of human pedigrees, and involves correlation of the segregation of physically assayable markers such as a restriction fragment length polymorphism (RFLP), or visible chromosomal alterations, with genetic traits. Some of these marker genes have already been cloned and fully sequenced. Many such markers, some representing disease genes, have been mapped along the 22 autosomes and the X and the Y sex chromosomes comprising the human genome (NIH/CEPH Collaborative Mapping Group, 1992; Davies, 1992). A genetic map aids the assignment of a biochemical trait to a certain region of a specific chromosome, thereby allowing the correlation of the nucleotide sequences of a region with a biochemical function. A physical map consists of assayable sequences at defined locations along the chromosomes separated by known nucleotide distances with no regard to association with a genetic trait. The points on a physical map represent oligonucleotide sequences that can be located to specific regions of a chromosome through hybridization to intact chromosomes. They are known as sequence-tagged sites or STSs, and can be traced on to DNA clones derived from the chromosome. STSs serve as landmarks for the ordered assembly of overlapping DNA fragments obtained from a chromosome by restriction endonuclease digestion, into a contiguous unit. The physical map is an essential prelude to the linear ordering of the actual sequence information obtained by sequencing of the DNA fragments, required to arrive at the complete sequence of a chromosome. To date, several genes, and many genetic and physical markers, have been identified along all of the human chromosomes (Davies, 1992; NIH/CEPH Collaborative Mapping Group, 1992 and Genome Map III in the same journal issue). Ultimately, individual fragments derived from all chromosomes will be sequenced to produce a complete map of the human genome. According to the current agenda of the HGP, the ultimate goal of sequencing the entire human genome is scheduled for the first decade of the twenty-first century (Yager *et al.,* 1991).

From a therapeutic standpoint, knowing the full sequence of the human genome is expected to permit rapid identification of the genetic basis for many diseases. The sequence of a newly isolated disease-causing gene can be compared to the gene sequences in the data base, and this may lead to the assignment of a function to the encoded protein based on common structural motifs (Hood, 1992; Gilbert, 1992). This information, combined with the understanding of the role of the gene product at a molecular and cellular level, would permit the development of new therapies, through methods described in the earlier chapters. Comparable information from the model systems, especially the mouse, would provide systems for the creation of experimentally manipulatable whole animal systems including disease models.

The human genome project has not been without its critics. Criticism is directed primarily at the cost of the project of about 200 million dollars annually in the US, and the resulting diversion of precious research funds towards producing a nucleic acid sequence of doubtful information value (Rechsteiner, 1991). Over 95% of the human genome is estimated to exist as pseudogenes, repeated sequences, and introns which do not encode proteins. Further, even in the case of functional genes, interruption of the coding sequences in the genome by large numbers of introns makes the deduction of the sequence encoding the protein product tentative (Farr and Goodfellow, 1992). It is also difficult to determine if short coding regions or "open reading frames" (ORFs) are relevant and are likely to be expressed into a protein (Bains, 1992a). The determination of sequences encoding proteins is further complicated by the occurrence of sequencing errors, especially base deletions and insertions, which shift the reading frame (Roberts, 1991). Therefore, the sequencing of expressed cDNAs has been proposed as a cost-effective alternative. However, proponents of the HPG argue that this approach would miss the information on the regulatory sequences that do not appear in the mRNA, and would also miss scores of mRNAs that are expressed transiently through development (Hood, 1992). Another criticism against HGP is that the availability of a protein sequence associated with a disease does not guarantee the biochemical understanding of the function. For instance, there are disease-associated proteins such as oncogenes and tumor suppressor genes whose sequences have been known for decades with little immediate insight into their function. These criticisms notwithstanding the HGP is in swing. The early results have appeared recently, with the complete sequencing of the 315,000 base pairs of yeast chromosomes III. Also, the complete physical maps of two human chromosomes have been determined. These results have generated considerable excitement and optimism about HGP. The sequence of yeast chromosome III has revealed over a hundred ORFs that may code for proteins not known to exist heretofore (Hodgson, 1992). The success of the physical mapping of human Y chromosome and chromosome 21 has provided a favorable assessment of the magnitude and the direction of the HGP effort. This has resulted in the redefinition of the approaches to HGP (Roberts, 1992b,c).

The current success of the HGP is a result of the technological developments of the past decades, including oligonucleotide synthesis, sequencing methods, PCR, and *in situ* hybridization techniques. In addition, cloning vectors derived recently from yeast artificial chromosomes, known as YAC vectors, permit the cloning of DNA fragments megabases in length, a size far beyond the capacity of earlier phage and cosmid vectors, which were limited to cloning fragments 10 to 40 kilobases in length (Judson, 1992; Roberts, 1992b). Beyond this present stage, the timely achievement of the goals of the HGP is also dependent on the fruition of other technical developments currently on the drawing board; the timely development of these enabling techniques is also one of the goals of the HGP. They include rapid, cost-effective sequencing methods, robotic techniques for the routine handling and manipulation of multiple clones, computer algorithms for data collection and verification, and the software for analysis of sequences to gauge their biological significance. Advances are occurring in these areas at a rapid pace. Several alternative sequencing approaches based on oligonucleotide hybridization and other techniques such as scanning-tip electron microscopy, dispensing with the need for the currently used costly gel-based techniques, are under development (Hood, 1992; Strezoska *et al.,* 1991; Bains, 1992b; Edgington, 1993). Further, robotic- and bio-information systems for the gathering sequence data and its analysis respectively are also under development (Bains, 1992a; Martin and Walmsley, 1990). Aside from the direct disease-related information provided by the sequence of the human genome, these technological developments will have a strong impact on the practice of medicine and on the conduct of research in molecular and cell biology as applied to pharmaceutical research and development (Caskey, 1992; Hood, 1992).

The developments in molecular biology and instrumentation techniques born of HGP and those developed independently as discussed in the foregoing sections, combined with the new insights gained through their application, will continue to influence the design and development of pharmaceuticals well into the twenty-first century in novel ways that are difficult to predict at this time.

REFERENCES

Adams, M.D., Dubnick, M., Kerlavage, A.R., Moreno, R., Kelley, J.M., Utterback, T.R., Nagle, J.W., Fields, C., and Venter, C.J. (1992). Sequence identification of 2,375 human brain genes. *Nature* **355,** 632–634.

Adams, M.D., Kelley, J.M., Gocayne, J.D., Dubnick, M., Polymeropoulous, M.H., Xiao, H., Merril, C.R., Wu, A., Olde, B., Moreno, R.F., Kerlavage, A.R., McCombie, W.R., and Venter, J.C. (1991). Complementary DNA sequencing: expressed sequence tags and human genome project. *Science* **252,** 1651–1656.

Adler, R.G. (1992). Genome research: fulfilling the public's expectations for knowledge and commercialization. *Science* **257,** 908–914.

Amato, I. (1992). Speeding up a chemical game of chance. *Science* **257,** 330–331.

Bains, W. (1992a). Sequence — so what? *Bio/Technology* **10,** 751–754.

Bains, W. (1992b). Setting a sequence to sequence a sequence. *Bio/Technology* **10,** 757–758.

Birenbaum, R. (1992). Scientists use bacteriophage to remodel proteases. *Genetic Engineering News* **12,** No. 7, May 1, 1–25.

Bluestone, M. (1991). Patenting human genes raises storm. *Bio/Technology* **9,** 1310–1312.

Brenner, S. and Lerner, R.A. (1992). Encoded combinatorial chemistry. *Proc. Natl. Acad. Sci. USA* **89,** 5381–5383.

Brown, K.D. (1992). Screening technology advances may enhance biotechnology process of drug discovery. *Genetic Engineering News* **19,** No. 12, December, 1–23.

Campbell, A.M. (1991). *Monoclonal Antibody and Immunosensor Technology* (New York: Elsevier).

Caskey, C.T. (1992). DNA-based medicine: prevention and therapy. In *The Code of Codes: Scientific and Social Issues in the Human Genome Project.* D.J. Kevles and L. Hood, eds. (Cambridge, MA: Harvard University Press), pp. 112–135.

Chait, B.T. and Kent, S.B.H. (1992). Weighing naked proteins: practical, high-accuracy mass measurements of peptides and proteins. *Science* **257,** 1885–1894.

Cull, M.G., Miller, J.F., and Schatz, P.J. (1992). Screening for receptor ligands using large libraries of peptides linked to the C terminus of the *lac* repressor. *Proc. Natl. Acad. Sci. USA* **89,** 1865–1869.

Davies, K. (1992). Mapping the way forward. *Nature* **353,** 798–799.

Dower, W.J. (1992). Phage power. *Curr. Biol.* **2,** 251–253.

Edgington, S.M. (1993). Breaking open the bottlenecks in genomic DNA sequencing. *Bio/Technology* **11,** 39–41.

Farr, C.J. and Goodfellow, P.N. (1992). Hidden messages in genetic maps. *Science* **258,** 49.

Fodor, S.P.A., Read, J.L., Pirrung, M.C., Stryer, L., Lu, A.T., and Solas, D. (1991). Light-directed, spatially addressable parallel chemical synthesis. *Science* **251,** 767–773.

French, D.L. (1992). Antibody production: fabulous Fabs from phage. *Curr. Biol.* **2,** 507–509.

Gilbert, W. (1992). A vision of the grail. In *The Code of Codes: Scientific and Social Issues in the Human Genome Project.* D.J. Kevles and L. Hood, eds. (Cambridge, MA: Harvard University Press), pp. 83–97.

Granzow, R. and Reed, R. (1992). Interactions in the fourth dimension. *Bio/Technology* **10,** 390–393.

Hodgson, J. (1992). Sequencing and mapping efforts in model organisms. *Bio/Technology* **10,** 760–761.

Hood, L. (1992). Biology and medicine in the twenty-first century. In *The Code of Codes: Scientific and Social Issues in the Human Genome Project.* D.J. Kevles and L. Hood, eds. (Cambridge, MA: Harvard University Press), pp. 136–165.

Houghten, R.A., Pinilla, C., Blondelle, S.E., Appel, J.R., Dooley, C.T., and Cuervo, J.H. (1991). Generation and use of synthetic peptide libraries for basic research and drug discovery. *Nature* **354,** 84–86.

Judson, H.F. (1992). A history of the science and the technology behind gene mapping and sequencing. In *The Code of Codes: Scientific and Social Issues in the Human Genome Project.* D.J. Kevles and L. Hood, eds. (Cambridge, MA: Harvard University Press), pp. 37–80.

Kiley, T.D. (1992). Patents on random complementary DNA fragments? *Science* **257,** 915–918.

Lam, K.S., Salmon, S.E., Hersh, E.M., Hruby, V.J., Kazmeirski, W.M., and Knapp, R.J. (1991). A new type of synthetic peptide library for identifying ligand-binding activity. *Nature* **354,** 82–84.

Lerner, R.A., Kang, A.S., Bain, J.D., Burton, D.R., and Barbas, III, C.F. (1992). Antibodies without immunization. *Science* **258,** 1313–1314.

Malmqvist, M. (1993). Biospecific interaction analysis using biosensor technology. *Nature* **361,** 186–187.

Martin, W.J. and Walmsley, R.M. (1990). Vision assisted robotics and tape technology in the life science laboratory: applications to genome analysis. *Bio/Technology* **8,** 1258–1262.

McConnell, H.M., Owicki, J.C., Parce, J.W., Miller, D.L., Baxter, G.T., Wada, H.G., and Pitchford, S. (1992). The cytosensor microphysiometer: biological applications of silicon technology. *Science* **257,** 1906–1912.

NIH/CEPH Collaborative Mapping Group (1992). A comprehensive genetic linkage map of the human genome. *Science* **258,** 67–86.

Rechsteiner, R.C. (1991). The human genome project: misguided science policy. *TIBS* **16,** 455–459.

Roberts, L. (1991). Finding DNA sequencing errors. *Science* **252,** 1255–1256.

Roberts, L. (1992a). Two strikes against cDNA patents. *Science* **257,** 1620.

Roberts, L. (1992b). Two chromosomes down, 22 to go. *Science* **258,** 28–30.

Roberts, L. (1992c). NIH takes a new tack on gene mapping. *Science* **258,** 1753.

Roberts, B.L., Markland, W., Ley, A.C., Kent, R.B., White, D.W., Guterman, S.K., and Ladner, R.C. (1992). Directed evolution of a protein: selection of potent neutrophil elastase inhibitors displayed on M13 fusion phage. *Proc. Natl. Acad. Sci. USA* **89,** 2429–2433.

Strezoska, Z., Paunesku, T., Radosavljevic, D., Labat, I., Drmanac, R., and Crkvenjakov, R. (1991). DNA sequencing by hybridization: 100 bases read by a non-gel-based method. *Proc. Natl. Acad. Sci. USA* **88,** 10089–10093.

Strimpel, H. (1992). Experts say patent squabbles affect NIH–industry relations. *Genetic Engineering News* **12,** No. 19, December, 1–29.

Swimmer, C., Lehar, S.M., McCafferty, J., Chiswell, D.J., Blattner, W.A., and Guild, B.C. (1992). Phage display of ricin B chain and its single binding domains: system for screening galactose-binding mutants. *Proc. Natl. Acad. Sci. USA* **89,** 3756–3760.

Yager, T.D., Nickerson, D.A., and Hood, L.E. (1991). The human genome project: creating an infrastructure for biology and medicine. *TIBS* **16,** 454–461.

Appendix (Chapter updates)

The rapid pace of movement of research in biotechnology has been a recurrent theme throughout the chapters of this book. In keeping with this trend, several interesting developments have occurred between the writing of the chapters and completion of editing of the book. The goal of this section is to provide an update on the relevant developments that have occurred during this period. These include some scientific advances and several articles of interest. With brevity in mind, I have presented the references grouped under appropriate chapter headings. Although the article titles are self-explanatory in most cases, I have included annotations where appropriate.

CHAPTER 1

New biological drug approval

Fox, J.L. (1993). FDA advisory panel okays beta interferon for MS. *Bio/Technology* **11**, 538–539. **(Should be added to Table 1.3, bringing the total number to 20.)**

The 10th anniversary issue of *Bio/Technology* (March 1993) contains the following articles which provide a review of the progress of biotechnology over the last decade.

Bud, R. (1993). 100 years of biotechnology. *Bio/Technology* **11,** S14–S15.

Drews, J. (1993). Into the 21st century. *Bio/Technology* **11,** S16–S20.

Rathmann, G.B. (1993). Knocking on opportunity's window. *Bio/Technology* **11,** S27–S32. **(A retrospective review of the birth and growth of the biotech industry from a financial perspective.)**

Klausner, A.D. (1993). Back to the future: product sales 1983–1993. *Bio/Technology* **11,** S35–S37.

Middleton, A. (1993). Lessons from the past. *Bio/Technology* **11,** S40–S43. **(Perspectives of individual biotech entrepreneurs.)**

Abrams, P. (1993). Analyzing biotech's past, present, and future. *Bio/Technology* **11,** 450–451.

Stone, R. (1993). Biotech sails into heavy financial seas. *Science* **260,** 908–910.

(Update on the financial aspects of the biotech industry.)

CHAPTER 2

In addition to the alpha, beta, and random coil motifs in the secondary structure of protein depicted in Fig. 2.2, a new motif known as parallel beta helix, with 22 amino acid residues per turn and a pitch of 0.22 Å per residue.

Cohen, F.E. (1993). The parallel β helix of pectate lyase C: something to sneeze at. *Science* **260,** 1444–1445.

Simplifications caused by recent advances in technology of producing recombinant baculoviruses combined with the ability to infect simultaneously with several different recombinant viruses allows for the production and analysis of multisubunit proteins.

Glaser, V. (1993). Biotechnology industry's interest grows in baculovirus expression systems. *Genetic Engineering News* **13,** March 15, 10–11.

CHAPTER 3

New biological drugs, and novel applications of known ones and their modified versions, continue to be discovered.

Weiss, R. (1993). Promising protein for Parkinson's. *Science* **260,** 1072–1073.

Mudge, A.W. (1993). New ligands for Neu? *Curr. Biol.* **3,** 361–364.

Fox, S. (1993). TNF mutants may pave way to cancer therapy. *Genetic Engineering News* **13,** March 15, 1–16.

Edgington, S. M. (1993). Molecular crosstalk. *Bio/Technology* **11,** 465–470.

Lasky, L.A. (1993). Combinatorial mediators of inflammation? *Curr. Biol.* **3,** 366–368.

The controversy surrounding the efficacy of t-PA over less expensive thrombolytics has taken a turn in favor of t-PA although the extent of the added benefit is debated, and cost issues continue to be a major factor. This turn of events may spark new life into the development of t-PA mutants and variants.

Potter, R. (1993). Genentech's t-PA finally wins. *Bio/Technology* **11,** 651–652.

Review of recent developments in delivery of protein drugs.

Wallace, B.M. and Lasker, J.S. (1993). Stand and deliver: getting peptide drugs into the body. *Science* **260,** 912–913.

A useful review of the considerations in multiuse protein manufacturing facility.

Hamers, M.N. (1993). Multiuse biopharmaceutical manufacturing. *Bio/Technology* **11,** 561–570.

CHAPTER 4

Molecular pharmacology continues to move rapidly, unravelling the molecular basis of several inherited and metabolic diseases, raising glimmers of hope for the therapy of devastating diseases. The gene for Huntington's disease has finally been identified. Huntington's disease patients show an increase in the number of certain trinucleotide sequences within the coding sequences of this gene, resulting in an altered protein. This phenomenon known as "triple repeat expansion", transmitted in a non-Mendelian fashion, has been shown to be involved in several other diseases.

Little, P. (1993). Huntington's disease: end of a beginning. *Nature* **362,** 408–409.

Morell, V. (1993). Huntington's gene finally found: gene discovery points to a better HD test. *Science* **260,** 28–30.

Morell, V. (1993). The puzzle of the triple repeats. *Science* **260,** 1422–1423.

Other articles of interest for drug development:

Marx, J. (1993). New colon cancer gene discovered. *Science* **260,** 751–752.

Marx, J. (1993). Learning how to suppress cancer. *Science* **261,** 1385–1387. **(An update on tumor suppressor genes.)**

Travis, J. (1993). Biotech gets grips on cell adhesion. *Science* **260,** 906–908.

Travis, J. (1993). Novel anticancer agents move closer to reality. *Science* **260,** 1877–1878. **(Inhibitors of protein farnesylation.)**

Chien, K.R. (1993). Molecular advance in cardiovascular biology. *Science* **260,** 916–917.

Brugge, J.S. (1993). New intracellular targets for therapeutic drug design. *Science* **260,** 918–919. **(Protein targets in the signal transduction pathways.)**

Lanzavecchia, A. (1993). Identifying strategies for immune intervention. *Science* **260,** 937–944.

Hodgson, J. (1993). Pharmaceutical screening: from off-the-wall to off-the-shelf. *Bio/Technology* **11,** 683–688. **(An update of screening methodologies.)**

Marx, J. (1994). New tumor suppressor may rival p53. *Science* 264, 344–345. **(Discovery of a new tumor suppressor gene which may be mutated or deleted in cancers more frequently than p53. A possible target for gene therapy.)**

Harris, C.C. (1993). p53: At the crossroads of molecular carcinogenesis and risk assessment. *Science* 262, 1980–1981. **(p53 named molecule of the year by *Science*.)**

Coughlin, S.R. (1994). Expanding horizons for receptors coupled to G proteins: diversity and disease. *Curr. Opinion in Cell Biol.* **6,** 191–197. **(Diseases caused by mutations in G proteins.)**

Exton, J.H. (1994). Messenger molecules derived from membrane lipids. *Curr. Opinion in Cell Biol.* **6,** 226–229.

Utermann, G. (1994). Alzheimer's disease: the apolipoprotein E connection. *Curr. Biol.* **4,** 362–365. **(A new twist in the susceptibility to Alzheimer's disease.)**

Wells, J.A. (1994). Structural and functional basis for hormone binding and receptor oligomerization. *Curr. Opinion in Cell Biol.* **6,** 163–173. **(How receptor oligomerization controls responses dependent on ligand concentration.)**

CHAPTER 5

An exciting example of structure-based design of inhibitors of viral replication.

Taylor, G. (1993). Drug design: a rational attack on influenza. *Nature* **363,** 401–402.

Structure of an important protein complex.

Ploegh, H. and Benaroch, P. (1993). Immunology: MHC class II dimer of dimers. *Nature* **364,** 16–17.

Tools for empirical structure determination.

Fetrow, J.S. and Bryant, S.H. (1993). New programs for protein tertiary structure prediction. *Bio/Technology* **11,** 479–484.

Edgington, S.M. (1993). Desktop molecular modeling: another look. *Bio/Technology* **11,** 472–473.

Other recent articles of significance:

Peters, R. and McKinstry, R.C. (1994). Three-dimensional modeling and drug development. *Bio/Technology* **12,** 147–150.

Bug, C.E., Carson, W.M., and Montogmery, J.A. (1993). Drugs by design. *Sci. Am.,* **269,** 92–98. **(Structure-based drug design.)**

SH2 and SH3 domains:

SH2 and SH3 domains are structural motifs found in proteins involved in signal transduction. SH2 domains are involved in binding of proteins which contain them to phosphorylated tyrosines on other proteins. The discovery of these structures has brought a new dimension to the understanding of signal transduction.

Pawson, R.B. and Schlessinger, J. (1993). SH2 and SH3 domains. *Curr. Biol.* **3,** 434–441.

Birge, R.B. and Hanafusa, H. (1993). Closing in on SH2 specificity. *Science* **262,** 1522–1524.

CHAPTER 6

Recent review.

Mulligan, R.C. (1993). The basic science of gene therapy. *Science* **260,** 926–932.

Industry trends.

Culotta, E. (1993). New startups move in as gene therapy goes commercial. *Science* **260,** 914–915.

Vectors and gene delivery.

Jiao, S., Cheng, L., Wolff, J.A., and Yang, N-S. (1993). Particle bombardment-mediated gene transfer and expression in rat brain tissues. *Bio/Technology* **11,** 497–502.

Neve, R.L. (1993). Adenovirus vectors enter the brain. *Trends in Neurosci.* **16,** 251–253.

Cell therapy.

Bjorklund, A. (1993). Better cells for brain repair. *Nature* **362,** 414–415. **(Genetically engineered cell for brain implants.)**

New antisense oligonucleotides.

Wagner, R.W., Matteucci, M.D., Lewis, J.G., Gutierrez, A.J., Moulds, C., and Froehler, B.C. (1993). Antisense gene inhibition by oligonucleotides containing C-5 propyne pyrimidines. *Science* **260,** 1510–1513.

A novel approach to vaccination by using the gene instead of the protein it encodes.

Cohen, J. (1993). Naked DNA points way to vaccines. *Science* **259,** 1689–1690.

Other developments of significance:

Barinaga, M. (1993). Ribozymes: killing the messenger. *Science* **262,** 1512–1514. **(An update of progress in therapeutic use of ribozymes.)**

Dutton, G. (1994). Gene therapy likely to target cancer patients on a large scale. *Genetic Engineering News* **14,** January 15, 1–14.

Ivinson, A.J. (1994). Righting an inherited wrong. *Nature* **368,** 665. (**Successful *ex vivo* gene therapy of familial hypercholestrolemia using LDL receptor gene is discussed.)**

CHAPTER 7

Commercial and ownership issues involving transgenic mice.

Fox, J.L. (1993). Transgenic mice fall far short. *Bio/Technology* **11,** 663.

Some recent mouse models and applications.

Marotti, K.R., Castle, C.K., Boyle, T.P., Lin, A.H., Murray, R.W., and Melchior, G.W. (1993). Severe atherosclerosis in transgenic mice expressing simian cholesteryl ester transfer protein. *Nature* **364,** 73–75.

Lane, D.P. (1993). A death in life of p53. *Nature* **362,** 786–787. **(p53 gene knockout mice.)**

Hyde, S.C., Gill, D.R., Higgins, C.F., Trezise, A.E.O., MacVinish, L.J., Cuthbert, A.W., Ratcliff, R., Evans, M.J., and Colledge, W.H. (1993). Correction of ion transport in cystic fibrosis transgenic mice by gene therapy. *Nature* **362,** 250–255. **(Application to gene therapy.)**

Useful reviews.

Breslow, J. (1994). Lipoprotein and heart disease: transgenic mice models helping in the search for new therapies. *Bio/Technology* **12,** 365–370. **(An overview of application of transgenic mice to the area of atherosclerosis.)**

Sedivy, J.M. and Joyner, A.L. (1992). *Gene Targeting* (New York: W.H. Freeman & Co.). **(An excellent text on the principles and practice of ES cell mediated gene targeting.)**

CHAPTER 9

Review of therapeutics development by evolution of nucleic acids and oligonucleotides which bind proteins, and of ribozymes.

Edgington, S.M. (1993). Shape space: biopharmaceutical discovery entering a new evolutionary stage? *Bio/Technology* **11,** 285–289.

Isolation of genes of importance to therapeutic and diagnostic development.

Morell, V. (1993). Huntington's gene finally found: gene discovery points to a better HD test. *Science* **260,** 28–30.

Marx, J. (1993). New colon cancer gene discovered. *Science* **260,** 751–752.

A useful text covering the recent advances in molecular genetics of the human genome.

McConkey, E.H. (1993). *Human Genetics: The Molecular Revolution.* Jones and Bartlett, New York.

Update on a patent controversy.

Fox, J.L. (1994). NIH mixes human DNA patents. What next? *Bio/Technology* **12,** 348. **(NIH drops the patent appliaction on the "EST" cDNA fragments.)**

Index